Essentials of Pharmacology and Therapeutics for Dentistry

Essentials of Pharmacology and Therapeutics for Dentistry

Frank J. Dowd DDS, PhD

Emeritus Professor
Department of Pharmacology
Creighton University School of Medicine and School of Dentistry
Omaha, NE
United States

Angelo Mariotti BS, DDS, PhD

Dean
School of Dentistry
LSU Health Science Center
New Orleans, LA
United States

ELSEVIER

Elsevier
3251 Riverport Lane
St. Louis, Missouri 63043

ESSENTIALS OF PHARMACOLOGY AND THERAPEUTICS FOR DENTISTRY

ISBN: 978-0-323-82659-4

Notice

Practitioners and researchers must always rely on their own experience and knowledge in evaluating and using any information, methods, compounds, or experiments described herein. Because of rapid advances in the medical sciences, in particular, independent verification of diagnoses and drug dosages should be made. To the fullest extent of the law, no responsibility is assumed by Elsevier, authors, editors, or contributors for any injury and/or damage to persons or property as a matter of products liability, negligence or otherwise, or from any use or operation of any methods, products, instructions, or ideas contained in the material herein.

Senior Content Strategist: Lauren Boyle
Senior Content Development Specialist: Shweta Pant
Publishing Services Manager: Deepthi Unni
Project Manager: Sheik Mohideen K
Design Direction: Ryan Cook

Printed in India

Last digit is the print number: 9 8 7 6 5 4 3 2 1

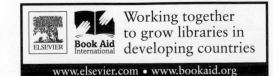

Preface

This is the first edition of *Essentials of Pharmacology and Therapeutics for Dentistry*. The purpose of this book is to identify several central areas in pharmacology and to prepare students in organizing their study of the discipline. This book should be viewed as a foundation for the textbook *Pharmacology and Therapeutics for Dentistry*, which presents a thorough treatment of pharmacology and is the major textbook for dental students. *Pharmacology and Therapeutics for Dentistry* also includes useful information presented in case studies and study aids, help with drug terminology, more general references, and many other features. Each chapter in the *Essentials* textbook is meant to reference the corresponding chapter(s) in *Pharmacology and Therapeutics for Dentistry* for a more complete and comprehensive study of pharmacology.

Pharmacology textbooks usually discuss, in their earlier chapters, the principles of how drugs act (pharmacodynamics), how drugs are handled by the body (pharmacokinetics), adverse effects of drugs, genetic influences on drug responses, and principles of therapeutic responses to drugs. This is then followed by a discussion of individual classes of drugs. This textbook, as well as *Pharmacology and Therapeutics for Dentistry*, follows the same sequence.

The editors (and authors) trust that, in the course of the student's study, *Essential of Pharmacology and Therapeutics for Dentistry* will fill the need for a quick reference and review. This briefer textbook will also help in organizing the extensive information in pharmacology, in addition to providing a road map for the course in dental pharmacology.

Acknowledgments

We thank all our textbook strategists and managers at Elsevier. It has been rewarding to work with them. We are grateful for the direction and help from Lauren Boyle, the Senior Content Strategist, who has been with us every step of the way. She has helped us with all our authoring and editing issues, providing us with continued and appropriate direction. Ranjana Sharma, our Content Development Manager, was crucial with her advice on editing procedures. Shweta Pant, Senor Content Development Specialist, provided needed advice and help with images and related issues. Sheik Mohideen K, as Project Manager, adroitly oversaw the final stages in the production of this book.

Contents

Contents

1

Pharmacodynamics: Mechanisms of Drug Action

KEY POINTS

- Most drugs bind to and act through receptors.
- There are five major types of receptors.
- The cellular effect of a drug (i.e., agonist) after binding to a receptor is called signal transduction.
- Drug agonists at a given receptor can be distinguished based upon affinity of binding, potency effective concentration$_{50}$ (EC$_{50}$), and intrinsic activity (i.e., maximal effect, ceiling effect, or E$_{max}$).
- Antagonists are drugs that bind to receptors and block the effects of agonists.

DEFINITIONS

- **Pharmacodynamics:** the study of how drugs act to achieve a response.
- **Receptor:** Proteins with highly ordered physiological and/or biochemical properties that permit specific compounds to combine with them to initiate a biological effect.
- **Ligand:** A molecule, such as a hormone, drug, etc., that binds to a receptor (Fig. 1.1).
- **Agonist:** A drug, neurotransmitter, or hormone that initiates a biological response when combined with a receptor.
- **Antagonist:** A drug, which when combined with a receptor, interferes with or inhibits a biological response of an agonist.
- **Dose Response Relationship:** The magnitude of drug exposure (dose) has a direct relationship to a specific magnitude of outcome (response) in an organism.

Drugs, Receptors, and Signal Transduction

Drugs are chemical substances that are administered to alter or modify existing physiological or pathological processes. In conventional doses, most therapeutic agents are generally selective in their action and influence a narrow spectrum of biological events.

Tissue proteins that bind drugs are called **receptors**. Receptors have highly ordered physiological/biochemical properties that permit only particular compounds to combine with them, while prohibiting all others from doing so. Once bound, the drug-receptor complexes initiate other events to occur at the cellular level. The existence of receptors that respond to exogenously administered drugs implies that drugs often mimic or inhibit the actions of endogenous ligands (i.e., naturally occurring chemicals in the body that bind to these receptors).

Usually drugs will activate cellular receptors to produce a response; however, there are drugs that do not require a receptor to act. Some examples of pharmacologic agents that do not require a receptor to act include chemically reactive drugs such as stomach antacids, antiseptic agents, and antidotes to heavy metals.

Characteristics of Signal Transduction

Drugs generally are not highly reactive compounds in the chemical sense; they exert their influences indirectly by altering, through their receptor attachment, the activity of an important regulator of biologic processes. Therefore, the drug-receptor complex begins the first event in a series of complex reactions that culminate in a pharmacologic effect. More specifically, the drug-receptor complex initiates a signal transduction, which is the transmission of molecular signals to the interior of the cell (Fig. 1.2).

Signal transduction or cell signaling, is a cascade of events that eventually results in an observable pharmacologic effect. These events constitute the **signal transduction pathway**, which is also called stimulus–response

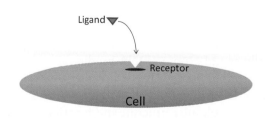

• **Fig. 1.1** A ligand binding to a membrane-bound receptor.

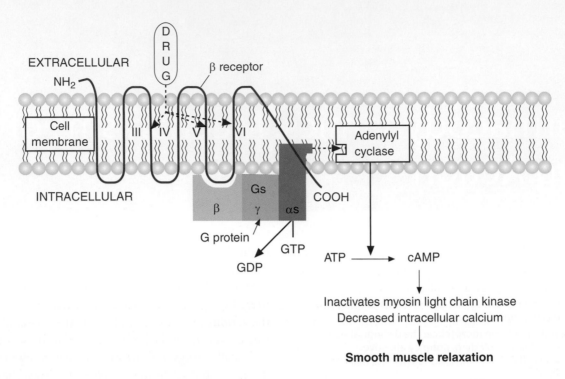

• **Fig. 1.2** Example of a signal transduction pathway. A drug called a beta adrenergic agonist stimulates its membrane receptor resulting in stimulation of an enzyme (adenylyl cyclase) that leads to an effector response inside the cell (smooth muscle relaxation). G protein, designated GS; *cAMP*, cyclic adenosine monophosphate; *ATP*, Adenosine triphosphate; *GDP*, guanosine diphosphate; *GTP*, guanosine triphosphate. (From Gardenhire DS. Rau's respiratory care pharmacology. 9th ed, St. Louis: Elsevier; 2016. pii:B9780323341363000354/f035-002-9780323341363.)

coupling. Different types of receptors have different signal transduction pathways, the general functional signal transduction pathways are linked to five major receptor classes: ion channel receptors, G protein–linked receptors, transmembrane receptors that have enzymatic cytosolic activity, transmembrane receptors that bind to a separate cytosolic enzyme, and intracellular (nuclear) receptors.

Receptor Classification and Signal Transduction

Receptors are complex macromolecules possessing a ligand-binding site to interact with specific drugs and an effector site to initiate the pharmacologic response. Most receptors are membrane bound and have one or more extracellular ligand-binding domain linked by one or more lipophilic membrane-spanning segments to an effector domain often, but not always, located on the cytoplasmic side of the membrane. Other receptors are intracellular and expose a DNA-binding site allowing the receptor to interact with DNA and alter transcription.

Receptors involved in physiologic regulation can be grouped by molecular structure and functional characteristics into five major classes.

Ion Channel–linked Receptors

There are two general classes of ion channels (Fig. 1.3):

1. **Voltage-gated ion channels** are activated by alterations in membrane voltage. For instance, voltage-gated Na^+ channels open when the membrane is depolarized to a threshold potential and contribute to further membrane depolarization by allowing Na^+ influx into the cell.
2. **Ligand-gated ion channels** are activated in response to the binding of specific ligands or drugs. Another name for ligand-gated ion channels is ionotropic receptors. Ion channel receptors react to drugs by either increasing or decreasing their conductance. Channels are usually selective for a single ion. The increase or decrease in conductance of an ion leads to a cell event, such as depolarization of the cell, hyperpolarization of the cell, or calcium signaling. Nicotinic receptors and chloride channel receptors are examples of this class of receptors.

G Protein–coupled Receptors

G protein–coupled receptors, sometimes referred to as metabotropic receptors, constitute a large family of integral membrane proteins, and collectively serve as targets for approximately half of all non-antimicrobial prescription drugs.

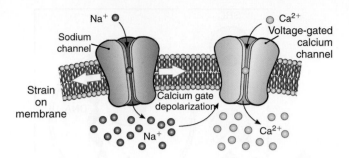

• **Fig. 1.3** Two ion channels are pictured (sodium channel and calcium channel). (From Sasso R., et al, Benzel's Spine Surgery: Techniques, Complication Avoidance, and Management. In: Belven OII, Denzel EC, Steinmetz MP, eds. Chapter 29 - Pathophysiology of Cervical Spondylosis, Radiculopathy, and Myelopathy. 5th ed. Elsevier; 2022. pii:B978032363668100029X/f29-04-9780323636681.)

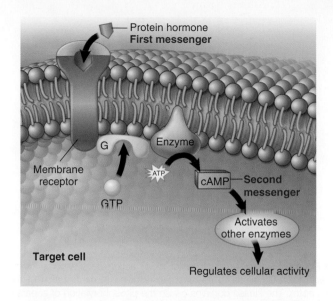

• **Fig. 1.4** A G protein-linked receptor and signal transduction. The ligand that binds to the receptor is called the "first messenger". In this pathway, cAMP is the "second messenger" which leads to regulation of cellular activity." *ATP*, Adenosine triphosphate; *cAMP*, cyclic adenosine monophosphate; *GMP*, guanosine triphosphate. (From Patton KT & Thibodeau GA. The human body in health and disease, chapter 18 - Mechanisms of Hormonal Regulation. In: Huether and McCance's Understanding Pathophysiology, Second Canadian Edition, 7th ed. Elsevier; 2018. pii:B9780323778848000185/f18-05-9780323778848.)

G proteins are molecules that bind guanine nucleotides, such as guanosine diphosphate (GDP) and guanosine triphosphate (GTP). G proteins are a complex system comprising heterotrimers consisting of α, β, and γ subunits. The basic structure of G-protein-coupled receptors includes a component on the inner surface of the cell plasma membrane and a seven-membered transmembrane domain. Generally, metabotropic receptors greatly amplify extracellular biologic signals because they activate G proteins, which in turn, stimulate effector enzymes (e.g., adenylyl cyclase) or less commonly, ion channels, leading to the introduction or formation of a host of internal second messengers for each extracellular signal (e.g., ligand) molecule detected (Figs. 1.2 and 1.4).

G protein–linked receptors encompass a wide variety of signaling pathways. G proteins are classified based on the nature of their α subunit. Generally, the G protein complex is inactive when GDP is bound to the α subunit, which happens when the receptor is not stimulated by an agonist. After the ligand binds to the receptor, dissociation of GDP from the α subunit takes place, and the replacement binding of GTP causes the α subunit to separate from the β–γ subunit complex. At this point, the α subunit, activated by ATP, affects the activity of a nearby enzyme, leading eventually to an effector response. The G proteins include G_s, G_i, and G_q, and their corresponding alpha subunits are α_s, α_i, and α_q.

One receptor subtype may activate different G proteins, several receptor subtypes may activate the same G protein, and the ultimate target proteins can exist in tissue-specific isoforms with differing susceptibilities to secondary effector systems. For example, depending on the receptor, a G protein–linked receptor can stimulate adenylyl cyclase, inhibit adenylyl cyclase, or activate phospholipase C depending on the subunit complex associated with the G proteins.

The different G protein pathways can also interact with one another. The complexity of G protein signal transduction provides a sophisticated regulatory system by which cellular responses can vary, depending on the combination of receptors activated and the cell-specific expression of distinct regulatory and target proteins.

Transmembrane Receptors That Have Enzymatic Cytosolic Function

These enzyme-linked receptors have only one transmembrane domain per protein subunit, with an enzymatic catalytic site on the cytoplasmic side of the receptor. The most important cytoplasmic sites have one of the following functions:
(1) tyrosine kinase activity,
(2) tyrosine phosphatase activity,
(3) serine or threonine kinase activity,
(4) guanylyl cyclase activity.

Enzymatic activity on the cytosolic aspect of the receptor catalyzes changes that lead to characteristic cell changes. For example, epidermal growth factor (EGF) binding stimulates signal transduction of intracellular tyrosine kinase, which causes the phosphorylation of separate substrates. Activation of several subsequent pathways

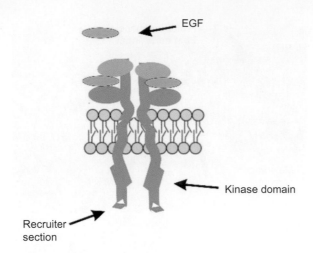

• **Fig. 1.5** Epidermal growth factor *(EGF)* acting on a tyrosine kinase receptor. EGF binds to its receptor, resulting in dimerization of the receptor. The kinase domains cause the phosphorylation of separate intracellular proteins, which are recruited to the cytoplasmic terminal of the receptor. This results in a cascade of downstream events.

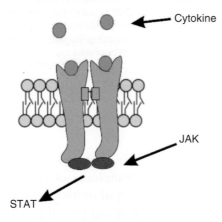

• **Fig. 1.6** Cytokine receptor and initial steps in signal transduction. Cytokines bind to the cytokine receptor shown as a dimer. Activation of Janus kinase *(JAK)* follows, leading to activation of signal transducers and activators of transcription *(STATs)*.

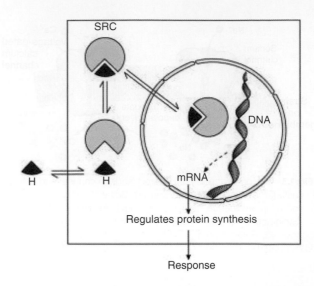

• **Fig. 1.7** Intracellular receptor and signal transduction. *SRC*, Steroid-receptor complex. (From Tara V, Shanbhag TV et al., Pharmacology for Dentistry. In: Chapter 10 - Endocrine Pharmacology. 4th ed. India: Elsevier; 2021. pii:B9788131258170000199/f10-05-9788131258170.)

by the kinase domain of the receptor leads to further molecular changes. These kinase substrates are recruited to the cytoplasmic terminal of the receptor (Fig. 1.5). Insulin acts through a similar receptor.

Transmembrane Receptors That Bind to a Separate Cytosolic Enzyme

Another type of transmembrane receptor is one that has a noncatalytic domain that activates a separate cytosolic tyrosine kinase, called Janus kinase (JAK). This receptor dimerizes after binding to the kinase and is the type of receptor to which cytokine molecules can bind (Fig. 1.6).

Typically, the JAK enzyme phosphorylates a group of proteins called; signal transducers and activators of transcription (STATs). Activated STATs migrate to the nucleus to induce transcription of selective genes. Activation of several subsequent pathways (e.g., mitogen-activated protein kinase [MAP kinase] pathway) leads to further molecular changes. Various cytokines act through these receptors.

Intracellular Receptors

Lipophilic substances capable of crossing the plasma membrane may activate intracellular receptors located in the cytoplasm or nucleus of the cell. More specifically, drugs that bind to these receptors diffuse into the cell and bind to intracellular receptors. Dimerization with a co-receptor protein usually occurs after drug binding, followed by movement of the entire complex into the nucleus, and induction of transcription of selective genes by binding to specific response elements (promoters/enhancers) on the DNA (Fig. 1.7).

Other steps are involved in the signaling pathways, and several other proteins, including co-activators and co-inhibitors, are involved in shaping the final transcription process. Binding of thyroid hormone to its receptor produces more than a 10-fold increase in receptor affinity for binding to DNA. Because this type of signal transduction requires protein synthesis, drugs that activate intracellular receptors typically have a delay of several hours before the onset of their pharmacologic effect. Sex steroids, mineralocorticoids, glucocorticoids, thyroid hormones, and vitamin D derivatives all activate specific nuclear receptors that initiate DNA transcription.

Drug-binding Forces

Implicit in the interaction of a drug with its receptor is the chemical binding of that drug to one or more specific sites on the receptor molecule. Multiple bond formation often accompanies the interaction between a drug and receptor. Four basic types of bond formation are hydrogen bonds, hydrophobic bonds, ionic bonds, and covalent bonds. Drug-binding forces vary in strength. For example, hydrophobic binding is often very weak, whereas covalent binding can be quite strong.

Most drugs reversibly bind to their receptors. The duration of action of drugs is related to how long an effective drug concentration remains in the vicinity of the drug–receptor complex. This time may vary from a few minutes to many days, but usually it is on the order of minutes to hours. If a drug irreversibly binds to a receptor, new receptor synthesis is often required to reverse the effect of the drug.

Structure–Activity Relationships

The study of structure–activity relationships (SARs) evaluates drug–receptor interactions. In SAR investigations, specific features of the structure of a drug molecule are identified and then altered systematically to determine their influence on pharmacologic activity. SAR studies of closely related agents (congeners) led to an understanding of the chemical prerequisites for pharmacologic activity and made possible the molecular modification of drugs to provide enhanced or even novel therapeutic effects, while reducing the incidence and severity of toxic reactions. In addition, SAR studies serve to illustrate how the combined action of the various binding forces are necessary for maximal drug activity.

Drug Size, Shape, and Isomerism

Most clinically useful drugs are organic compounds that have molecular weights less than 1000 and greater than 100 daltons. Selectivity of a drug for a receptor is dependent on the three-dimensional structure of the drug. Thus, conversion of a d- to an l- conformation of a drug can have dramatic effects on affinity. Optical isomers of drugs often have very different affinities for the same receptor (Fig. 1.8).

Concentration-Response Relationships

Drug Ligands

Agonists

An agonist has affinity for the receptor while also possessing **intrinsic activity** and **potency**.

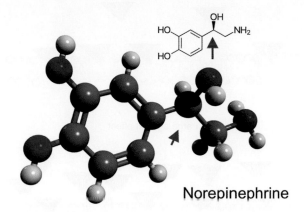

Norepinephrine

• **Fig. 1.8** Structure of norepinephrine (NE) showing the stick drawing (top) and the ball and stick drawing (bottom). The red arrows point to the chiral carbon atom which accounts for the optical isomerism giving either the d-, of l- conformation of norepinephrine. The optical isomers are mirror images of one another. The difference between isomers corresponds to about a 10-fold difference in clinical effect. (Modified from: Dreamstine.com ID 198717164 © Volodymyr Dvornyk.)

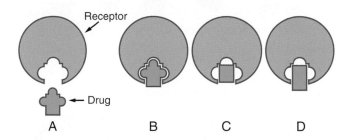

• **Fig. 1.9** (A) Receptor and agonist. (B) Agonist binding to receptor. (C) Antagonist blocking effect of agonist. (D) Partial agonist binds but has a lower Emax. (Modified from Clayton BD, Willihnganz MJ. Basic pharmacology for nurses. 17th ed. St. Louis: Elsevier; 2017. pii:B9780323642477000003X/f03-09-9780323642477.)

1. **Full agonist**: an agonist that, given sufficient drug, results in the maximal effect (E_{max}) possible from stimulating that receptor. (The E_{max} **of a drug is a measure of the intrinsic activity of that drug.**)
2. **Partial agonist**: an agonist that has a lower E_{max} than the E_{max} of a full agonist.
3. **Indirect agonist**: an agonist that increases the concentration of a direct agonist at the receptor.

Antagonists

The antagonist has affinity for the receptor but no intrinsic activity. Importantly, the antagonist blocks the effect of the agonist (Fig. 1.9).

1. **Competitive antagonist:** an antagonist whose inhibition of the effect of an agonist can be overcome by adding sufficient agonist (Fig. 1.10).
2. **Noncompetitive antagonist:** an antagonist whose inhibition of the effect of the agonist **cannot** be

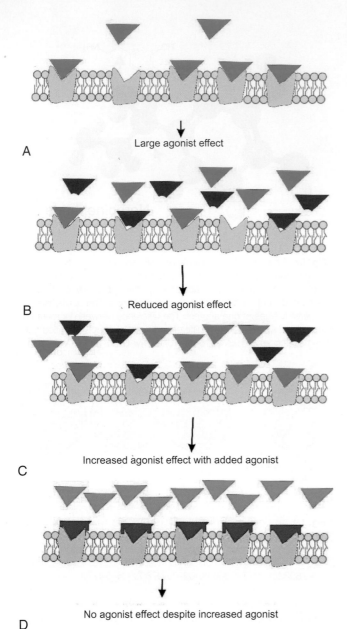

A   Large agonist effect

B   Reduced agonist effect

C   Increased agonist effect with added agonist

D   No agonist effect despite increased agonist

• **Fig. 1.10** Effect of antagonists on response to an agonist. (A) Agonist molecules shown in green bind to receptors, leading to a large response. (B) Addition of a competitive antagonist, in *red*, leads to a reduced response to the agonist. (C) The addition of more agonist is able to overcome the inhibitory effect of the competitive antagonist. (D) Addition of a noncompetitive antagonist is able to remove the effect of the agonist, despite excess numbers of agonist molecules. In this case, the noncompetitive nature of the antagonist results from covalent binding of the antagonist to the receptor.

overcome by adding high concentrations of the agonist (see Fig. 1.10).

Receptor Binding and Effects

The higher the drug dose, the greater is the concentration of the drug at its receptor. Likewise, there is a positive correlation between the dose of a drug and the magnitude of the response to the drug. However, several factors determine the effect of a given dose of the drug on the actual magnitude of the response to the drug.

Examine what happens when a drug agonist binds to (occupies) its receptor.

$$D + R \leftrightarrow DR$$

The strength of the binding of a drug to its receptor is called **affinity**. The greater the affinity, the greater the number of receptors occupied by the drug at a given concentration of the drug.

This binding alone, however, is not sufficient to explain the magnitude of its effect. DR needs to be converted to an effect.

$$D + R \leftrightarrow DR \rightarrow Effect$$

Graphing Graded Responses to Drugs

Drug Agonists

When one graphs the response to a drug **agonist** (notice the log scale on the "*x*" axis) one gets a sigmoid curve (Fig. 1.11). Thus, the magnitude of the drug response depends on the concentration of the drug at its receptor. It also assumes that there is an effect of the drug resulting from its binding to its receptor (more about that later). Since the range of the drug effect is shown in the graph, this graph is called a **graded** concentration-response curve. The effect of increasing the drug concentration results in a greater response until the maximum effect is reached, after which further increases in drug concentrations do not lead to an increased effect (see Fig. 1.11).

The maximum response to a drug is termed, E_{max} or **ceiling effect** and, as indicated above, is a measure of the **intrinsic activity** of the drug. The concentration of a drug that results in a half-maximal effect is termed, the effective concentration$_{50}$ or EC_{50}. The EC_{50} is a useful measure of the **potency** of a drug. The E_{max} and EC_{50} render useful information about drugs (Fig. 1.12). Notice that affinity and potency are not the same (Fig. 1.13). Affinity is a measure of the attractiveness of the drug to its receptor. Potency implies affinity to a receptor, but potency also encompasses the signal transduction pathway and how robust that pathway is. The same is true for intrinsic activity (see Fig. 1.13).

Drug Agonist Plus Antagonists

When one adds an antagonist with an agonist, the effect of the agonist is inhibited. If that antagonist is a **competitive antagonist**, the inhibition of the effect of an agonist

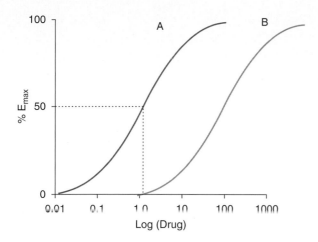

• **Fig. 1.11** Concentration effect curves for two drugs (A and B) differing in potency by a factor of 100.

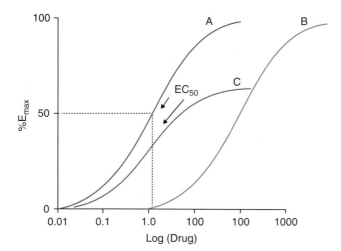

• **Fig. 1.12** Theoretical concentration-response curves for three agonists acting at the same receptor. Drugs A and B have the same intrinsic activity (E_{max}), but B has less potency than A. Drug C has a lower intrinsic activity than either A or B, but it has the same potency as drug A (as measured by the EC_{50}). Affinity relates solely to drug binding, whereas intrinsic activity and potency encompass both binding and the events that follow, leading to an effect.

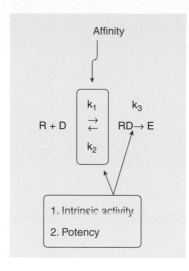

• **Fig. 1.13** Depiction of drug characteristics. Affinity relates solely to drug binding, whereas intrinsic activity and potency encompass both binding and the events that follow leading to an effect. The left panel shows the effect of a competitive antagonist. Note that the EC50 values for the agonist increase with increasing concentrations of the antagonist. The right panel shows the effect of a noncompetitive antagonist. Note that the EC50 values for the agonist do not change with the antagonist.

can be overcome by adding sufficient agonist. (See the parallel shift to the right of the curves and a shift to the right in the apparent EC_{50} in Fig. 1.13.)

When the antagonist is a **noncompetitive antagonist**, the inhibition of the effect of the agonist cannot be fully overcome by adding high concentrations of the agonist. (See the profile in Fig.1.13 with no shift in the EC_{50}.) When sufficient noncompetitive antagonist is added, the effect of the agonist will be completely inhibited despite adding a large excess of the agonist.

From the conditions of the above discussion, an antagonist, if it is a pure antagonist, has affinity for the receptor but neither potency nor intrinsic activity. Its pharmacological action is limited to preventing the effect of the agonist.

Spare Receptors

Spare receptors (receptor reserve) are the number of receptors in a tissue or organ that are more than the number of receptors needed for the maximal effect of the full agonist in that tissue or organ.

Pharmacodynamic Tolerance

Pharmacodynamic tolerance is the reduction in the response to a drug despite a constant concentration of the agonist at the receptor.

Mechanisms:
1. **Desensitization:** a reversible loss of response due to a physical or chemical change in the receptor. The binding of an agonist may eventually cause the receptor to be uncoupled from the signaling pathway.
2. **Down-regulation:** a reversible loss of response to a drug due to internalization of the receptor, thus decreasing the presence of the receptor on the cell surface. The binding of an agonist may lead to the removal of the receptor from the plasma membrane.

Further information on pharmacodynamics can be found in Chapter 1 in "Pharmacology and Therapeutics for Dentistry" 8th edition with updates on the Elsevier website.

2

Pharmacokinetics: The Absorption, Distribution, and Fate of Drugs

KEY POINTS

Each route of drug administration has its own absorption characteristics.

The liver is the most important organ for drug metabolism, employing many key enzymes, most notably the cytochrome P450 enzymes.

The kidneys are the most important organs for excreting drugs.

Drugs differ from one another in their volumes of distribution, elimination of half-lives, and clearances.

The characteristics that determine the transit of free drugs in the body include volumes of distribution, half-lives, clearance values, and steady-state plasma concentrations (for multiple dosing).

DEFINITIONS

- Pharmacokinetics deals with the movement of drugs through the body.
- Absorption is the transfer of a drug from its administration site into the bloodstream.
- Distribution is the movement of drugs through various body compartments.
- Metabolism is a means of chemical modification of drugs, a major pathway for the alteration of pharmacologic effects of drugs and is often a prerequisite for the excretion of lipid-soluble chemicals.
- Excretion is the removal of the drug from the body.
- Active transport is a carrier-mediated transfer of a drug against its electrochemical gradient.
- Total drug concentration in the blood refers to the sum of the bound and free drug concentration in the serum or plasma.
- Free drug refers to a drug not bound to proteins in the serum or plasma. Only the free drug is biologically active and can be absorbed, distributed, metabolized, and excreted.
- Bound drug refers to the drugs attached to plasma proteins or tissues. It is an inactive form of the drug and can act as a reservoir for the release of the free drug.
- Drug carriers are proteins that selectively combine with drugs for transport across a membrane.
- Zero-order kinetics refers to a process (e.g., elimination of a drug) in which a constant amount of drug is eliminated per unit of time.
- First-order kinetics refers to a process (e.g., elimination of a drug) in which a constant percentage of drug is eliminated per unit of time.

The effect of a drug is directly related to the concentration of the free drug at the relevant receptors. However, when a drug is administered, several factors contribute to achieving the drug concentration at the receptors. Drug concentrations are rarely static since they increase and decrease as dictated by the processes of absorption, distribution, metabolism, and excretion (Fig. 2.1).

Passage of Drugs Across Membranes

For a drug to be absorbed, reach its site of action, and eventually be eliminated, it must cross one or more biologic membrane barriers. Because such barriers to drugs behave similarly, the cell membrane (i.e., a bimolecular sheet of lipids with proteins interspersed) can serve as an example of all membrane barriers.

Diffusion of Drugs Across Cell Membranes

The passage of drugs across biologic membranes can involve several different mechanisms, including passive diffusion, simple diffusion, and facilitated diffusion. Of these, passive diffusion is the most commonly encountered.

Passive Diffusion

The defining characteristic of passive diffusion is that the drug moves down its electrochemical gradient when crossing the membrane. The gut epithelial barrier is a good example of how drugs can permeate cell barriers.

Simple Diffusion

One way that hydrophilic drugs penetrate a cell barrier is by aqueous diffusion, by permeating between tight epithelial junctions, or through aqueous pores. This avoids the lipid barrier of the cell membrane but is limited by drug size and other restrictions. More commonly, lipophilic drugs will diffuse directly through the lipid barrier of the cell membrane (lipid diffusion) (Fig. 2.2).

Facilitated Diffusion

Water, small electrolytes, and hydrophilic molecules of biologic importance generally move across plasma membranes much more readily than would be predicted by simple diffusion. In these instances, transmembrane proteins serve to circumvent the lipid bilayer and facilitate diffusion (see Fig. 2.2). The simplest mechanism involves a transmembrane pore.

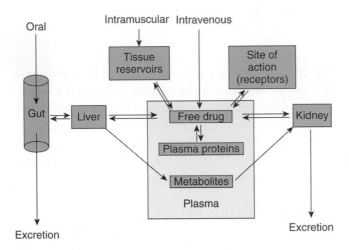

• **Fig. 2.1** Outline of the major pathways of absorption, distribution, metabolism, and excretion of drugs. Compounds taken orally must pass through the liver before reaching the systemic circulation. When in the bloodstream, agents are distributed throughout the body and come in contact with their respective sites of action. Drugs are filtered by the kidney, only to be reabsorbed if lipid soluble. Metabolism of many drugs occurs primarily in the liver, after which the metabolites are excreted in bile or in the urine. Some agents eliminated in the bile are subject to reabsorption and may participate in an enterohepatic cycle.

The movement of specific ions (e.g., Na^+, K^+, and Ca^{++}) across the cell membrane is facilitated by the presence of transmembrane channels.

Numerous substances are shuttled across plasma membranes (**carriers** or **transporters**) by a number of transporter molecules which are finite in number and can be saturated.

Active Transport

Active transport requires the expenditure of energy and may be blocked by inhibitors of cellular metabolism. Active transport requires an energy source, often adenosine triphosphate (ATP) (see Fig. 2.2).

Endocytosis and Exocytosis

The processes of endocytosis and exocytosis are together the most complex methods of drug transfer across a biologic membrane. The term *endocytosis* refers to a series of events whereby a substance is engulfed and internalized by the cell.

Endocytosis usually begins with the binding of a compound to be absorbed, often a macromolecule, by its receptor on the membrane surface and absorbed by invagination of its membrane to form a vacuole. The process of exocytosis occurs when vesicles, such as those produced by the Golgi apparatus, fuse with the plasma membrane and discharge their contents outside the cell.

Absorption

Absorption refers to the transfer of a drug from its administration site into the bloodstream. The particular route of administration selected greatly influences the rate and

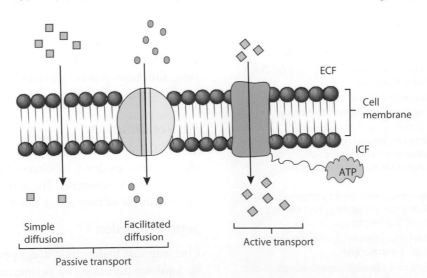

• **Fig. 2.2** Drug transfer across membranes. Facilitated diffusion requires a macromolecule to assist in the transport. In addition, active transport requires an energy source. ATP, Adenosine triphosphate; ECF, extracellular fluid; ICF, intracellular fluid. (Taken from Singh H, Singh I, Yadav M, Cellular Physiology. In: Chapter 2, *Fundamentals of Medical Physiology*. India: Elsevier; 2018. pii:B978813125409700002X/f02-08-9788131254097.)

perhaps the extent of drug absorption. Table 2.1 summarizes the characteristics of various routes of drug administration. The different routes provide a variety of choices for drug delivery depending on the drug's characteristics and clinical situation.

Distribution

Distribution refers to the movement of drugs throughout the body. The rate, sequence, and extent of distribution depend on many factors: the physicochemical properties of the drug, cardiac output, and regional blood flow, anatomic characteristics of membranes, transmembrane electrical and pH gradients, and binding to plasma proteins and tissue reservoirs, and carrier-mediated transport. For all but very few drugs that act intravascularly, the capillary membrane constitutes the first tissue barrier to be crossed in the journey of a drug from the bloodstream to its site of action.

The effect of pH on drugs that are weak acids or weak bases has important effects on the ability of these drugs to cross the membrane. This can be demonstrated by examining absorption across the gastric mucosa. Fig. 2.3 shows that aspirin, a non-charged drug, readily crosses the gastric membrane, whereas codeine, a weak base, does not.

Capillary Penetration

After a drug gains access to the systemic circulation, it becomes diluted by the plasma volume of the entire vascular compartment. For a compound administered intravenously, this process requires only several minutes for completion; however, for drugs given by other routes, intravascular distribution occurs concurrently with absorption. The transfer of drugs out of the bloodstream is governed by the same factors that control its entrance. Lipophilic drugs diffuse across the capillary membrane extremely rapidly.

TABLE 2.1 Characteristics of Routes of Drug Administration

Route of Administration	Absorption Characteristics	Advantages	Disadvantages
Oral	Variable depends on the rate of gastric emptying; dosage forms affect the rate of absorption.	Convenient, economical, self-administration, low cost, relatively safe	Requires patient compliance, unsuitable for poorly absorbed drugs, rapid inactivation for some drugs,
Sublingual, buccal	Rapid for some drugs	Avoids first-pass metabolism, predictable effect for some drugs	Drug must be kept in contact with the absorption site.
Intravenous	Immediate	Ideal for emergencies, rapid titration is possible, the fastest way to achieve predictable plasma drug concentrations; large volumes can be given over time.	Adverse effects appear rapidly and are difficult to reverse. Suspensions cannot be given. Adverse effects: pain, vasculitis, extravasation. Not usually for self-administration
Intramuscular	Rapid for aqueous solutions, slow for suspensions or depot forms	More predictable response than for oral drugs. The rate of absorption can be manipulated. Useful for non-compliant patients.	Painful, may cause muscle damage, bleeding risk with patients on anticoagulants, may interfere with some diagnostic tests that measure organ or tissue damage
Inhalation	Rapid absorption for anesthetics, some inhaled drugs (e.g., antiasthma drugs) stay in the respiration tract.	Useful for bronchodilators and inhaled steroids, useful for gaseous or volatile liquid anesthetics, and titration of anesthetic.	Coughing, Bronchodilator, and steroid self-administration require patient education.
Subcutaneous	Rapid for aqueous solutions, slow for suspensions or depot forms	Aqueous or depot forms can be used.	Pain, tissue necrosis
Topical	Patches have been developed to render a near continuous release of drugs.	Transdermal absorption is useful for certain drugs such as nitroglycerine and nicotine.	Local irritation is possible limited to certain drugs

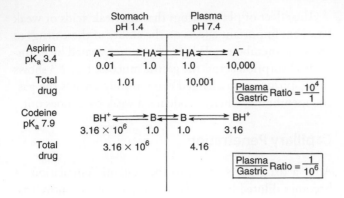

	Stomach pH 1.4		Plasma pH 7.4	
Aspirin pK_a 3.4	A⁻ ⇌ HA	→	HA ⇌	A⁻
	0.01 1.0		1.0	10,000
Total drug	1.01		10,001	

$$\frac{Plasma}{Gastric} \, Ratio = \frac{10^4}{1}$$

	Stomach pH 1.4		Plasma pH 7.4	
Codeine pK_a 7.9	BH⁺ ⇌ B	→	B ⇌	BH⁺
	3.16×10^6 1.0		1.0	3.16
Total drug	3.16×10^6		4.16	

$$\frac{Plasma}{Gastric} \, Ratio = \frac{1}{10^6}$$

• **Fig. 2.3** Gastric absorption of aspirin, a weak acid, and codeine, a weak base. The absorption of aspirin is promoted by ion trapping within the plasma; the low pH of stomach fluid favors gastric retention of codeine. (The actual 3.49 pK_a of aspirin is truncated to 3.4 for illustration purposes.)

Entry of Drugs Into Cells

The cell membrane acts as a semipermeable barrier, admitting some drugs into the cell while excluding others. Nonpolar, lipid-soluble compounds distribute evenly across plasma membranes, but the distribution of weak electrolytes at equilibrium is more complex. Charged drugs that do gain access to the cell by passive diffusion are distributed at equilibrium according to their electrochemical gradient across the membrane.

Restricted Distribution

In some tissues or organs, anatomic relationships and membrane transporters sequester interstitial or transcellular fluids from the general extracellular space and restrict intracellular access to drugs.

Central Nervous System

Entry of drugs into the central nervous system (CNS) is unusually dependent on lipid solubility. Most drugs with high lipid/water partition coefficients are taken up very quickly. Drugs that are sparingly lipid soluble are largely excluded from the interstitial space of the brain. There are four reasons for an added barrier in the brain constituting the **blood-brain barrier**. These characteristics include: (1) The capillaries of the brain do not have fenestrations and are characterized by tight junctions. (2) A cellular sheath composed of processes extending from connective tissue astrocytes surrounds the capillaries. (3) P-Glycoproteins actively transport drugs out of the brain. (4) Choroid plexus cells provide an avenue to pump drugs out of the cerebrospinal fluid. This is illustrated in Fig. 2.4.

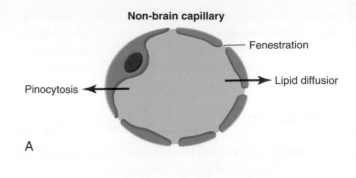

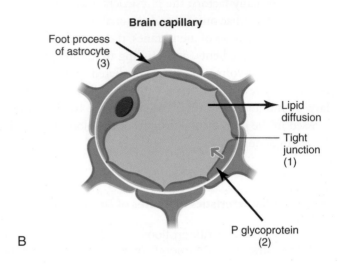

• **Fig. 2.4** The contributors to the blood-brain barrier. The following four factors are shown. A brain capillary is compared to capillaries elsewhere in the body. (1) Tight junctions characterize the capillaries in the brain. (compare A vs B). (2) P-Glycoproteins pump drugs into the capillary lumen (B). (3) Astrocytes (glial cells) surround brain capillaries, providing an additional lipid barrier (B). (4) The third illustration (C) shows cells of the choroid plexus surrounding a capillary. These cells have SLC pumps (active transport), that transport drugs from the CSF into the capillary lumen. *CSF*, Cerebrospinal fluid; *SLC*, solute carrier transporters.

Volume of Distribution

Drugs are not distributed equally throughout the body. Although lipophilic substances tend to penetrate all tissue compartments, hydrophilic compounds are often disseminated more restrictively. The **volume of distribution** (V_d) is a useful indicator of how drugs are dispersed among the various body compartments. In its simplest form, the V_d is calculated from the equation: $D = V_d \cdot Cp_0$, where D is the quantity of drug administered in a single dose, and Cp_0 is the plasma concentration of the drug extrapolated to zero time. In summary, the V_d is the *hypothetical* amount of water by which a particular dose would have to be diluted to produce a given plasma concentration, assuming that no drug has been lost through incomplete absorption or by metabolism or excretion. The volumes of distribution of various drugs are given in Table 2.2. The higher numbers in Table 2.2 are only possible if there is an unequal distribution of the drug. Fig. 2.5 indicates that numbers of around 40 L or below may more closely approximate near equal distribution of drugs in the three body compartments.

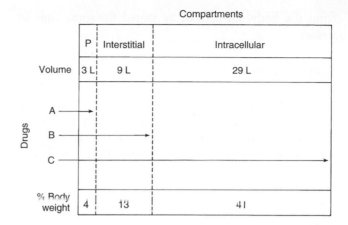

• **Fig. 2.5** Body water compartments. The membrane barriers that separate plasma from interstitial fluid and interstitial fluid from intracellular water are indicated by *dashed lines*. The upper set of figures represent the respective volumes for a 70-kg man; the lower set are percentages of total body weight. Of the drugs shown, *A* is restricted to the plasma, *B* is distributed within the extracellular compartment (plasma + interstitial fluid), and *C* is disseminated throughout the total body water.

TABLE 2.2	Apparent Volumes of Distribution of Various Agents	
Agent	V_d (L)[a]	Corresponding Fluid Compartment
Evans blue	3	Plasma water
Iodine 131–albumin	3	
Mannitol	12	Extracellular water
Amoxicillin	15	
Na+	18	
Enalapril	40	
Urea	41	Total body water
Lidocaine	77	
Tetracycline	100	
Atropine	120	
Meperidine	300	
Chlorpromazine	1,500	
Propofol	4,000	
Chloroquine	13,000	

[a]For a 70 kg male. Several drugs have an apparent volume of distribution that is higher than that of total body water. This is due to non-homogeneous distribution, resulting from concentration in one or more non-vascular compartment(s).

Drug Binding and Storage

The sojourn of drugs in the body is considerably influenced by binding to proteins and other tissue components. Reducing the concentration of **free** drugs causes a decrease in the rate of passage across membrane barriers and may alter drug distribution at equilibrium, as reflected in V_d determinations. Drug sequestration can also affect the processes of absorption, metabolism, and elimination.

Plasma Protein Binding

Numerous drugs bind to plasma proteins, especially albumin. A second plasma protein, α_1-acid glycoprotein, binds basic drugs.

Two potential clinical concerns related to plasma protein binding involve patient variability in binding efficacy and the possibility of a drug interaction. Individual differences in drug binding affect the concentration of free drugs within the bloodstream and may lead to insufficient therapy in one patient and toxicity in another. Inasmuch as the attachment of drugs to plasma proteins is generally less selective than are drug-receptor associations, competition between drugs for plasma protein binding sites is relatively common.

Tissue Binding

Drugs bind to tissue proteins to varying degrees. This binding is determined by the drug and its characteristics. For instance, generally, lipophilic drugs bind to fat and muscle tissue to a greater degree than those that are more hydrophilic. Such binding slows the rate of elimination from the body. Drugs can be stored for some time in tissues.

Redistribution

Strongly lipophilic drugs, especially when administered intravenously in bolus form, characteristically go through several phases of distribution: an initial transfer into vessel-rich organs (brain, heart, kidneys, liver, and lungs) followed by progressive redistribution to less highly vascularized tissues (muscle, skin, and eventually fat).

Saliva

The transfer of drugs into saliva can be considered a form of redistribution because the drugs may regain access to the systemic circulation after the saliva is swallowed. Although not involved in drug elimination, the entry of agents into the saliva is of pharmacologic interest. Salivary drug determinations may provide a noninvasive measure of the free plasma concentration of certain drugs. Because the free drug concentration in plasma is normally the primary determinant of patient response, the benefit of salivary drug quantitation has therapeutic potential (Table 2.3).

Drugs may enter the oral fluids from several sources: (1) passive diffusion across the alveolar and ductal cells of salivary glands, (2) active transport into saliva, (3) passive diffusion across the oral epithelium, and (4) bulk flow of fluid from the gingival crevice. Of these avenues, passive diffusion across the alveolar and ductal cells of salivary glands is the greatest contributor.

Gingival Crevicular Fluid

The gingival sulcus or gingival crevice is the anatomic space between tooth enamel and/or cementum, junctional epithelium, and sulcular epithelium (Fig. 2.6). The fluid that is secreted from the gingival sulcus has been designated gingival crevicular fluid. In general, it is a combination of serum from the systemic circulation and locally generated materials secreted from the gingiva and bacteria. More specifically, the gingival crevicular

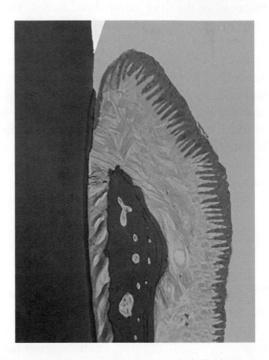

• **Fig. 2.6** Anatomical representation of the gingival sulcus.

TABLE 2.3	Saliva/Plasma Values for Seven Representative Drugs			
Drug	AUC (Saliva/ Plasma)	C_{max} (Saliva/ Plasma)	T_{max} (Saliva/ Plasma)	Correlation Coefficient
Sitagliptin	0.16	0.19	4.00	0.99
Tolterodine	0.21	0.31	1.53	0.99
Hydrochlorothiazide	0.41	0.79	1.12	0.83
Metformin	0.11	0.12	2.23	0.87
Cloxacillin	1.76	2.61	1.00	0.99
Azithromycin	5.61	16.89	1.03	0.99
Rosuvastatin	0.08	0.17	1.05	0.89

The data in columns 2 to 4 are ratios (drugs in saliva/drugs present in the plasma). *AUC*, Area under the curve (see later discussion of AUC); C_{max}, peak concentration of drug; T_{max}, time to peak concentration of the drug. The correlation coefficients are the degree of linear relationship between drug concentration in saliva and drug concentration in plasma up to T_{max} for plasma. Data were taken from Idkaidek N, Arafat T. Saliva versus plasma pharmacokinetics: theory and application of a salivary excretion classification system. *Mol Pharm.* 2012;9:2358–2363.

fluid contains cellular elements (e.g., epithelial cells, leukocytes, bacteria, etc.), electrolytes (e.g., sodium, potassium, etc.), proteins (e.g., immunoglobulins, cytokines, collagens, etc.), hormones (e.g., cortisol, etc.), drugs (e.g., tetracycline, etc.) and metabolic products from gingival tissues and bacteria (e.g., amino acids, hormones, etc.) In the past 25 years, numerous studies have suggested the diagnostic potential of gingival crevicular fluid as well as for the pharmacologic management of periodontal diseases.

Regarding pharmacokinetics, the gingival crevicular fluid has a significant influence on drugs locally delivered into the gingiva sulcus. To begin, during periods of gingival inflammation (i.e., gingivitis or periodontitis), the gingival flow rate is much higher that at healthy rates. This high rate of fluid flow will cause the rate of fluid turnover (or complete replacement) of gingival crevicular fluid to be many times per hour. As a result, the substantivity of most agents is quite low. Second, since the fluid in the sulcus contains many proteins, ionized drugs are easily bound to these proteins and excreted into the saliva by the relatively high rate of flow of the gingival crevicular fluid. Finally, the subgingival biofilm, which is highly resistant to drug penetration, creates problems in getting a drug to the site of action in the gingival sulcus. As a result of these factors, the efficacy of the locally delivered agents to the gingival sulcus will be dramatically affected by gingival crevicular clearance, availability of free drugs, and difficulty of a therapeutic drug concentration reaching the site of action.

Metabolism

Metabolism is a major pathway for the alteration of pharmacologic effects of drugs and is often a prerequisite for the excretion of lipid-soluble chemicals. Typically, compounds are rendered **pharmacologically inactive** by metabolic attack. However, this is not always the case. Numerous drugs yield metabolites with full or partial activity, and some provide derivatives with novel or highly toxic drug effects. An increasing number of agents require chemical activation to be of therapeutic benefit. The other typical effect of drug metabolism is the conversion of the parent drug to polar, relatively **lipid-insoluble compounds** that are susceptible to renal or biliary excretion or both.

Drug metabolism can be categorized according to the types of reactions involved and where they occur. Nonsynthetic reactions include the various transformations of molecular structure: oxidation, reduction, and hydrolysis. These events are also called **phase I reactions** because they often represent the initial stage of biotransformation. **Phase II reactions** consist of the conjugation

of drugs or their metabolites with functional groups provided by endogenous cofactors. Drugs may be metabolized by virtually any organ of the body, but quantitatively the most important enzyme systems for the biotransformation of exogenous substances are located in the **liver**.

Hepatic Microsomal Metabolism

Each hepatocyte contains an extensive network of **smooth endoplasmic reticulum** that catalyzes the metabolism of various endogenous chemicals (e.g., bilirubin, thyroxine, and steroids). Studies of fragmented reticular elements isolated along with other membrane structures in the form of **microsomes** have shown that numerous drugs are also chemically altered by enzymes located within this subcellular organelle. The greatest number of reactions involve oxidation; however, reduction, hydrolysis, and conjugation with glucuronic acid also occur.

Oxidation

The oxidation of drugs results in compounds that tend to be more polar, relatively more hydrophilic, and less likely to penetrate cells and bind to tissue elements. Of particular significance to microsomal oxidation is the enzyme that actually binds the drug during metabolism, **cytochrome P450 (CYP)**. There are several distinct cytochromes involved in drug metabolism. Three cytochromes that constitute most of these drug-metabolizing cytochromes are listed in Table 2.4.

Reduction

The microsomal reduction of drugs is limited to molecules with nitro or carbonyl groups or azo linkages. Similar reactions may also be mediated by nonmicrosomal enzymes of the body, but most reductions of this variety seem to result primarily from the action of enteric bacteria.

Hydrolysis

The hydrolysis of ester or amide compounds resulting in the production of two smaller entities, each with a polar end, occasionally depends on microsomal enzymes.

Dehalogenation

Various compounds are dehalogenated by microsomal enzymes. The reactions are complex, may involve both oxidative and reductive steps, and may result in the formation of potentially toxic metabolites.

Glucuronide Conjugation

The combination of compounds with glucuronic acid is the only phase II reaction catalyzed by microsomal enzymes (in this case, by a group of glucuronosyltransferases).

TABLE 2.4	Three Major Cytochrome P450 Enzymes and Representative Substrates, Inhibitors, and Inducers of These Cytochromes		
CYP	Substrates	Inhibitors	Inducers
2C8/9	Amitriptyline, celecoxib, fluoxetine, fluvastatin, losartan, nonsteroidal anti-inflammatory drugs, oral hypoglycemics, phenobarbital, phenytoin, sulfaphenazole, S-warfarin, tamoxifen	Amiodarone, azole antifungals, fluvastatin, lovastatin, metronidazole, paroxetine, ritonavir, sertraline, trimethoprim, zafirlukast	Barbiturates, dihydropyridines, ifosfamide, rifampin
2D6	Amphetamine β-adrenergic blockers, chlorpheniramine, clomipramine, clozapine, codeine, dextromethorphan, flecainide, fluoxetine, haloperidol, hydrocodone, metoclopramide, mexiletine, ondansetron, oxycodone, paroxetine, propoxyphene, risperidone, selegiline, thioridazine, tramadol, tricyclic antidepressants, venlafaxine	Amiodarone, antipsychotics, celecoxib, cimetidine, cocaine, fluoxetine, methadone, metoclopramide, paroxetine, quinidine, ritonavir, sertraline, terbinafine, ticlopidine, venlafaxine	Dexamethasone, rifampin
3A4/5/7	Acetaminophen, alfentanil, alprazolam, amiodarone, atorvastatin, buspirone, chlorpheniramine, cocaine, cortisol, cyclosporine, dapsone, diazepam, dihydroergotamine, dihydropyridines, diltiazem, dronabinol, ethinyl estradiol, fentanyl, indinavir, lidocaine, lovastatin, macrolides, methadone, miconazole, midazolam, mifepristone, modafinil, ondansetron, paclitaxel, progesterone, quinidine, ritonavir, saquinavir, sildenafil, spironolactone, sufentanil, sulfamethoxazole, tacrolimus, tamoxifen, testosterone, trazodone, triazolam, verapamil, zaleplon, zolpidem	Amiodarone, chloramphenicol, cimetidine, ciprofloxacin, clarithromycin, dihydroergotamine, diltiazem, doxycycline, erythromycin, felodipine, fluoxetine, fluvoxamine, glucocorticoids, grapefruit juice, HIV antivirals, itraconazole, ketoconazole, nefazodone, sildenafil, verapamil	Barbiturates, carbamazepine, glucocorticoids, ifosfamide, modafinil, nevirapine, phenytoin, rifampin, St. John's wort, troleandomycin

TABLE 2.5	Example of Phase I and Phase II Reactions
Drug	Metabolite
Phase I Example: Oxidation	
Codeine →	Morphine
Phase II Example: Glucuronidation	
Aspirin (to Salicylic acid) →	Salicyl-glucuronides

The **glucuronide conjugate** produced is excreted, often with the help of active secretion, into the bile or urine. In contrast to many phase I reactions, conjugation with glucuronic acid almost invariably but, with a few exceptions, results in a total loss of pharmacologic activity. An example of phase I and a phase II reaction is given in Table 2.5.

Nonhepatic Metabolism

Although focusing on the liver when considering biotransformation is appropriate generally, other organs contain drug-metabolizing enzymes (including members of the CYP family) and contribute to the microsomal and nonmicrosomal metabolism of drugs. Almost every tissue has some metabolic activity; however, by virtue of location and blood supply, the kidney, intestine, and lung play special roles in drug metabolism.

Factors Affecting Drug Metabolism

The rate of drug biotransformation depends on numerous variables, including access to the site of metabolism, the concentration and phenotype of the enzyme present, and the effect of certain agents on enzymatic activity. Because most drugs are metabolized in the liver, attention is centered on factors influencing hepatic drug biotransformation.

Enzyme Inhibition

Drug-metabolizing enzymes are subject to competitive and noncompetitive antagonism. This is a common mechanism of drug-drug interactions, with sometimes dramatic effects on a drug's half-life. The CYP system is commonly involved.

Enzyme Induction

Microsomal CYP drug-metabolizing enzymes are inducible and under an appropriate chemical stimulus, catalytic activity increases. Many chemicals, including therapeutic agents and environmental toxins, are capable of stimulating their own biotransformation and the biotransformation of closely related compounds. In addition, some chemicals can augment the breakdown of a host of diverse substances.

Regardless of the pattern of induction, the rate of metabolism of affected compounds may be enhanced by seven times the baseline. Enzyme induction has many important therapeutic ramifications. It is another cause of drug interactions. Examples of inhibitors and inducers at a CYP enzyme are shown in Table 2.4.

Genetic Factors

Individuals vary in their ability to metabolize drugs. Although differences can result from the environmental induction of microsomal enzymes (as seen in chemical factory workers and cigarette smokers), studies comparing identical and fraternal twins have conclusively established the preeminent influence of heredity on the rate of biotransformation.

Age

Neonates, especially premature infants, often lack certain functional drug-metabolizing systems. The relative inability to conjugate bilirubin with glucuronic acid and the resultant development of hyperbilirubinemia is a commonly observed example of this deficiency in biotransformation. In contrast to newborns, children are often more adept at metabolizing drugs on a weight basis than are young adults. Thereafter, biotransformation capacity seems to diminish with age; elderly individuals may often exhibit retarded rates of drug metabolism. Table 2.6 lists disease and other factors that can affect liver metabolism.

Excretion

Foreign substances, including therapeutic medications, are prevented from building up in the body by the combined action of metabolism and excretion. Drugs and their metabolites may be eliminated by numerous routes, including urine, bile, sweat, saliva, gastrointestinal secretions, pulmonary exhalation, tears, and breast milk. The kidney is the major organ of drug excretion.

TABLE 2.6 Conditions That Can Affect Hepatic Drug Metabolism

Condition		Effect on Drug Metabolism	Mechanism
Disease			
	Uremia	Increase	Reduces binding capacity of albumin—increases free drug delivery to liver
	Stress -inflammation	Decrease	Increases α_1-acid glycoprotein—reduces free drug delivery for some basic drugs
	Cirrhosis	Decrease	Reduces hepatic blood flow and damages hepatic cells
	Cardiac insufficiency	Decrease	Reduces hepatic blood flow
	Some infections	Decrease	Reduce hepatic blood flow
	Hypothyroidism	Decrease	Reduces synthesis of metabolic enzymes
	Hyperthyroidism	Increase	Increases synthesis of metabolic enzymes
Other Factors			
	Reduced hepatic blood flow from drugs and other factors	Decrease	Reduces hepatic blood flow
	Neonatal—elderly Population	Decrease	Reduced liver enzymes in both age groups
	Genetic factors	Increase or decrease	Increase or decrease in liver enzyme activity

Renal Excretion

Three processes, glomerular filtration, tubular reabsorption, and active transport, control the urinary elimination of drugs. Although all drugs are subject to filtration, the percentage filtered is inversely related to the degree of plasma protein binding. Once filtered, drugs tend to be reabsorbed in relation to their lipid/water partition coefficients. These considerations favor the renal excretion of highly polar compounds, but the exact rate of elimination also depends on whether active transport into (or, rarely, out of) the tubular fluid occurs (Fig. 2.7).

Glomerular Filtration

Most drugs, including small proteins, pass through the glomerulus on their way to excretion.

Tubular Reabsorption

Because of the kidney's ability to concentrate tubular fluid, a chemical gradient is set up for the diffusion of drugs back into the systemic circulation. Agents with a favorable lipid/water partition coefficient readily traverse the tubular epithelium and return to the bloodstream (see Fig. 2.7).

Active Secretion

Numerous organic anions and cations are actively secreted into the urine by cells of the proximal convoluted tubule.

Clearance

Clearance of drugs from the body is the sum of removal from every organ (renal clearance + hepatic clearance + clearance from other organs). The kidney is the major organ for removing drugs from the body. The rate of drug removal from the body is often calculated as the volume of plasma water "cleared" of drug per unit time, referred to as **"clearance" (CL)**. Therefore the unit of clearance is expressed as volume/time (e.g., liters per hour).

Biliary Excretion

Numerous cationic, anionic, and steroid-like molecules are selectively removed from the blood for excretion into the bile and eventually the feces. Generally, these substances have molecular weights exceeding 500 Da. The transport process is an active one in which the dissolved substance is transferred from the plasma to the hepatocytes and then to the bile. The bile is also a route of excretion for metabolized drugs, especially drugs that have undergone phase II reactions such as glucuronidation.

Biliary excretion is responsible for all but a small portion of the fecal elimination of drugs. The feces may also contain a variable amount of unabsorbed drugs. Reabsorption of molecules excreted through the bile can occur, known as enterohepatic recycling. It can prolong the duration of action of a drug. Interestingly, some glucuronide conjugates secreted via bile into the gut can be metabolized, by gut bacterial enzymes, back to the active parent drug, which can then be reabsorbed (Fig. 2.8).

Other Routes of Excretion

Pulmonary excretion is a primary route for the elimination of gases and some volatile compounds. Elimination of drugs by breast milk is important, not because of any

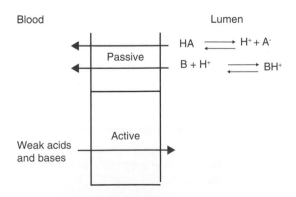

• **Fig. 2.7** Enterohepatic recirculation. The drug released by the action of glucuronidase can be reabsorbed into the liver. (Taken from Bardal SK, Waechter JE, Martin DS: Drug Interactions, in Applied Pharmacology, 2011, Elsevier.pii:B978143770310800004X/f4)

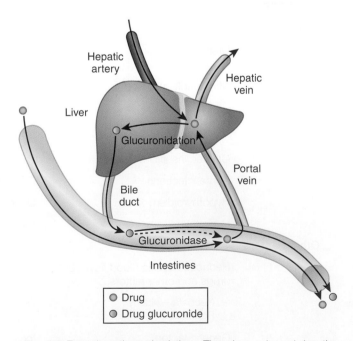

• **Fig. 2.8** Enterohepatic recirculation. The drug released by the action of glucuronidase can be reabsorbed into the liver. (Taken from Bardal SK, Waechter JE, Martin DS. Drug Interactions. In: *Applied Pharmacology*, Elsevier; 2011.)

quantitative significance, but because it represents a potential danger to the nursing infant. The primary variable influencing the passage of drugs into milk is lipid solubility.

Other minor routes of excretion include sweat, tears, saliva, and gastric/pancreatic/intestinal secretions. In all cases, excretion is limited by the lipid/water partition coefficient. For saliva and related gastrointestinal fluids, drugs are deposited into the gastrointestinal tract after secretion and are available for reabsorption into the systemic circulation.

Time Course of Drug Action

A temporal description of drug concentration based on pharmacokinetic principles is useful in illustrating how absorption, distribution, metabolism, and excretion influence drug effects in concert and provide guidance for adjusting dosage schedules to achieve therapeutic results with a minimum of drug toxicity.

Kinetics of Absorption and Elimination

The rates of most biologic events involving the fate of drugs can be described in simple kinetic terms, i.e., either zero-order or first-order kinetics. Most emphasis is on the rate of **drug elimination** from the body.

A key dynamic of drug elimination is whether the body can keep up with the amount of drug absorbed into the body. Most of the time, at the doses of drugs used clinically, the body can increase the amount of drug eliminated as the dose of the drug increases. That means that a constant fraction (or first order) of the remaining drug in the body is removed per unit of time. In this situation, plotting the reduction in the plasma concentration after a single dose of the drug gives a straight line on a semilog plot. Fig. 2.9 compares the expected drug disappearance curve when the "Y" axis is linear to that of a plot when the "Y" axis is on a log scale. The latter plot can be used to determine values such as the plasma concentration of a drug at a given time after drug administration and the elimination half–time of the drug. In reality, when a drug is administered, it goes through a distribution phase (α phase) before it reaches a straight line disappearance curve (β phase) (Fig. 2.10). The β phase is most useful in measuring drug kinetic values.

In dentistry, therapeutic agents are often administered in single doses. Whether the drug is lidocaine injected for regional anesthesia, atropine to control salivation, or

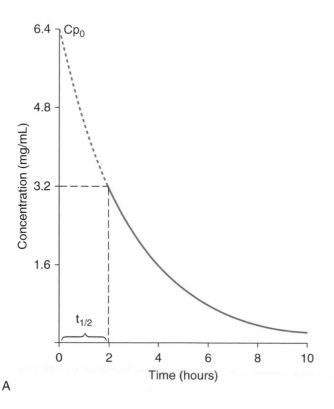 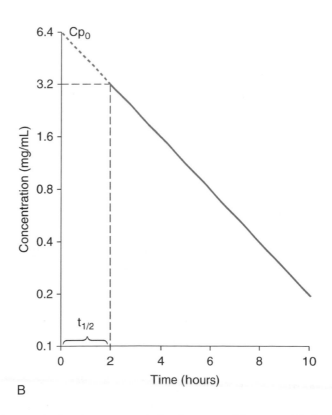

• **Fig. 2.9** First-order elimination of a drug given as an intravenous bolus. In this example of a plasma concentration-time curve, it is assumed that the body behaves as a single compartment and that the distribution of the drug is essentially instantaneous. (A) The plasma concentration is plotted on an arithmetic scale. (B) A logarithmic scale is used to yield a straight line. The elimination half-life (T½) is determined by the time interval required (2 hours in this case) for the plasma concentration to decrease by 50%. The Cp0 indicates the interpolated concentration of drug (from line extension of drug disappearance trace in B) immediately after drug injection.

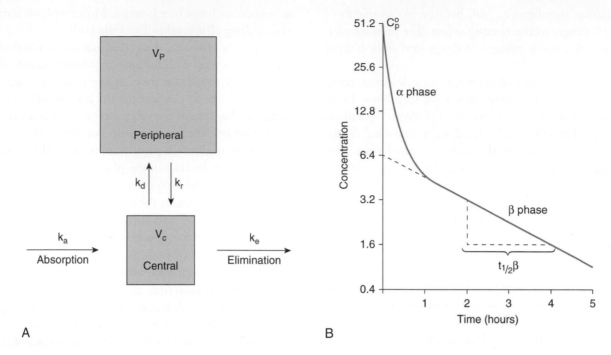

• **Fig. 2.10** A model of drug kinetics. (A) In this model, drugs are absorbed into and eliminated from a central compartment that is linked by distribution processes (having rate constants of k_d and k_r) to a second, peripheral compartment. The central compartment is the blood, from which drug determinations are taken. (B) The plasma concentration-time curve consists of two phases: an early distribution or α phase, during which the concentration decreases largely as a result of distribution out of the central compartment, and a late elimination or β phase, during which metabolism and excretion predominate. The terminal half-life (T½ β) is calculated from the log-linear portion of the elimination curve. The Cp_0 (C_p^0) is determined from the extension of the β phase line to the "y" axis. The Cp_0 is, therefore, an extrapolated value since direct measurement of Cp_0 is impossible.

triazolam to provide preoperative sedation, the plasma concentration increases to a peak during the absorptive phase and subsequently decreases, eventually to zero, as the drug is eliminated from the bloodstream.

On the other hand, with repeated doses of a drug under first-order elimination conditions, it is easier to maintain an acceptable blood level (plateau or steady-state plasma level) with repeated doses of the drug. (Fig. 2.11) compares intermittent dosing, such as with oral administration, to continuous dosing by intravenous administration. With an equal amount of drug absorbed by each route, the general pattern is similar, except for fluctuations with oral dosing. This curve is instructive for some key reasons:
1. The plateau steady state condition is reached after about four elimination half-times of the drug if dosing is the same and continuous.
2. Oral dosing leads to predictable fluctuations in plasma concentrations for reasons given in Fig. 2.11.
3. The steady-state plasma concentration is directly dependent on the dose absorbed and inversely dependent on the rate of drug elimination. (Drug elimination is measured by clearance which varies inversely with the half-life of the drug.)

The elimination half-life of a drug is a commonly used characteristic of a drug. This value can be used to determine the rate of drug removal from the body and how long it takes to reach the plateau phase with constant dosing (a little over four half-lives). It also is useful in determining the dosing regimen, including the dosing interval. Table 2.7 lists the half-lives of several drugs.

Sometimes it is desirable or necessary to get a more rapid effect of the drug rather than wait for the plateau steady state to be reached. In that case, a higher initial dose, loading dose, can be given, followed by the maintenance dose.

What if for a given drug, the body's ability to remove the drug is saturated and cannot match the drug dosing with an equal percentage of elimination of the drug? In this case (zero order kinetics) it is much easier to produce drug toxicity because the amount of drug removed from the body has reached a maximum. Therefore added care must be taken to avoid exceeding the drug dosing rate.

Fig. 2.11 shows a time course of changes in plasma concentrations combining absorption and elimination under different conditions. The three panels show the effects of various doses, rates of absorption of drugs, and rates of elimination. An important pharmacological measure of

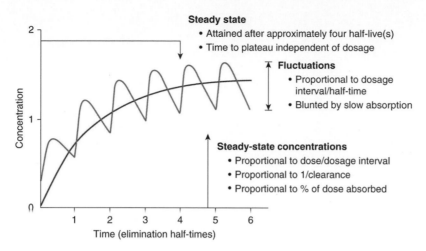

• **Fig. 2.11** Time course of plasma concentration involving drug accumulation. The blue wavy line reflects the pattern of accumulation observed during the repeated administration of a drug at intervals equal to its elimination half-life when drug absorption is 10 times as rapid as elimination. The smooth line depicts drug accumulation during the administration of an equivalent dosage by continuous intravenous infusion. (Adapted from Buxton ILO, Benet LZ. Pharmacokinetics: The Dynamics of Drug Absorption, Distribution, Metabolism, and Elimination. In: Brunton LL, Chabner BA, Knollmann BC, eds., Goodman & Gilman's the Pharmacological Basis of Therapeutics. 12th ed. New York: McGraw-Hill; 2011.)

TABLE 2.7	Approximate Half-Lives of Common Drugs
Drug	**Elimination Half-Life (h)**
Antibiotics	
Amoxicillin	1.7
Clindamycin	3
Erythromycin	1.5
Penicillin G	0.5
Tetracycline	10
Analgesics	
Acetaminophen	3
Aspirin (as salicylate)	3–20[a]
Codeine	3[b]
Meperidine	3
Morphine	2[b]
Local Anesthetics	
Articaine	0.4
Bupivacaine	2.4
Lidocaine	1.8[b]
Procaine	0.01
Sedative Agents	
Ethyl alcohol	1.4–20[a]
Diazepam	45[b]
Pentobarbital	30
Triazolam	3

[a]Capacity-limited metabolism at higher doses.
[b]Converted to an active metabolite.

clinical activity is the **area under the curve (AUC)**. The AUC is used to compare the effect of different factors on the magnitude of drug effect and can be seen as the area under each plasma concentration curve. Changing the dosage amount or rate of elimination has a predictable effect on the AUC. The AUC also indicates the effectiveness of different routes of administration. Notice also the dramatic effect of reducing the clearance of a drug on the AUC, whereas the rate of drug absorption of the drug does not affect the AUC given equal oral doses.

Suggested Readings

Duckworth RM. Pharmacokinetics in the oral cavity: fluoride and other active ingredients. *Monogr Oral Sci.* 2013;23:125–139.

Dowd F Pharmacokinetics: The Absorption, Distribution, and fate of Drugs. Pharmacology and Therapeutics for Dentistry. St. Louis: Elsevier; 2021. In: Dowd FJ, Mariotti AJ, eds. 8th ed. In preparation.

3

Pharmacotherapeutics: The Clinical Use of Drugs

KEY POINTS

- Quantal dose-response curves are used to measure responses to drugs in populations.
- Body weight, age, biologic sex, genetic factors, disease status, pregnancy, and lactation are important factors in a patient's response to drugs and in the occurrence of adverse effects.
- Drug-drug interactions can lead to unexpected adverse effects.
- Adverse drug effects include extensions of the therapeutic effect, side effects, idiosyncratic reactions, and allergies, carcinogenesis, poisoning, teratogenesis, and/or poisoning.
- Pharmacogenetics will be used to personalize selection of drugs for optimal effects.

DEFINITIONS

- Potency is the measure of drug activity expressed as the amount required to produce a given effect. It is expressed as the concentration or dose required to produce 50% of a drug's maximal effect.
- Clinical efficacy is the effectiveness of a drug to achieve a clinical response.
- Tolerance describes the reduced reaction to a drug following repeated use.
- An idiosyncratic reaction may be defined as a genetically determined abnormal response to a drug.
- Teratogen refers to a drug that causes malformation of the embryo or fetus.
- Pharmacogenetics is the branch of pharmacology that seeks to understand the genetic basis for differences in drug responsiveness among the human population.
- Genotype is a genetic trait defined by the DNA sequences (i.e., alleles) inherited from the mother and the father.
- Phenotype is a biologic or measurable expression of the genetic trait. Phenotypes are dependent upon the level of penetrance of the gene, the accuracy and selectivity of the method used to measure it, and the influence of environmental factors in the expression of the trait.
- Genetic polymorphism refers to two or more variants of the DNA sequence of a particular gene. The genetic expression (phenotypes) of a drug may results from variants of one gene (mongenic), or multiple genes (polygenic).

Numerous factors that complicate the attainment of therapeutic responses and the avoidance of unwanted effects should be considered when drugs are properly selected and administered. Drugs are often selective in the effects they produce because they stimulate or inhibit specific drug receptors. However, even the most selective agents generally evoke a spectrum of reactions rather than a single pharmacologic outcome. There are several reasons why this occurs. First, a drug is often used to target a given receptor in a particular organ, but these same receptors are usually located in other tissues and organs as well. Second, although a drug is selective, it often is not specific and may have effects at another receptor(s), especially at higher doses. Third, the drug may have non-selective effects, such as gastrointestinal upset. Fourth, a therapeutic dose of drug for one person may be ineffective for a second person and toxic to a third person. Therefore it becomes necessary to measure the effects of drugs in populations to determine the range of responses and to gauge their levels of safety.

Measuring Drug Responses in Populations; Quantal Dose-Response Curves

A **quantal dose-response** graph represents the percentage of subjects responding to an agent as a logarithmic function of the dose (Fig. 3.1). The graph is constructed by counting the number of patients exhibiting a specified effect at various doses. With low amounts of drug, very few individuals within the population react and as the dose is increased more are affected until a dose is reached at which the response is universal. Although similar in appearance, this quantal dose-effect relationship must not be confused with the graded dose-response curve. Although potency is represented in quantal and graded relationships by the position of the curve on the abscissa, intrinsic activity is apparent only in graded responses (Chapter 1). On a quantal dose-response curve,

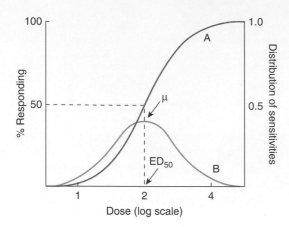

• **Fig. 3.1** Quantal dose-response curves (log scale). Curve *A* represents the cumulative distribution, and curve *B* represents the frequency distribution of patient responses in a normal population. As shown, the mean *(μ)* and median (50% responding) sensitivities fall on the same dose (median effective dose, *ED$_{50}$*). (Adapted from Goldstein A, Aronow L, Kalman SM. *Principles of Drug Action: The Basis of Pharmacology.* 2nd ed. New York: John Wiley & Sons; 1974.)

the **median effective dose (ED$_{50}$)** is the amount of drug required to produce a particular effect in 50% of treated individuals.

Patients who are unusually sensitive to a drug are said to be **hyperreactive** or **hypersusceptible**, or perhaps **drug intolerant**. Individuals unexpectedly resistant to conventional doses of drug are referred to as being **hyporeactive**. Many variables influence the responsiveness of individuals to drugs. Because it is impossible to predict how a given patient will respond to a particular agent, appropriate monitoring of drug effects is usually necessary to achieve optimal therapy.

Factors Influencing Drug Effects

Differences between patients in reaction to a therapeutic agent may arise from disparities in drug concentration obtained with a standardized dose (**pharmacokinetic differences**), from variations in individual responsiveness to a given drug concentration (**pharmacodynamic differences**), or from secondary factors, such as the failure of patients to take their medication as prescribed (e.g., **noncompliance**).

Patient Factors

Many factors that can influence drug effects clinically are highly variable in individual patients. Size, age, and genetic makeup must be taken into account whenever drug therapy is planned.

Body Weight and Composition

Adults may differ three times or more in weight. Because the volume of distribution of a drug is a function of

body mass, extremes in patient size may result in significant differences in plasma concentration when drugs are administered in the form of a "standard adult dose." Body composition is also an important variable. Two equally heavy patients, one obese and the other muscular, may react quite differently to certain agents.

Age

Pediatric patients generally cannot be given adult dosages of drugs. The primary reason is their smaller body size, and various formulas have been devised to calculate pediatric fractions of the adult dose. For the following reasons, however, children must not be thought of as merely miniature adults. First, even with the size differential taken into account, neonates display an unusual hyperreactivity to drugs. Table 3.1 gives a summary of how one's age group can influence a drug response.

Geriatric patients are frequently hyperreactive to drugs, thus careful selection of drug and dosage schedules is necessary, especially with drugs of low safety.

Genetic Influences

Genetic variables contribute greatly to the differences in drug responsiveness. Although the importance of heredity is underscored by the evolution of pharmacogenetics into a recognized field of study, the elucidation of multigenetic factors that lead to normal distributions in drug reactivity has proven difficult. Nonetheless, genetic differences in a single enzyme, for instance, have been shown to dramatically affect a patient's response to a drug (see below.)

Biologic Sex, Pregnancy, and Lactation

Dosage adjustments may be necessary for some drugs simply because women tend to be smaller than men and to have a higher percentage of body fat. Hepatic disposition of drugs seems not to be influenced as much by biologic sex when variables such as age, size, body composition, and drug use are taken into account.

Pregnancy is a major concern in pharmacotherapeutics. Alterations in liver function are common, and the hepatic toxicity of tetracycline and certain other compounds is markedly accentuated by pregnancy. The metabolism of numerous drugs is increased because of the ability of the high estrogen and progesterone concentrations to stimulate the pregnane X receptor and cause enzyme induction. Renal excretion is likewise increased because of the elevated cardiac output and glomerular filtration. When present, pregnancy toxemia may increase drug effects by reducing the binding capacity of albumin, which is already reduced in a healthy pregnancy.

Of primary importance are the actions of drugs on the fetus. Spontaneous abortion, teratogenesis, mental

TABLE 3.1	Age Effects on Responses to Drugs		
Age Group	**Effect**	**Mechanism**	**Examples**
Neonates	Drug Accumulation	Immature livers and kidneys	Benzocaine toxicity, Grey baby syndrome with chloramphenicol
	Greater effects from drugs entering the CNS	Immature blood-brain barrier	Penicillin G
Children	Abnormal growth effects (Up to age 8 yrs.)	Staining of teeth	Tetracyclines
	Impairment of growth	Hormonal effects	Hormones especially steroids
Children through young adults	Reye syndrome	Mitochondrial damage has been proposed	Aspirin and other salicylates
Geriatric patients*	Hyperreactive to drugs	Reduced ability to eliminate drugs, existing pathologies, drug-drug interactions	Sedative hypnotics

*65 years and older.
CNS, Central nervous system.

retardation, drug dependence, and cancer have resulted from drug administration during pregnancy. Because few, if any, agents have been proven to be totally safe for the fetus, it is best to avoid all medications when possible. Drug administration should also be conservative in women of childbearing age because pregnancy is often undiagnosed during the first trimester, the most critical period of fetal development. In the lactating mother, many drugs (e.g., methadone) are excreted in the milk. Because some of these agents may cause unwanted effects in the nursing infant, it is advisable to review carefully drug exposure during lactation as well. For example, nursing is contraindicated in women taking anticancer drugs, immunosuppressants, radioactive chemicals, ergot alkaloids, drugs of abuse, lithium salts, gold, and various antibiotics.

Environmental Factors

Factors such as ambient temperature, sunlight, and altitude are capable of influencing responses to certain drugs. Children given atropine on a warm day are especially susceptible to drug-induced hyperthermia, toxic skin reactions to sulfonamides increase with exposure to sunlight, and nitrous oxide loses efficacy in mountainous regions. Probably the most important environmental factor influencing drug effects is diet. The timing of meals and the types of food eaten can markedly affect drug absorption. The gastrointestinal absorption of most tetracyclines is impaired when taken with milk or other dairy products. Furthermore, numerous chemicals that are ingested, inhaled, or absorbed through the skin can influence the body's disposition of, or response to, various drugs.

The indigenous microflora represents a special kind of environmental variable. Several drugs given orally are metabolized by bacterial enzymes to such an extent that absorption may be significantly impaired.

Physiologic Variables

Numerous physiologic factors can modify clinical responses to drugs. Fluctuations in gastric, plasma, and urinary pH may alter the pharmacokinetics of weak electrolytes. Salt and water balance, exercise, sleep, body temperature, blood pressure, and many other factors also influence patient reactions. The effects of drug inhibitors are particularly sensitive to variations in physiologic or biochemical events.

Pathologic Factors

Diseases may influence pharmacotherapeutics by modifying drug disposition or tissue responsiveness. Pathologic states most commonly associated with altered patient reactivity involve the organs of absorption, distribution, metabolism, and excretion. Hepatic dysfunction and renal disease can create major changes in the pharmacokinetics of a drug. As examples, Table 3.2 list the dosage consequences of renal impairment for three drugs.

Drug Factors

In addition to individual variations in patient reactivity, certain drug factors, namely the formulation and dosage regimen of an agent and the development of tolerance, can markedly influence the success of drug therapy.

TABLE 3.2   Dosage Adjustments of Three Drugs in Renal Failure

Drug	Route of Elimination	DOSE INTERVAL IN HOURS AND (PERCENTAGE OF NORMAL DOSE) ACCORDING TO DEGREE OF RENAL FAILURE[a]		
		Normal Function	Moderate Impairment	Severe Impairment
Penicillin G	Mainly renal	4–6	4–6 (50%)	8 (33%–50%)
Acetaminophen	Hepatic	4	6	6
Lisinopril	Mainly renal	24	24 (50%–75%)	24 (25%–50%)

[a]The degree of renal failure as defined by creatinine clearance: normal function to minimal impairment, >50 mL/min; moderate impairment, 10 to 50 mL/min; severe impairment, <10 mL/min.
Data from St. Peter WL, Halstenson CE. Pharmacologic approach in patients with renal failure. In Chernow B, ed. *The Pharmacologic Approach to the Critically Ill Patient*. 3rd ed. Baltimore: Williams & Wilkins; 1994.

TABLE 3.3   Types of Tolerances to Drugs

Type	Mechanism	Examples
Pharmacodynamic	Cell tolerance due to receptor change and/or other cell changes	Down-regulation of the β-adrenergic receptor, decrease in response to mood-changing drugs
Immune	Antibodies bind to drug	Antibodies to digoxin reduce its effect
Pharmacokinetic (drug disposition)	Induction or inhibition of enzymes of metabolism	Decreased half-life of carbamazepine with continued use due to induction
Cellular distribution	Therapy results in changes in cells that make up a tissue	Anticancer drug therapy leads to cell resistance due to overexpression of P-glycoprotein
Learned tolerance	Individual uses coping skills to compensate for drug effects	Ability of alcoholics to disguise the effects of ethanol

Variables in Drug Administration

Depending on variables in drug administration (e.g., the route of administration, dose, drug formulation, drug accumulation, time of administration, and duration of therapy), the clinical efficacy and toxicologic effects of a drug may be affected.

Drug tolerance

Two major categories of tolerance are recognized: **pharmacokinetic or drug-disposition tolerance**, in which the effective concentration of the drug is diminished, and **pharmacodynamic or cellular tolerance**, in which the reaction to a given concentration of the drug is reduced. Specific mechanisms of tolerance have been established for certain drugs that evoke a rapidly developing form of tolerance termed **tachyphylaxis**. The types of drug tolerance are listed in Table 3.3.

Factors Associated With the Therapeutic Regimen

Some factors influencing drug effects are related to the therapeutic context in which the agent is administered or prescribed. Attitudes toward the drug regimen or practitioner may determine whether an agent proves effective in a patient (or even if the drug is taken). Concurrent use of other medicines may alter drug effects directly through pharmacologic mechanisms or indirectly by promoting errors in drug administration.

Placebo Effects

A placebo effect is any effect attributable to a medication or procedure that is not related to its pharmacodynamic or specific properties. In pharmacotherapeutics, a placebo is a preparation that is pharmacologically inert (e.g., a lactose tablet). Placebo responses to drugs arise from expectations by the patient concerning their effects and from a wish to obtain benefit or relief. There is no justification for the therapeutic use of placebo medication in routine dental practice.

Patient Noncompliance

The reasons for noncompliance are varied. They include a lack of understanding of the drug; the purpose for which it was prescribed; how it is to be administered; economic factors; negative feelings toward the drug, prescriber, or medical care in general; development of adverse reactions; forgetfulness or carelessness; perceived resolution of the problem before the drug regimen is complete; or, conversely, failure to notice any therapeutic benefit.

Drug Interactions

The effect of a drug may be increased, decreased, or otherwise altered by the concurrent administration of another compound. Because agents routinely used in dental practice have been implicated in drug interactions, the topic is of considerable interest to the clinician.

Adverse Drug Reactions

The introduction of new, highly efficacious compounds into pharmacotherapy during the past few decades has led to a disturbing increase in the incidence of adverse reactions. As a result, drug toxicity is now considered a major cause of iatrogenic disease. Reductions in mortality rates associated with certain drugs (e.g., aspirin) show, however, that toxic responses to therapeutic agents can be minimized through concerted efforts by health professionals, the pharmaceutical industry, government, and lay public.

Classification of Adverse Drug Reactions

Drug toxicity may come in many forms: acute versus chronic, mild versus severe, predictable versus unpredictable,

and local versus systemic. Therapeutic agents also differ widely in their tendency to elicit adverse reactions. Agents that are safe for some individuals may be life threatening to others. Although no classification of adverse drug reactions is universally accepted, a taxonomy based on mechanism of toxicity is the most useful in promoting the recognition, management, and prevention of untoward responses to drugs.

Extension Effects

Many drugs are used clinically in dosages that provide an intensity of effect that is submaximal. The reason for this is clear: increasing drug effects beyond a certain point (extension effects) may be dangerous. Adverse responses arising from an extension of the therapeutic effect are dose related and predictable (Table 3.4). Theoretically, they are the only toxic reactions that can be avoided without loss of therapeutic benefit by properly adjusting the dosage regimen.

Side Effects

Predictable, dose-dependent reactions unrelated to the goal of therapy, and often at therapeutic doses, are referred to as side effects. As illustrated in Table 3.5, drugs can produce a huge array of deleterious side effects. Although many such reactions are associated with only a single agent or class of drugs, others seem to be almost universal in occurrence. It is questionable, however, whether frequently noted side effects, such as nausea and drowsiness, are always drug related; similar symptoms are also commonly observed in patients after placebo administration and are reported by individuals receiving no medication whatsoever.

Side effects may be produced by the same drug-receptor interaction responsible for the therapeutic effect, differing only in the tissue or organ affected. In these instances, the categorization of drug responses as toxic

TABLE 3.4 Examples of Drug Toxicity as an Extension of the Therapeutic Effect

Drug	Medical Indication	Therapeutic Effect	Toxic Extension of Therapeutic Effect
Furosemide	Edema	Diuresis	Hypovolemia
Heparin	Thromboembolic disorders	Inhibition of coagulation	Spontaneous bleeding
Insulin	Diabetes mellitus	Reduction of blood glucose concentration	Hypoglycemia
Modafinil	Narcolepsy	Wakefulness	Insomnia
Vecuronium	Abdominal surgery	Skeletal muscle relaxation	Prolonged respiratory paralysis
Zolpidem	Insomnia	Hypnosis	Unconsciousness

TABLE 3.5   Examples of Side Effects of Drugs

Drug	Effect
	Oral Cavity
Diphenhydramine	Xerostomia
Griseofulvin	Black hairy tongue
Phenytoin	Gingival enlargement
Tetracycline	Pigmentation, hypoplasia of the teeth
	Skin and Hair
Amoxicillin	Dermatitis
	Bone and Joints
Ciprofloxacin	Arthralgia
Phenobarbital	Osteomalacia
Prednisolone	Osteoporosis
	Sensory Apparatus
Baclofen	Blurred vision
Gentamicin	Ototoxicity
	Blood
Prilocaine	Methemoglobinemia
	Metabolic Effects
Aspirin	Metabolic acidosis
	Neuromuscular System
Chlorpromazine	Tardive dyskinesia
Lidocaine	Convulsions
	Central Nervous System
Dexamethasone	Mental depression
Diazepam	Confusion
	Cardiovascular System
Bupivacaine	Bradycardia
Propofol	Hypotension
	Respiratory System
Isoflurane	Cough
Ketamine	Laryngospasm
Meperidine	Respiratory depression
	Gastrointestinal Tract
Aspirin	Melena
Erythromycin	Diarrhea
Morphine	Constipation

or therapeutic may depend on the purpose of treatment. Xerostomia induced by atropine is a side effect during the management of gastrointestinal hypermotility but is a desired effect when the drug is used to control excessive salivation. Side effects unrelated pharmacodynamically to the therapeutic action are also quite common, and they too may occasionally be useful.

Many side effects, particularly the more dangerous forms, develop only with drug overdose. Careful alteration of the administration regimen usually resolves these problems while maintaining effective treatment. Many other side effects occur at therapeutic or even subtherapeutic concentrations and cannot be avoided by dosage adjustment without loss of drug benefit. Such reactions can be tolerated, however, if they are mild, brief in duration, reversible, and compatible with therapy. Occasionally, even disturbing side effects are accepted if the need for medication is great. Drugs used in the treatment of various cancers often produce severe toxic effects that must be tolerated because no therapeutic alternative is available.

When two drugs share a common desired effect but cause different side effects, it is sometimes possible to limit toxic responses by using reduced doses of each agent when used in combination. Another pharmacologic approach to avoiding side effects is to add a secondary agent that is capable of blocking or otherwise compensating for the unwanted activity of the principal drug. These strategies presuppose that no additional toxicity will be generated by the combination over that produced by a single effective drug. The most fruitful pharmacologic approach to eliminating undesired side effects is through the development of more selective drugs. Studies of structure-activity relationships have proved invaluable in removing side effects unrelated to therapeutic actions and in reducing side effects that are related.

Idiosyncratic Reactions

An **idiosyncratic reaction** may be defined as a genetically determined abnormal response to a drug. Often a genetic abnormality has been identified and an enzyme change occurs (Table 3.6). Although dose dependent, such reactions are unpredictable in most instances because very few patients given an agent respond idiosyncratically and because the genetic trait responsible for an atypical reaction may be completely "silent" in the absence of drug challenge. When confronted with an unexpected response to a drug, it is a common, although erroneous, practice to describe the event as an idiosyncrasy. Most responses lying outside the normal range of drug reactivity are not truly idiosyncratic in nature but represent allergic manifestations or reflect extension or side effects in patients intolerant to the drug by virtue of factors such as age, weight, or existing disease. In dentistry, most falsely described "idiosyncratic" reactions to

TABLE 3.6	Some Idiosyncratic Reactions to Drugs	
Genetic Abnormality	**Some Drugs Affected**	**Idiosyncratic Response**
NADH-methemoglobin reductase deficiency	Benzocaine, prilocaine	Methemoglobinemia
Glucose-6-phosphate dehydrogenase deficiency	Aspirin, primaquine, sulfonamides	Hemolytic anemia
Abnormal heme synthesis	Barbiturates, sulfonamides	Porphyria
Low plasma cholinesterase activity	Procaine and other ester local anesthetics, succinylcholine	Local anesthetic toxicity, extended paralysis
Altered muscle calcium homeostasis	Volatile inhalation anesthetics, succinylcholine	Malignant hyperthermia
Prolonged QT interval	Cisapride, some antipsychotics and antiarrhythmics	Torsades de pointes

NADH, Reduced nicotinamide adenine dinucleotide.

local anesthetics are the result of accidental intravascular injections or anxiety reactions to the process of injection.

Drug Allergy

Adverse responses of immunologic origin account for approximately 10% of all untoward reactions to drugs. **Allergy** can be distinguished from other forms of drug toxicity in several respects. First, prior exposure to the drug or a closely related compound is necessary to elicit the reaction. Second, the severity of response is seemingly dose independent. Third, the unfavorable effect is due to the drug eliciting an immune response. Finally, the reaction is unpredictable; it usually occurs in a small portion of the population, sometimes in patients who had been previously treated with the inciting drug on numerous occasions without mishap.

Four types of drug allergies have been differentiated on the basis of the immune reactions that cause them and the loci of their actions. The four different types of allergic reactions are recognized as **Type I reactions**, **Type II (cytotoxic, reactions)**, **Type III (immune complex, reactions)**, and **Type IV reactions** (Fig. 3.2).

Although drug allergies cannot always be prevented, their frequency of occurrence can be minimized by observing the following precautions:
1. *Take an adequate medical history.*
2. *Avoid the offending drug and likely cross-reactors.*
3. *Avoid inappropriate drug administration.*
4. *Promote oral use and limit topical exposure.*
5. *Request allergy testing when appropriate.*

Adherence to these recommendations will reduce the incidence of allergic reactions to drugs.

Pseudoallergic and Secondary Reactions

Pseudoallergic reactions are adverse drug responses caused by mediators of allergy that are released through antibody-independent processes. As with true allergies, these reactions are unpredictable, however, they seem to be dose dependent, do not require prior sensitization, and may occur on initial exposure to the drug.

Secondary reactions are indirect (and often unpredictable) consequences of a drug's primary pharmacologic action. For example, antibiotic administration may cause the development of superinfection, a secondary microbial disease made possible by the antibiotic-induced suppression of the normal microflora.

Carcinogenesis

Virtually any agent capable of altering the structure of DNA is a potential carcinogen. Agents known to be carcinogenic include radioactive substances, alkylating agents, nitrosamines, and various aromatic amines and polycyclic aromatic hydrocarbons. Neoplastic transformation occurs when mutations develop in genes regulating cellular growth. Cancer is normally a multistage phenomenon involving multiple genetic mutations such as in **oncogenes** (promote growth and development) and mutations in **tumor suppressor genes** (inhibit cell grow).

Special Problems

Hazards of medication pertaining to abuse, poisoning, and effects on the unborn child warrant special comment because the individuals affected are generally not exposed to the agent for therapeutic purposes. In these

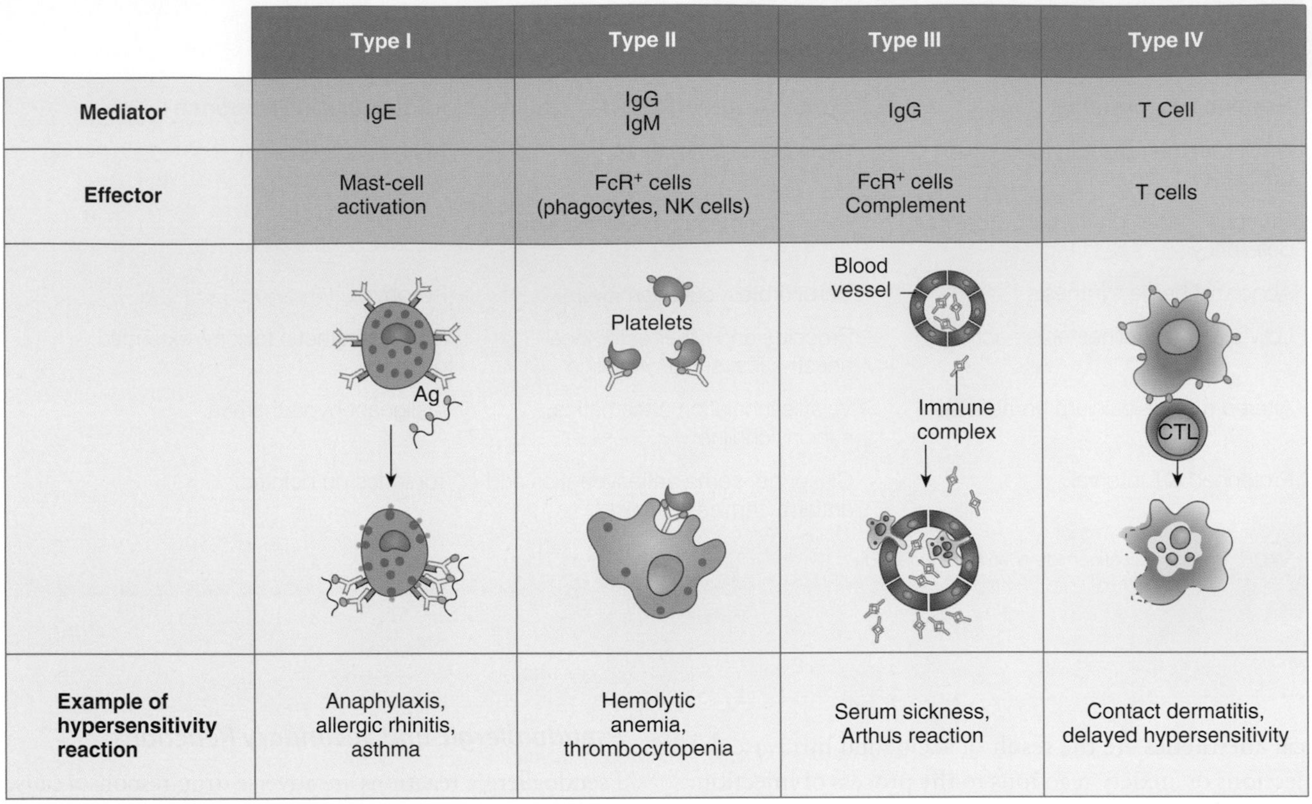

	Type I	Type II	Type III	Type IV
Mediator	IgE	IgG IgM	IgG	T Cell
Effector	Mast-cell activation	FcR⁺ cells (phagocytes, NK cells)	FcR⁺ cells Complement	T cells
Example of hypersensitivity reaction	Anaphylaxis, allergic rhinitis, asthma	Hemolytic anemia, thrombocytopenia	Serum sickness, Arthus reaction	Contact dermatitis, delayed hypersensitivity

• **Fig. 3.2** Major types of allergic reactions. Type I: The antigen cross-links antibodies attached to mast cells leading to release of histamine and other mediators. These are immediate reactions. Type II: Antigen attaches to circulating components such as platelets (shown) or red blood cells. Cytotoxic T cells and complement are involved in lysis of platelets and/or red blood cells. Type III: Antigen-antibody complexes form within blood vessels and then are deposited in tissues leading to macrophage and complement-mediated attack. Type IV: Langerhans cells (antigen presenting cells) bind the antigen, then migrate to lymph nodes. Here they activate the T cell response which is delayed. Other types of Type IV allergic reactions are not shown. *FcR+ cells*, cells possessing the receptor for the tail region of the antibody. *CTL*, Cytotoxic T lymphocytes; *NK*, natural killer; *IgE, IgG, IgM*, immunoglobulins E, G, and M, respectively. (Modified from Pichler WJ. Immune mechanism of drug hypersensitivity. *Immunol Allergy Clin North Am* 2004; 24: 373–397, with permission from Elsevier.)

situations, the prevention and management of adverse reactions can be complicated by matters such as the intent of the person taking the drug, an inability to identify the offending agent, and the unique susceptibility of the embryo to drug toxicity.

Drug Abuse

Typified by persistent and excessive self-administration, drug abuse refers to the inappropriate and deviant use of any drug, despite the knowledge that it will do harm. Drug abuse presents a special problem in toxicology because of the hazards of taking pharmacologically active agents in questionable doses without proper medical supervision. Prevention and treatment of drug abuse, through various strategies, are important. The dentist has a role in preventing and monitoring drug abuse among the dentist's patients.

Drug Poisoning

Drugs most commonly implicated in fatal poisonings are analgesics, antidepressants, alcohol, central nervous system (CNS) stimulants, and cardiovascular agents.

Children younger than 5 years of age account for most poisonings with approximately 2% of the deaths from poisoning. Aspirin, historically the leading cause of drug toxicity in small children, provides a noteworthy example of how unintentional poisoning can be controlled.

Drugs and Pregnancy

Certain compounds have been implicated in the development of congenital abnormalities. These teratogens disturb organogenesis in the developing embryo so that defects in one or more structures are produced. Laboratory experiments in animals and investigations of accidental teratogenesis in humans have found that drug-induced malformation is governed by the sequential pattern of embryonic and fetal development. If the defects are incompatible with life, fetal death and either resorption or spontaneous abortion ensues whereas if they are less severe, the result is a malformed child.

Despite uncertainties concerning most drugs and the unborn child, many pharmacologic agents have been

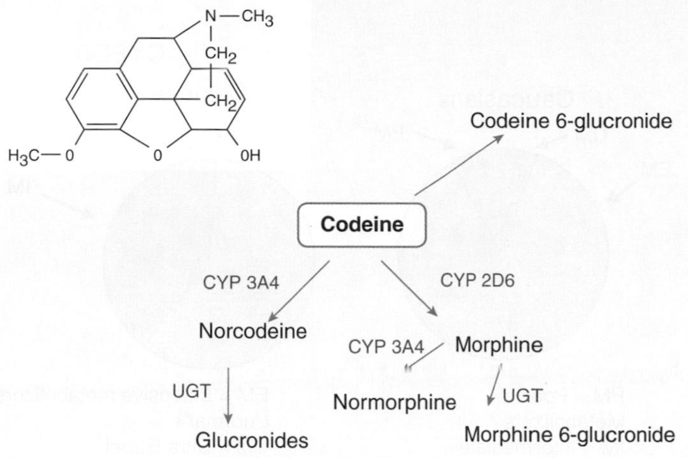

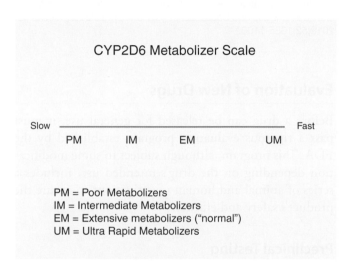

• **Fig. 3.3** Metabolism of Codeine. *UGT,* Uridine diphosphate glucuronosyl transferase.

CYP2D6 Metabolizer Scale

Slow ———————————————————————— Fast

PM   IM   EM   UM

PM = Poor Metabolizers
IM = Intermediate Metabolizers
EM = Extensive metabolizers ("normal")
UM = Ultra Rapid Metabolizers

• **Fig. 3.4** Genetic variants (polymorphisms) in CYP2D6 enzyme activity and the effect on codeine metabolism by the enzyme.

used extensively by pregnant women. The major drug categories include iron supplements, analgesics, vitamins, sedative-hypnotics, diuretics, antiemetics, antimicrobials, cold remedies, hormones, "tranquilizers," bronchodilators, and appetite suppressants. However, a risk-versus-benefit analysis should be done before taking any drug during pregnancy.

Pharmacogenetics

Pharmacogenetics is the branch of pharmacology that investigates the genetic basis for differences in drug responsiveness among the human population. The ability to select the safest and most effective drug and dose for a patient based on the patient's pharmacogenetic profile should simplify the process of adjusting the therapeutic

regimen to achieve the desired clinical response. In fact, clinicians, including dentists, must be aware of the potential for differences in patient responses to the drugs that are prescribed by that clinician. Pharmacogenetics is defined by the FDA as the investigation of the role of variations in DNA sequence on drug response.

The influence of an individual's genetic makeup can have a dramatic effect on the response to a drug. An example is the difference that can exist in a cytochrome P_{450} (CYP) drug metabolizing enzyme within a population. Sometimes this can be due to variants in a single gene (**monogenetic**). These variants are called **polymorphisms**. Different polymorphisms in a drug metabolizing enzyme can lead to variations in the rate of drug metabolism among individual patients.

In Fig. 3.3 notice that several enzymes are involved in the metabolism of codeine. However, it is only cytochrome P450 2D6 (CYP2D6) that converts codeine to morphine. The conversion of codeine to morphine accounts for the analgesic effect of codeine. The activity of this enzyme can vary greatly in the population and among various ethnic populations. If the activity of the enzyme is very high, higher levels of morphine are produced and toxicity may result. Likewise, a very low activity of CYP 2D6 would result in minimal analgesia from codeine.

Fig. 3.4 shows the distinct categories of polymorphisms in CYP2D6 enzyme activity and the effect they have on the rate of metabolism. Fig. 3.5 shows a comparison of two populations of patients. Notice in both populations, extensive metabolizers predominate. Also notice that the two populations vary greatly in the percentages of the polymorphisms. Thus, ethnicity may play a role in the patient's enzyme profile. Furthermore, even within each population, there are some patients who are either poor

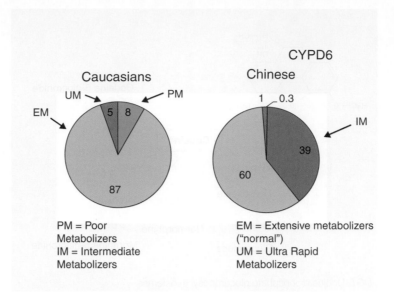

• **Fig. 3.5** The percentage of four different polymorphisms of CYP2D6 in two ethnic populations tested. (Modified from Barter ZE, Tucker GT, Rowland-Yeo K. Differences in cytochrome p450-mediated pharmacokinetics between Chinese and Caucasian populations predicted by mechanistic physiologically based pharmacokinetic modelling. *Clin. Pharmacokinetics*. 2013;52:1085-1100.)

metabolizers or ultra-rapid metabolizers. Poor metabolizers would be expected to have a poor analgesic effect from codeine, whereas ultra-rapid metabolizers would be expected to have a heightened, perhaps toxic, effect.

CYP 2D6 can also be affected by several drugs that can induce or inhibit the enzyme (see Chapter 2). Coadministration of one or more of these other drugs with codeine is likely to increase the conversion to morphine (inducer) or decrease the conversion to morphine (inhibitor).

Since these drug-drug interactions occur at the level of drug metabolism, this and the genetic characteristics of CYP2D6 combine to further challenge the clinician to choose an acceptable drug and at the correct dosage. The results of testing for gene variants are becoming part of the patient record. These tests are becoming more rapidly available, which will aid in deciding on suitable drugs and dosages.

Polygenetic inheritance (i.e., complex inheritance) affecting drug response is more common than **monogenetic inheritance (Mandelian inheritance)** affecting drug response. In a situation of complex inheritance, pharmacologic management of the disease requires dealing with the effects of several genes that contribute to the patient's response to a drug. As discussed above, genetic polymorphisms can not only affect drug metabolism, but they can also affect drug distribution, receptor response, and other events. Thus the complexity of the role of multiple genes adds significantly to variations in patient responses.

Evaluation of New Drugs

Before a drug can be released for general use, it must pass a rigorous evaluation program established by the FDA. This program, although subject to some modification depending on the drug's intended use, includes a series of animal and human investigations to ensure the product's safety and efficacy.

Preclinical Testing

The first step in evaluating a newly discovered compound is to ascertain its pharmacologic activity in animals. Initially, laboratory animals such as rats may be given several different doses of the chemical and observed for any disturbances that may occur in physiology or behavior. If the drug is being developed for a given purpose (e.g., to reduce blood pressure), it would be tested for that particular effect as well. Agents that seem to have a useful action are enrolled in more extensive examinations. When a specific therapeutic effect is identified, quantal dose-effect relationships are drawn to estimate the compound's relative safety.

All drugs are capable of a lethal effect. The dose causing death in 50% of the test animals in a given period is designated as the **median lethal dose (LD_{50})**. The ratio of this dose to the **median effective dose (ED_{50})** defines the **therapeutic index (LD_{50}/ED_{50})**, a crude but useful measure of drug safety in humans. This is shown graphically in Fig. 3.6. (Remember that Fig. 3.6 shows **quantal dose-response curves**.)

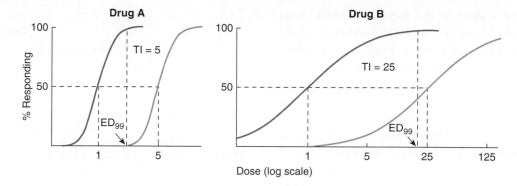

• **Fig. 3.6** Quantal dose-response relationships (log scale) of two drugs, A and B. For each drug, the curve on the left reflects a therapeutic response and the curve on the right represents a toxic reaction. ED_{99}, Dose effective in 99% of the population; *TI*, therapeutic index. Drug B shows one limitation of the TI. The large overlap of the two curves for drug B makes the TI of little use for predicting safety.

Regardless of the number, size, or sophistication of animal tests used, studies in humans are necessary to establish the clinical worth of any drug. Primarily because of unpredictable differences in biotransformation, pharmacokinetic studies in animals cannot be relied on to determine the correct dose or the duration of action of a drug in humans. Of even greater importance is the inability of preclinical studies to detect many forms of drug adverse effects that occur in humans.

Clinical Trials

If an agent seems sufficiently promising on the basis of its preclinical evaluation to warrant testing in humans, the drug sponsor (generally a large pharmaceutical company) must first submit an application to the FDA in the form of a **Notice of Claimed Investigational Exemption for a New Drug (IND application)** detailing, among other things, (1) the identity of the drug and how it is prepared; (2) all results of preclinical investigations to date; (3) the intended use of the agent, dosage form, and route of administration; and (4) the procedures to be followed in assessing the drug's safety and effectiveness in humans. Upon FDA approval of the IND application, the first phase of clinical evaluation can begin. Fig. 3.7 is a summary of the drug development and approval process from preclinical studies to postmarketing surveillance.

Impact of FDA Regulations on the Development of New Drugs

Regulations by the FDA governing the development and marketing of therapeutic agents exist largely as a result of public concern over the adverse effects of drugs.

A primary objective of the FDA is safety. Nevertheless, there have been strategies instituted within the FDA to speed the review process. The Modernization Act of

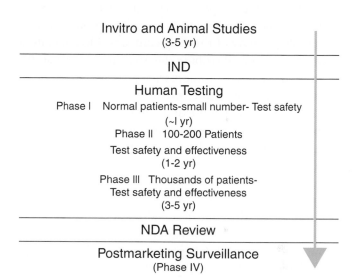

• **Fig. 3.7** Overview of the development of new drugs and drug approval. *IND*, Investigational new drug (application); *NDA*, New drug application.

1997 allowed patients to receive investigational drugs targeted against serious or life-threatening disease outside clinical trials when no satisfactory alternative therapy was available.

The Covid-19 pandemic brought speed-to market-to a whole new level. In the space of less than one year, vaccines against the virus were ready for clinical use. This was due to several factors, including the early sequencing of the virus genome, the recent development of new strategies and methods as applied to vaccine development, and a concerted effort to begin to mass-produce the vaccines before the approval process was finished.

Drug Nomenclature

During the course of development and marketing, a drug acquires various names or designations. The first identification of a drug is the formal chemical name. Although descriptive of the molecular structure of the compound, the chemical name is usually too unwieldy for practical purposes. A newly synthesized drug is often given a simple code name by the parent pharmaceutical firm to denote the agent during the various stages of drug evaluation. If the drug manufacturer intends to request approval by the FDA for distributing the agent, a **nonproprietary name**, or United States Adopted Name, is assigned to the drug by the United States Adopted Name Council (USANC), an organization jointly sponsored by the United States Pharmacopeia, the American Medical Association, and the American Pharmacists Association. A **trade, or proprietary, name** is given to a drug by the manufacturer when the agent is approved for general release. In contrast to the nonproprietary name, which is publicly owned, a trade name receives copyright protection and is the sole property of the drug company. Occasionally, a manufacturer may distribute the agent under several different trade names to promote separate uses of the drug. In addition, the manufacturer may arrange with other pharmaceutical firms to sell the drug, each using its own trade name. A profusion of trade names may develop when the drug patent expires, and other companies are permitted by law to produce the agent. Assignment of trade names to drug combination products contributes yet further to the proliferation of drug names. Fig. 3.8 applies these different names to the same drug, lidocaine.

Note: For further information on the subjects in this chapter, please consult Chapters 3 and 4 of *Pharmacology and Therapeutics for Dentistry*.

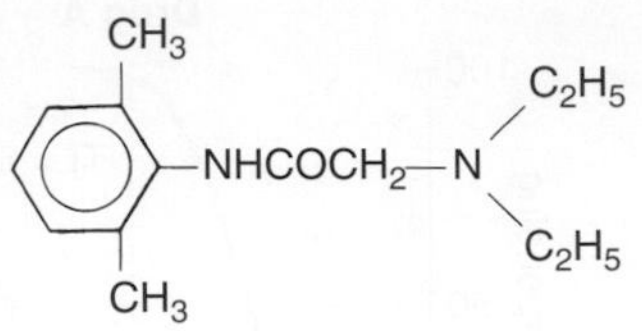

Chemical name (IUPAC):	2-(diethylamino) N-(2,6-dimethylphenyl acetamide)
Code name (Astra):	LL 30
Nonproprietary name (USANC):	Lidocaine
Official name (USP):	Lidocaine
Nonproprietary name (BAN)	Lignocaine
Trade names (selected):	Xylocaine, Dilocaine, Lignospan, Nervocaine, Octocaine

• **Fig. 3.8** Full nomenclature of a local anesthetic. *BAN*, British Adopted Name; *IUPAC*, International Union of Pure and Applied Chemistry; *USANC*, United States Adopted Name Council; *USP*, United States Pharmacopeia.

Suggested Readings

Garcia I, Kuska R, Sommerman MJ. Expanding the foundation for personalized medicine: implications and challenges for dentistry. *J Dent Res*. 2013;92:S3–S10.

Glick A, Sista V, Johnson C. Oral manifestations of commonly prescribed drugs. *Am Fam Physician*. 2020;102(10):613–621.

Zheng LY, Rifkin BR, Spielman AI, et al. The teaching of personalized dentistry in North American dental schools: changes from 2014 to 2017. *J Dent Educ*. 2019;83(9):1065–1075.

4

Introduction to Autonomic Nervous System Drugs

KEY POINTS

- The autonomic nervous system regulates the function of smooth muscles, the heart, and certain secretory glands.
- Sympathetic division nerve pathways originate in thoracic and lumbar regions of the spinal cord.
- Parasympathetic division nerve pathways originate in cranial and sacral regions of the spinal cord.
- Norepinephrine is the neurotransmitter released from most postganglionic sympathetic nerves, whereas both norepinephrine and epinephrine are released from the adrenal medulla.
- Acetylcholine is the neurotransmitter released from all nerves in the parasympathetic nervous system.
- Norepinephrine and epinephrine produce their effects by activating α- and/or β-adrenergic receptors on organs and tissues.
- Acetylcholine produces its effects by activating muscarinic or nicotinic receptors on nerves, organs, or tissues.

DEFINITIONS

- The **autonomic nervous system** is a component of the peripheral nervous system that regulates involuntary physiologic processes including heart rate, blood pressure, respiration, digestion, etc.
- The **parasympathetic nervous system (PSNS)** is one of two major divisions of the autonomic nervous system, which includes nerve pathways from the craniosacral regions of the cerebrospinal axis.
- The **sympathetic division** includes nerve pathways that originate in the thoracolumbar regions of the spinal cord.

Autonomic Nervous System

The **autonomic nervous system (ANS)** and the endocrine system are the major regulatory systems for controlling homeostatic functions. These two systems collectively regulate and coordinate the cardiovascular, respiratory, gastrointestinal, renal, reproductive, metabolic, and immunologic systems. An understanding of the pharmacology of agents affecting the ANS rests on two basic foundations: a knowledge of the structural and functional organization of the ANS, and an understanding of where certain neurotransmitters are located and how these neurotransmitters affect cellular function.

The ANS, also referred to as the visceral, vegetative, or involuntary nervous system, regulates the function of smooth muscle, the heart, and certain secretory glands. Most of our knowledge of the ANS is restricted to efferent nerve fibers (nerves that conduct from the central nervous system [CNS] to the periphery); much less is known about the afferent nerve fibers (sensory nerves that conduct from the periphery to the CNS). Sensory afferent fibers carry impulses that are received and organized centrally, often at an unconscious level. A person is unaware of impulses generated at the baroreceptors, although these impulses may trigger a generalized body response, such as a **reflex** decrease in blood pressure, which the person may sense. It has been estimated that approximately 80% of the vagus nerve consists of primary afferent fibers; nevertheless, most currently available ANS drugs influence efferent activity.

Anatomy

In contrast to the somatic nervous system, the ANS consists of a two-neuron system in which preganglionic nerves emanate from cell bodies in the cerebrospinal axis and synapse with postganglionic nerves originating in autonomic ganglia outside the CNS (Fig. 4.1).

The ANS is divided into two parts on the basis of the anatomic characteristics of each division. The **sympathetic division** includes nerve pathways that originate in the thoracolumbar regions of the spinal cord, whereas the **parasympathetic division** includes nerve pathways from the craniosacral regions of the cerebrospinal axis.

The wider organizational anatomy of the two divisions of the ANS is shown in greater detail in Fig. 4.2.

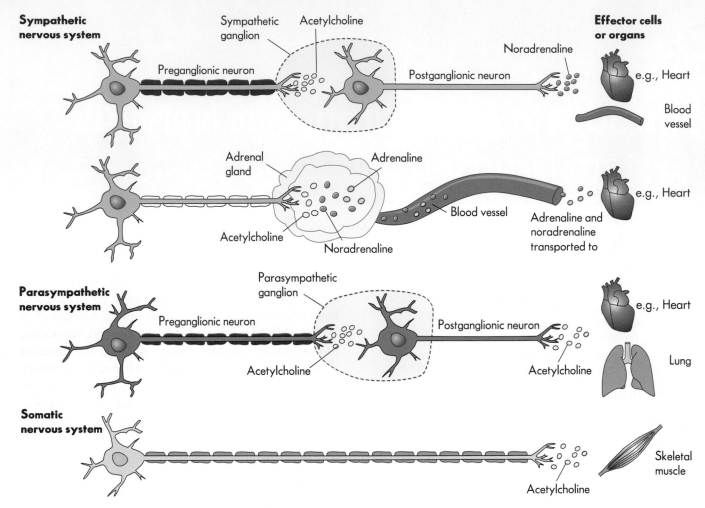

• **Fig. 4.1** Comparison of the autonomic and somatic nervous systems. *CNS*, Central nervous system; *PNS*, peripheral nervous system. (Source: Craft, J et. al: *Understanding Pathophysiology*, Australian adaptation, ed. 2, Merrickville, Australia: Elsevier, 2015, Elsevier.)

Parasympathetic Nervous System

The parasympathetic nervous system (PSNS), or craniosacral division of the ANS, has its origin in neurons with cell bodies located in the brainstem nuclei of four cranial nerves—the oculomotor (cranial nerve III), the facial (cranial nerve VII), the glossopharyngeal (cranial nerve IX), and the vagus (cranial nerve X)—and in the second, third, and fourth segments of the sacral spinal cord. Postganglionic nerves, very short in length, arise from these ganglia to terminate in the aforementioned structures. Neurons originating from sacral segments form the pelvic nerves, which synapse in terminal ganglia lying near or within the uterus, bladder, rectum, and sex organs. In contrast to the arrangement in the sympathetic nervous system, there is little divergence in postganglionic neurons and more focused responses. The postganglionic nerves are very short, and the ganglia are usually buried in the tissues that are innervated.

Sympathetic Nervous System

The sympathetic division originates from neurons with cell bodies located in the **spinal cord**, extending from the first thoracic to the third lumbar segments. The myelinated preganglionic fibers emerge with the ventral roots of the spinal nerves and synapse with second neurons in one of three possible types of ganglia: paravertebral, prevertebral, or terminal. The paravertebral ganglia are composed of ganglia lying on either side of the spinal cord. The superior cervical ganglia (the topmost pair) innervate structures in the head and neck, including the submandibular glands, whereas the superior, middle, and inferior cervical ganglia all innervate the heart. The prevertebral ganglia are located in the abdomen and pelvis and include the celiac, superior mesenteric, and inferior mesenteric, whose postganglionic nerves innervate the stomach, the small intestine, and the colon. The few terminal ganglia

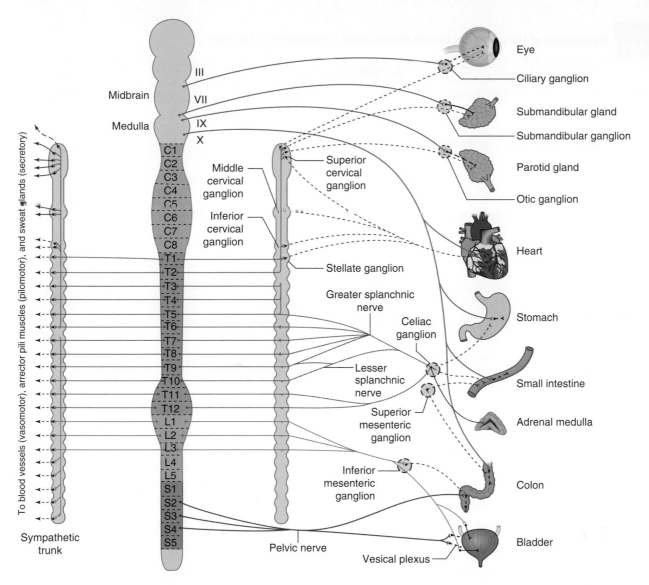

• **Fig. 4.2** The Autonomic Nervous System. Note the cranial-sacral origin of the parasympathetic division and the thoraco-lumbar origin of the sympathetic division. The figure also includes the organs and tissues innervated by the autonomic nervous system. (Reprinted with permission from Copenhaver: Bailey's Textbook of Histology 17e, Williams & Wilkins; 1978.)

lie near the organs they innervate, principally the urinary bladder and rectum.

A striking anatomic aspect of the sympathetic nervous system, and one that has great functional significance, is that a **single preganglionic nerve may contact 20 or more postganglionic nerves**. This arrangement provides an additional basis for the widespread effects of the sympathetic nervous system.

Functional Characteristics

Most organs are dually innervated by the sympathetic and PSNSs, such as most salivary glands, the heart, and abdominal and pelvic viscera, whereas other organs receive innervation from only one division. The **sweat glands, adrenal medulla, piloerector muscles**, and most **blood vessels** receive innervation from only the **sympathetic nervous system**. The parenchyma of the parotid, lacrimal, and nasopharyngeal glands are supplied only with parasympathetic nerves. Table 4.1 lists the organs to which nerve fibers of the parasympathetic and sympathetic nervous systems are distributed, the effects of stimulation of these nerves, and the autonomic receptors that are activated by neurotransmitters released from autonomic nerves.

To understand or predict the effects of autonomic drugs on a specific organ, it is necessary to know how each division of the ANS affects that organ, whether the

TABLE 4.1   Responses of Various Effectors to Stimulation by Autonomic Nerves

| Effector | Sympathetic | | Parasympathetic Response[a] |
	Response	Receptor	
Eye			
Radial muscle of the iris	Contraction (mydriasis)	α_1	—
Sphincter muscle of the iris	—		Contraction (miosis)
Ciliary muscle	Slight relaxation (far vision)	β_2	Contraction (near vision)
Heart[b]			
Sinoatrial node	Increase in rate	β_1, β_2	Decrease in rate
Atria	Increased contractility and conduction velocity	β_1, β_2	Decreased contractility, usually increased conduction velocity
Atrioventricular node	Increase in automaticity and conduction velocity	β_1, β_2	Decrease in conduction velocity
Ventricles	Increased contractility, conduction velocity, and automaticity	β_1, β_2	—
Blood Vessels[c]			
Coronary	Functional significance doubtful due to metabolic autoregulation	$\alpha_1, \alpha_2, \beta_2$	—
Skin and mucosa	Constriction	α_1, α_2	Dilation, but of questionable significance
Skeletal muscle	Constriction; dilation	$\alpha, \beta_2{}^d$	—
Abdominal viscera	Constriction; dilation	α_1, β_2	—
Salivary glands	Constriction	α_1, α_2	Dilation
Erectile tissue	Constriction	α	Dilation
Lungs			
Bronchial smooth muscle	Relaxation	β_2	Contraction
Bronchial glands	Decreased secretion; increased secretion	α_1, β_2	Increased secretion
Gastrointestinal Tract			
Smooth muscle	Decreased motility and tone	$\alpha_1, \alpha_2, \beta_1, \beta_2$	Increased motility and tone
Sphincters	Contraction	α_1	Relaxation
Secretion	Inhibition	α_2	Stimulation
Salivary glands	Protein-rich secretion[e]	$\alpha_1, \beta_1, \beta_2$	Profuse, watery secretion
Spleen capsule			
	Contraction; mild relaxation	α_1, β_2	—
Urinary Bladder			
Detrusor	Relaxation	β_2, β_3	Contraction
Trigone and sphincter	Contraction	α_1	Relaxation

Continued

TABLE 4.1	Responses of Various Effectors to Stimulation by Autonomic Nerves—cont'd			
	Sympathetic			
Effector	**Response**	**Receptor**	**Parasympathetic Response**[a]	
Ureter				
Motility and tone	Increased	α_1	Increased (?)	
Uterus				
	Variable, depending on species, endocrine status	α_1, β_2	Variable	
Miscellaneous				
Pilomotor muscles	Contraction	α_1	—	
Sweat glands	Secretion[f]		—	
Liver	Glycogenolysis, gluconeogenesis	α_1, β_2	Glycogen synthesis	
Adipose tissue	Lipolysis	α_1, β_1, β_3	—	

[a]All parasympathetic responses are mediated by activation of muscarinic receptors. Most responses are mediated by predominantly M_3-muscarinic receptors, except in the heart where M_2-muscarinic receptors dominate.
[b]Norepinephrine released from sympathetic nerves activates primarily β_1 receptors; epinephrine released from the adrenal medulla stimulates β_1 and β_2 receptors. The predominant adrenergic receptor in the heart is β_1.
[c]In most smooth muscles, including blood vessels, α_1 receptors contract (constrict), whereas β_2 receptors relax (dilate). Prejunctional α_2 receptors on sympathetic nerve terminals inhibit norepinephrine release, which relaxes blood vessels and causes vasodilation; postjunctional α_2 receptors cause vasoconstriction.
[d]Blood vessels in skeletal muscle are innervated by some sympathetic nerves that release acetylcholine, which acts on muscarinic receptors to cause vasodilation. However, their functional significance is doubtful.
[e]The human parotid glands do not receive sympathetic innervation.
[f]The sweat glands receive sympathetic innervation, but with few exceptions (e.g., the sweat glands of the palms of the hands, which are activated by α_1 receptor stimulation), the transmitter is acetylcholine, and the receptors activated are muscarinic.

organ is singly or dually innervated, and if dually, which of the two systems is dominant in the organ. In most circumstances, one or the other of the two divisions of the ANS will provide the dominant influence, but often neither division is totally dominant in many of the dually innervated organs.

The sympathetic nervous system can produce a **"fright, fight, or flight"** response. The parasympathetic division is primarily concerned with the **conservation and restoration of bodily resources**.

Neurotransmitters

Acetylcholine is the primary neurotransmitter released from preganglionic nerves and from postganglionic nerves in the PSNS. Norepinephrine is the neurotransmitter released from most postganglionic sympathetic nerves, whereas norepinephrine and epinephrine are released after sympathetic stimulation of the adrenal medulla. See Figs. 4.1–4.3 to visualize these anatomical locations.

Cholinergic Characteristics

Cholinergic Receptor Location

Fig. 4.3 shows the location of both muscarinic and nicotinic receptors.

Synthesis, Release, Neurotransmission, and Fate of Acetylcholine

The general concept of transmitter synthesis, storage, and removal applies to acetylcholine at cholinergic junctions of the ANS (Fig. 4.4). Notice the role of **choline acetyltransferase**. The newly synthesized acetylcholine is transported into and stored in vesicles. Like the adrenergic neurotransmitter release process described later, depolarization of the nerve terminal triggers a Ca^{++}-dependent vesicular transport to the prejunctional membrane to make contact with specialized docking proteins, and releases the contents of the vesicles by exocytosis. Acetylcholine crosses the junctional cleft and attaches reversibly to the postjunctional receptors, but it is also subject to rapid metabolism by **acetylcholinesterase**

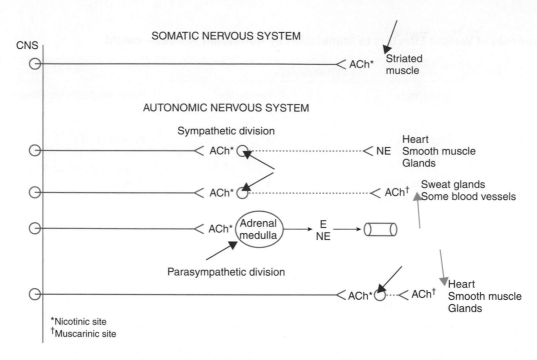

• **Fig. 4.3** Sites of muscarinic cholinergic *(blue)* and nicotinic cholinergic *(red)* receptors. *ACH,* Acetylcholine; *NE,* norepinephrine.

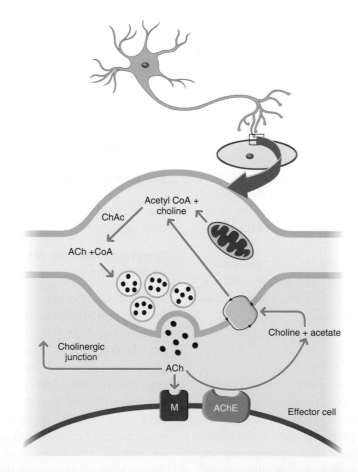

• **Fig. 4.4** Cholinergic nerve terminal and its effector, in which are shown the intraneuronal synthesis of acetylcholine *(ACh),* the vesicles containing ACh, the release of ACh into the junctional cleft, its removal by the action of acetylcholinesterase *(AChE)* and diffusion, and the subsequent reuptake of choline back into the nerve terminal. *CoA,* Coenzyme A; *ChAc,* choline acetyltransferase; *M,* muscarinic receptor. (Adapted from Hubbard JI. Mechanism of transmitter release from nerve terminals. *Ann N Y Acad Sci.* 1971;183:131–146.)

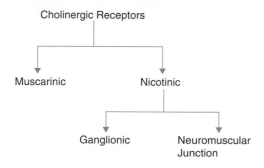

• **Fig. 4.5** Classification of cholinergic receptors.

(AChE). Notice also the role of neuronal uptake of choline (see Fig. 4.4). Nonspecific pseudocholinesterase can also metabolize acetylcholine outside the nerve.

Cholinergic Receptors

Acetylcholine receptors are classified in two major categories: nicotinic and muscarinic. The anatomic distribution and functional significance of these receptors have been described (Figs. 4.1 and 4.2). Nicotinic receptors outside the CNS are located on postganglionic nerves in autonomic ganglia, on chromaffin cells in the adrenal medulla, and on skeletal muscle in neuromuscular junctions. In contrast to adrenergic receptors and muscarinic receptors, nicotinic receptors are ion channel receptors in the plasma membrane.

Muscarinic receptors of the ANS are located primarily on effector cells—smooth muscle, the heart, and secretory glands—that are innervated by postganglionic parasympathetic nerves. As with adrenergic receptors, muscarinic receptors all have seven transmembrane-spanning domains and are G protein-linked. A summary of the classification of cholinergic receptors is shown in Fig. 4.5.

Signal Transduction and Second Messengers

The binding of an autonomic neurotransmitter to its receptor on the plasma membrane surface of a target cell initiates a signaling cascade that alters the physiologic activity of the cell. The exact response elicited depends on the type of receptor activated. In summary, there are two general classes of membrane-bound receptors that interact with autonomic drugs: (1) ion channel–linked and (2) G protein–linked seven transmembrane-spanning domain receptors (see below).

Adrenergic Neurotransmission

Catecholamines (A Chemical Term Referring to Structures Like Epinephrine and Norepinephrine)

Norepinephrine (noradrenaline) and epinephrine (adrenaline) are the primary neurotransmitters and hormones released from effector sites after stimulation of the sympathetic nervous system. In the adrenergic nerve terminal and adrenal medulla, the enzyme **tyrosine hydroxylase** is the rate-limiting enzyme in the synthesis of catecholamines. The enzyme **phenylethanolamine N-methyltransferase**, which catalyzes the conversion of norepinephrine to epinephrine, occurs almost exclusively in the chromaffin cells of the adrenal medulla and is missing in peripheral nerve terminals. Norepinephrine is the final product in most adrenergic nerves, whereas mainly epinephrine (80%), with some norepinephrine (20%), is produced in normal adrenal chromaffin cells in humans.

Catecholamine Release

About 95% of intracellular norepinephrine is stored in vesicles, where it is protected from intracellular enzymatic destruction until it is released by depolarization of the nerve; the other 5% is found in the cytoplasm. Membrane depolarization causes release of transmitter from the vesicles (also called granules). A diagrammatic representation of the adrenergic nerve terminal is shown in Fig. 4.6.

When the nerve is stimulated, extracellular Ca^{++} enters into the nerve terminals. Norepinephrine is then released into the junctional cleft by the process of exocytosis. After crossing the junctional cleft by passive diffusion, the transmitter binds to receptor sites on the effector organ and elicits an appropriate response.

Fig. 4.7 shows the classification of adrenergic receptors. Notice that the two major types are alpha (α) and beta (β). Both are further subdivided as shown. The α_1 adrenergic receptor is a postjunctional receptor, whereas the α_2 adrenergic receptor is located both prejunctionally and postjunctionally.

Location of Adrenergic Receptors

The locations of adrenergic receptors are shown in Fig. 4.8.

Responses of Tissues to Parasympathetic and Sympathetic Stimulation

Table 4.1 contrasts the effects of sympathetic and parasympathetic stimulation and the receptors involved where the nerves innervate various effectors. Notice that some organs express only one type of adrenergic receptor, whereas others have several types. The following statements apply the information in Table 4.1 to individual receptors.

α_1-Adrenergic receptors mediate smooth muscle contraction and glandular secretion and are often excitatory. The function of α_2 receptors at postjunctional sites includes regulation of several metabolic functions (e.g., glycogenolysis, lipolysis) and vascular smooth muscle

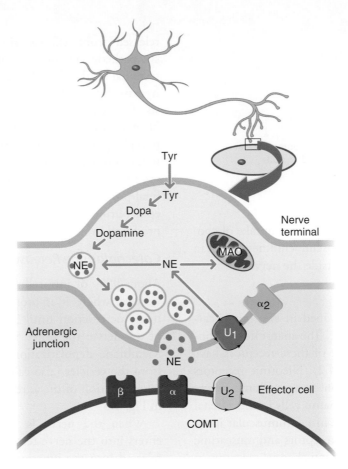

• **Fig. 4.6** Adrenergic Nerve Terminal and its Effector Cell. Shown are the precursors of norepinephrine *(NE)*, the sites of synthesis and storage of dopamine and NE, and the location of prejunctional and postjunctional adrenergic receptors (α_2, α, β). It also shows the enzymatic (catechol-O-methyltransferase [COMT], monoamine oxidase [MAO]), neuronal (uptake-1, U1), and extraneuronal (uptake-2, U2) mechanisms by which the action of NE is terminated. *Dopa*, Dihydroxyphenylalanine; *Tyr*, tyrosine.

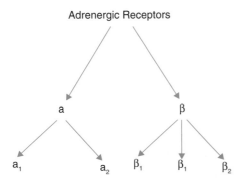

• **Fig. 4.7** Classification of adrenergic receptors.

contraction. Norepinephrine acts on prejunctional α_2 receptors to inhibit neurotransmitter release. Centrally, α_2 receptors are known to be involved in the regulation of blood pressure. β_1-Adrenergic receptors are often associated with excitatory cellular responses, and β_2 receptors are often associated with relaxation of smooth muscle. β_3 Receptors stimulate lipolysis in fat cells and relax the detrusor muscle in the bladder.

Fate of Catecholamines

The fate of the released catecholamines and systems responsible for termination of their action are quite different from mechanisms of neurotransmitter termination at cholinergic junctions. At adrenergic junctions, **uptake** of the transmitter accounts for the greatest proportion of transmitter loss, with enzymatic breakdown and diffusion away from the junction responsible for only a small percentage of the total. As depicted in Fig. 4.6, uptake can be neuronal (**uptake-1, U1**) or extraneuronal (**uptake-2, U2**). Neuronal uptake is by the **norepinephrine transporter**. Amphetamines, tyramine, and levonordefrin (α-methylnorepinephrine) are examples of other drugs that are taken up by this transporter system. Inhibitors of neuronal uptake include cocaine and imipramine. Extraneuronal uptake by the *extraneuronal transporter* has a greater capacity but lower affinity than neuronal uptake. At high concentrations of norepinephrine, extraneuronal uptake results in the rapid removal of the transmitter. Extraneuronal uptake is not sensitive to neuronal uptake inhibitors such as cocaine. Within the

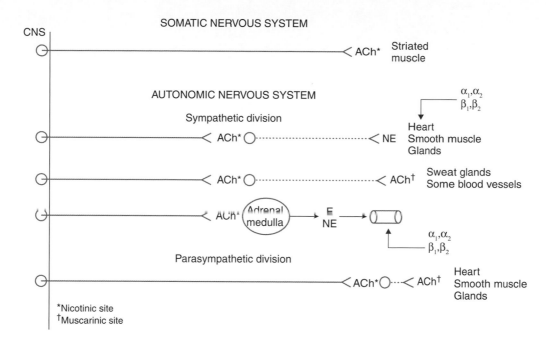

SOMATIC NERVOUS SYSTEM

*Nicotinic site

†Muscarinic site

• **Fig. 4.8** Location of Adrenergic Receptors in the Autonomic Nervous System. Notice that epinephrine and norepinephrine, released by the adrenal gland into the blood, stimulate adrenergic receptors in blood vessels as well as the heart, smooth muscle, and glands. *ACH*, Acetylcholine.

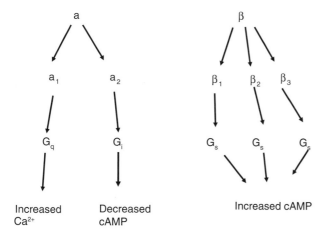

• **Fig. 4.9** Simplified organization of autonomic receptor signaling. *cAMP*, Cyclic adenosine triphosphate.

Receptor Signaling

The receptors and the signaling pathways for autonomic drugs are shown in Fig. 4.9. Refer to Chapter 1 for a more detailed description of each type of receptor and its pathway(s). Nicotinic receptor stimulation leads to opening of ion channels leading to an influx of Na^+ and membrane depolarization (not shown in Fig. 4.9).

Summary of Neurotransmission

The foregoing discussion in this chapter has shown that neurotransmission in the ANS, and normal function of the two divisions of the ANS, depends on many integrated steps:

• Synthesis of neurotransmitter
• Release of neurotransmitter
• Stimulation of receptor by neurotransmitter
• Termination of the effect of the neurotransmitter by either:
  • Metabolism of neurotransmitter or
  • Reuptake of neurotransmitter

Virtually all levels of the CNS contribute significantly to the regulation of the ANS; these include the spinal cord, brain stem, and higher centers.

nerve terminal, uptake of norepinephrine into the storage vesicles also takes place.

Although uptake into the nerve terminal is the major means by which the action of catecholamines is terminated, two enzymes are involved in the metabolism of catecholamines: **monoamine oxidase (MAO)**, which is located largely in the adrenergic nerve; and **catechol-O-methyltransferase (COMT)**, which is widely distributed in extraneuronal tissue.

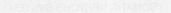

5

Cholinergic Agonists and Muscarinic Receptor Antagonists

KEY POINTS

Cholinergic agonists primarily stimulate muscarinic receptors, and a few cholinergic drugs may stimulate nicotinic receptors.

The metabolism of acetylcholine is inhibited by cholinesterases, principally acetylcholinesterase.

Acetylcholinesterase inhibitors increase the level of acetylcholine.

Agonists at cholinergic receptors are either acting directly on the muscarinic receptor or indirectly by inhibiting acetylcholinesterase.

A number of tissues respond to muscarinic receptor agonists.

DEFINITIONS

- Cholinergic agonists are drugs that stimulate muscarinic or nicotinic receptors.
- Cholinergic receptors are transmembrane proteins activated by acetylcholine. The two types of cholinergic receptors include nicotinic acetylcholine receptors (responsive to nicotine) and the muscarinic acetylcholine receptors (responsive to muscarine).
- Cholinomimetics are drugs that cause parasympathetic effects by stimulating muscarinic receptors.

Introduction

Most cholinergic drugs produce parasympathetic responses by stimulating muscarinic receptors located on tissues innervated by the postganglionic fibers of the parasympathetic nervous system. These drugs are often referred to as **muscarinic** or **parasympathomimetic** agonists. A few cholinergic agonists produce a nonselective stimulation of the parasympathetic and sympathetic branches of the autonomic nervous system by activating ganglionic nicotinic receptors located on the cell bodies of postganglionic fibers. In addition, some cholinergic agonists excite skeletal muscle by activating a separate group of nicotinic receptors located on the motor endplate of the neuromuscular junction. Finally, those synapses in the central nervous system (CNS) that contain nicotinic and muscarinic receptors can be stimulated by cholinomimetic agonists capable of crossing the blood–brain barrier. (Review Figs. 4.1 and 4.2 for important information on the anatomy and physiology of the autonomic nervous system and somatic nerves innervating skeletal muscles.)

Drugs that inhibit the hydrolysis of **acetylcholine (ACh)** by the enzyme **acetylcholinesterase (AChE)** produce their cholinomimetic effects indirectly (Fig. 5.1). They are therefore called **indirectly acting cholinergic** drugs. These anticholinesterases prolong the effective life of ACh released from cholinergic nerves. As a group, the anticholinesterases are less selective in effect than many directly acting cholinomimetics, and they are largely without activity in denervated tissues. Nevertheless, their dependence on ACh release confers the potential advantage of retaining neural control over their effects.

Cholinomimetic Agonists (Directly Acting)

Drugs

The cholinomimetic agonists directly stimulate cholinergic receptors (i.e., muscarinic or nicotinic or both) to cause a pharmacologic response in an effector tissue. These cholinergic drugs are classified into three groups: ACh (Fig. 5.2) and its synthetic congeners, the naturally occurring alkaloids, including **muscarine, pilocarpine, and nicotine**, and synthetic drugs, **cevimeline** being a major example. With few exceptions (e.g., nicotine), these agents exert predominately **muscarinic** effects (Table 5.1).

Mechanism of Action

ACh is capable of stimulating both muscarinic and nicotinic receptors when administered systemically; however

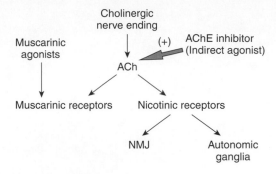

• **Fig. 5.1** Effects of release of acetylcholine (ACh) from cholinergic nerve endings, muscarinic agonists, and increase of ACh by inhibitors of acetylcholinesterase *(AChE)* inhibitors. *NMJ,* Skeletal neuromuscular junction.

$$(CH_3)_3\overset{+}{N}-CH_2-CH_2-O-\overset{\overset{\displaystyle O}{\|}}{C}-CH_3$$

Acetylcholine

• **Fig. 5.2** Structural formula of acetylcholine.

TABLE 5.1   **Summary of Some Cholinergic Agonists**

Drug	Receptor Stimulated	Metabolized by AChE
Acetylcholine	Muscarinic, Nicotinic	++++
Muscarine	Muscarinic	—
Pilocarpine	Muscarinic	—
Cevimeline	Muscarinic	—
Carbachol	Muscarinic, Nicotinic	—
Nicotine	Nicotinic	—

AChE, Acetylcholinesterase.

other drugs, **excluding nicotine, selectively stimulate muscarinic receptors** located on autonomic effector tissues (especially in smooth muscle and glandular tissues) and on the cell bodies of unique populations of CNS neurons. Parasympathomimetic responses to cholinergic drugs are mediated by the stimulation of several populations of muscarinic receptors.

Pharmacologic Effects of Acetylcholine and Other Muscarinic Receptor Agonists

The pharmacologic effects produced by directly acting cholinergic drugs vary according to the receptors they stimulate, their distribution throughout the body, and their mode of inactivation. The duration of action of ACh and its congeners is determined by their susceptibility to hydrolysis by **AChE** and **pseudocholinesterase**. Methacholine, with some susceptibility only to AChE, has a longer duration of action than ACh. Bethanechol, carbachol, cevimeline, and the natural alkaloids are not affected by the cholinesterases at all and therefore also have longer durations of action than ACh.

Cholinergic agonists that stimulate muscarinic receptors produce end-organ responses that mimic parasympathetic nervous system stimulation. Table 4.1 in Chapter 4 outlines several of the physiologic responses produced by direct electrical stimulation of parasympathetic nerves. Most major cholinergic events induced by cholinergic drugs at **muscarinic receptors** are shown in Fig. 5.3A–G.

The effects of muscarinic receptor stimulation at the following organs or tissues are reviewed. (In each box, clinical indications for muscarinic stimulation are given in parentheses.)

Eye

Intraocular pressure (IOP) is decreased as a result of miosis, particularly if the pressure was elevated initially. In addition, there may be a transient hyperemia of the conjunctiva (see Fig. 5.3A).

Heart

The direct muscarinic effects on the heart, as shown in Fig. 5.3D are subject to autonomic modification. For example, a baroreceptor-mediated increase in sympathetic nervous system activity may occur if the muscarinic drug produces a significant fall in blood pressure.

Vascular Smooth Muscle

The stimulation of muscarinic (M3) receptors on the intact **vascular endothelium** is unique because it produces a profound vasodilation by stimulating the production and release of nitric oxide, an important endothelium-derived relaxing factor (see Fig. 5.3C). **Nitric oxide** stimulates guanylyl cyclase located in vascular smooth muscle, which in turn catalyzes the formation of cyclic guanosine 3′,5′-monophosphate. This cyclic nucleotide reduces intracellular calcium concentrations, leading to vascular smooth muscle relaxation and vasodilation. The effect of agonists on the muscarinic receptors of endothelial cells accounts for the vasodilatation when these drugs are administered systemically, especially intravenously. This occurs despite the lack of nerve innervation to these receptors on endothelial cells.

Bronchial Smooth Muscle

The smooth muscle of the bronchioles is constricted by muscarinic receptor agonists and secretion is increased (see Fig. 5.3E).

Gastrointestinal Tract

Motility, peristaltic contractions, amplitude of contraction, and tone are all increased by muscarinic receptor agonists. Conversely, sphincter muscles are relaxed (see Fig. 5.3E).

Exocrine Glands

All glands that are innervated by cholinergic fibers are potentially stimulated by cholinergic drugs. These include the salivary, lacrimal, bronchial, sweat, gastric, intestinal, and pancreatic glands (see Fig. 5.3B). It should be noted again that the secretion by sweat glands is controlled by sympathetic nerves, which in this case have cholinergic postganglionic fibers.

Urinary Bladder

Muscarinic receptor agonists stimulate contraction of the detrusor muscle, which results in decreased bladder capacity and opening of the urethral orifice in the fundus of the bladder. The sphincter and trigone muscles are relaxed with muscarinic receptor stimulation (see Fig. 5.3F).

Organ or tissue and effect‡ (indications)

Eye

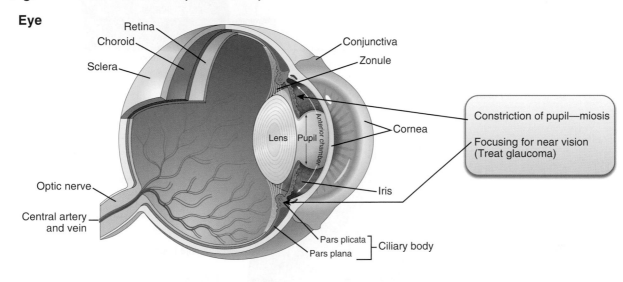

A

Exocrine gland

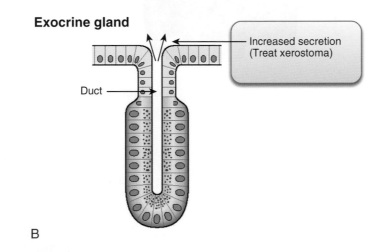

B

• **Fig. 5.3** (A–F) Effects of muscarinic receptor stimulation on various tissues. (**Eye,** Modified from Kumar V, Abbas AK, Aster JC. *Robbins and Cotran: Pathologic Basis of Disease.* 9th ed. Philadelphia: Saunders; 2015. **Exocrine Glands,** Modified from Waugh A, Grant A. *Ross and Wilson, Anatomy and Physiology in Health and Illness. 11th ed. Edinburgh: Churchill Livingstone;* 2010. **Blood Vessels,** Modified from Mahan LK, Stump SE, Raymond JL. *Krauses's Food and the Nutrition Care Process.* 13th ed. St. Louis: Saunders; 2011. **Heart,** Modified from Patton KT, Thibodeau GA. *The Human Body in Health and Disease.* 6th ed. St. Louis: Mosby; 2014. **Bronchus,** Modified from Standring F. *Gray's Anatomy: The Anatomical Basis of Clinical Practice.* 41st ed. Edinburgh: Churchill Livingstone; 2016. **Stomach and Intestines,** Modified from Bontrager KL, Lampignano JP. *Textbook of Radiographic Positioning and Related Anatomy.* 8th ed. St. Loius: Mosby; 2014. **Urinary Bladder,** Modified from Patton KT, Thibodeau GA. *Anatomy and Physiology.* 9th ed. St. Louis: Mosby; 2016.)

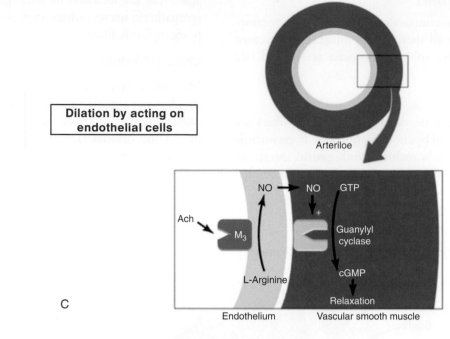

Dilation by acting on endothelial cells

C

Endothelium   Vascular smooth muscle

Heart

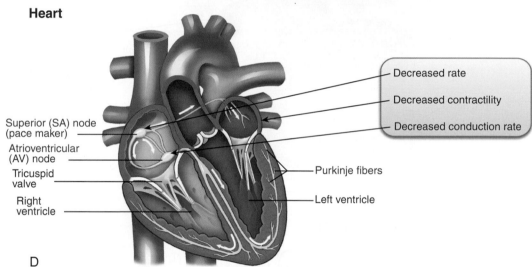

Superior (SA) node (pace maker)

Atrioventricular (AV) node

Tricuspid valve

Right ventricle

Decreased rate

Decreased contractility

Decreased conduction rate

Purkinje fibers

Left ventricle

D

Bronchus

Contraction; increased secretion

(Diagnostic test for hyperactive airway)

E

Stomach and intestines

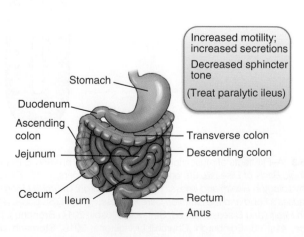

Increased motility; increased secretions

Decreased sphincter tone

(Treat paralytic ileus)

Stomach

Duodenum

Ascending colon

Jejunum

Cecum

Ileum

Transverse colon

Descending colon

Rectum

Anus

• **Fig. 5.3** Cont'd

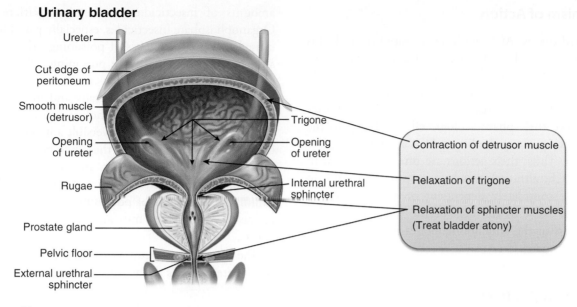

Urinary bladder

- Ureter
- Cut edge of peritoneum
- Smooth muscle (detrusor)
- Opening of ureter
- Rugae
- Prostate gland
- Pelvic floor
- External urethral sphincter
- Trigone
- Opening of ureter
- Internal urethral sphincter

Contraction of detrusor muscle

Relaxation of trigone

Relaxation of sphincter muscles (Treat bladder atony)

F

• **Fig. 5.3** Cont'd

• **BOX 5.1   Adverse Effects of Muscarinic Receptor Stimulation[a]**

Salivation
Sweating
Lacrimation
Urination
Defecation
Bronchospasms
Hypotension
Increases gastric secretion and motility

[a]Patients with increased risk of adverse responses include those with asthma, cardiovascular disease, and peptic ulcer.

Central Nervous System

As previously mentioned, there are both muscarinic and nicotinic receptors in the CNS. Central cholinergic systems have been implicated in central regulation of most physiologic systems (i.e., cardiovascular, respiratory, gastrointestinal, and somatomotor systems) and influence cognition and emotion.

Absorption

Most cholinergic receptor agonists are absorbed after administration by both oral and parenteral routes. Pilocarpine is well absorbed after oral, subcutaneous, or topical administration. It also gains ready access to the CNS, and it is well distributed through the tissues and organs of the body. A large fraction is excreted unchanged by the kidneys, with an elimination half-life of 0.75 to 1.5 hours. Cevimeline is also well absorbed after oral administration, with peak blood concentrations

occurring in 1.5 to 2 hours. Most of the drug is metabolized to sulfoxides and glucuronic acid conjugates, with an elimination half-life of about 5 hours.

Adverse Effects

In general, adverse reactions to the cholinomimetic drugs are predictable consequences of the stimulation of cholinergic receptors, as listed in Box 5.1.

Anticholinesterases (Indirect Agonists)

Summary and Classification

Anticholinesterases are drugs that stimulate cholinergic transmission indirectly by inhibiting the enzyme AChE, which hydrolyzes and inactivates ACh in the synaptic and junctional clefts of the autonomic nervous system, the CNS, and the neuromuscular junction of the somatic nervous system. Agents in this class derive their pharmacologic effects from their ability to prolong the life of ACh at receptor sites. These cholinesterase inhibitors are sometimes referred to as **indirectly acting** cholinergic drugs.

Anticholinesterases can be subclassified as either **reversible** or **irreversible** cholinesterase inhibitors. Reversible inhibitors (e.g., **neostigmine** and **physostigmine**) temporarily inactivate the enzyme by forming noncovalent associations with the enzyme or covalent bonds that are readily hydrolyzed. Irreversible cholinesterase inhibitors (**organophosphates**) inactivate the enzyme by forming a permanent covalent bond with the enzyme.

Mechanism of Action

AChE hydrolyzes ACh with great rapidity and this enzyme is localized in the region of cholinergic receptors. There is also a nonselective plasma cholinesterase, or pseudocholinesterase (butyrylcholinesterase).

The anticholinesterases, whether reversible or irreversible, owe their pharmacologic effects chiefly to the fact that they prolong the life of ACh at sites where it is a mediator. Thus, their actions are often identical with those of ACh, although much more prolonged and, in most cases, completely dependent on the presence of endogenous ACh in the area of the effector. For this reason, most of the anticholinesterases are ineffective in denervated organs.

Pharmacologic Effects

The cholinesterase inhibitors produce muscarinic effects similar to those elicited by the directly acting cholinergic agonists (described earlier and outlined in Chapter 4). These effects are mediated by increasing the concentration of ACh at the autonomic neuroeffector junctions. Nicotinic effects result from increasing ACh at skeletal muscle neuromuscular junctions and at ganglia.

An important disparity in action between **anticholinesterases** and direct-acting muscarinic drugs is that the former **do not cause significant muscarinic receptor–mediated vasodilation** because many blood vessels receive no parasympathetic innervation, and, thus, no ACh is available to be protected against hydrolysis. Instead, vascular effects of high doses of anticholinesterases are largely mediated through their effects on autonomic ganglia and on medullary vasomotor centers. As is the case with cholinomimetic drugs, certain anticholinesterases are also known to evoke CNS actions.

Absorption, Fate, and Excretion

Physostigmine is readily absorbed after oral, subcutaneous, and topical administration, and it is destroyed principally through hydrolysis at the ester linkage by esterases, including pseudocholinesterase. The other reversible cholinesterase inhibitors listed in this chapter, such as neostigmine and pyridostigmine, are quaternary ammonium compounds, which means they do not readily pass through biologic membranes.

Adverse Effects

In humans, intoxication from anticholinesterases has resulted from overdosage with drugs used in the treatment of myasthenia gravis, from exposure to toxic amounts of insecticides or chemical warfare agents. Organophosphate insecticides, especially parathion, have caused thousands of cases of poisoning. The symptomatology of anticholinesterase poisoning reflects the role of ACh as a neuromediator at muscarinic and nicotinic receptors located both peripherally and in the CNS. In high doses, the reversible anticholinesterases can produce the same symptoms as the irreversible anticholinesterases; the chief difference between these two groups lies in the ready access to the circulation and the longer duration of action of the irreversible anticholinesterases. Table 5.2 summarizes the signs of poisoning with the anticholinesterases according to muscarinic, nicotinic, and CNS effects.

The treatment of acute intoxication from an organophosphate includes the actions in Box 5.2.

Therapeutic Uses for Directly and Indirectly Acting Cholinergic Agonists

The esters of choline, pilocarpine, cevimeline, and reversible anticholinesterases are the main drugs used as therapeutic agents.

Glaucoma

Therapy in glaucoma is directed at stimulating the musculature of the iris and ciliary body, increasing the facility of outflow of aqueous humor, reducing its formation, or removing liquid from the eye. Although historically the cholinergic agents (in this application called *miotics*) have been the initial and principal drugs used in the treatment of chronic open-angle glaucoma, a number of other drugs are currently used, either alone or in conjunction with the cholinergic miotics. In fact, β-adrenergic receptor blockers and prostaglandin preparations are now more commonly used for first-line therapy.

Pilocarpine and other drugs that stimulate muscarinic receptors lower intraocular pressure by decreasing resistance to aqueous humor outflow. Pilocarpine is available for topical administration in various solutions and in a long-acting gel formulation. Carbachol, a slightly longer-acting drug, is now only occasionally used.

The long-acting miotic, the anticholinesterase demecarium, is occasionally used for patients with chronic open-angle glaucoma who are refractory to the short-acting miotics.

Xerostomia

Both **pilocarpine** and **cevimeline** have been approved for the treatment of xerostomia in certain patients. The saliva-stimulating effect depends on residual salivary gland

TABLE 5.2	Some Manifestations of Overdosage With Anticholinesterases		
Muscarinic Effects (Peripheral)	**Nicotinic Effects[a]**	**CNS Effects**
Miosis, frontal headache (brow ache), conjunctival hyperemia, blurred vision Rhinorrhea, nasal hyperemia Lacrimation, salivation, sweating Increased bronchial secretions, tightness of chest, bronchoconstriction, wheezing Anorexia, nausea, vomiting, cramps, diarrhea, involuntary defecation Urinary urgency, involuntary micturition Bradycardia, hypotension	Muscular weakness, twitching, fasciculations Tachycardia Elevation or depression of blood pressure Death from respiratory failure	Restlessness, giddiness, tension, anxiety, nausea Tremors, electroencephalographic changes Confusion, ataxia, convulsions Depression of respiratory and circulatory centers, cyanosis, coma, respiratory and circulatory collapse Death from respiratory failure

[a]Nicotinic effects include both stimulation and inhibition of synaptic and junctional transmission.
CNS, Central nervous system.

• BOX 5.2　Treatment of Organophosphate Poisoning

Remove the organophosphate from the victim.
Administer atropine.
Maintain the airway and give artificial respiration if necessary.
Administer diazepam or other benzodiazepine if convulsions are not relieved by atropine.
Administer pralidoxime (reserved only for organophosphates).

---

function. Generally, at these doses, there is no significant effect on blood pressure, heart rate, or cardiac function. Sweating is a common side effect; chills, nausea, and dizziness have also been reported. The dentist must carefully determine whether muscarinic receptor agonists should be used to treat dry mouth. Therapy for xerostomia must not compromise other therapy the patient may be receiving. Moreover, risk factors for muscarinic receptor agonists need to be considered.

Oral fluids, including saliva substitutes, may be added for the relief of dry mouth and should be substituted for pilocarpine and cevimeline if the drugs are not well tolerated in patients at risk such as those with uncontrolled asthma, in patients for whom pilocarpine or cevimeline would compromise existing therapy, or where there is a complete loss of salivary function

Myasthenia Gravis

Myasthenia gravis (MG) is an autoimmune disorder in which there is continuous production of antibodies to the **acetylcholine receptor (AChR)** at the neuromuscular junction.

Treatment for MG is now fairly standardized. After a positive diagnosis, six methods of treatment are available. At first, reversible anticholinesterases (such as **neostigmine**) are used to enhance neuromuscular transmission. Also sometimes employed are the following: thymectomy, adrenal corticosteroid therapy, immunosuppressant drugs, plasmapheresis, to remove offending antibodies, and high-dose intravenous immunoglobulins. A recent treatment is the use of an antibody fragment directed against ACHR autoantibodies present in patients with MG.

Therapy with an anticholinesterase is likely to be complicated by side effects resulting from the accumulation of ACh at cholinergic receptor sites. Some of these effects are characteristically muscarinic (e.g., abdominal cramps, diarrhea, sweating, salivation, lacrimation) and can be well controlled by the **administration of atropine** and related drugs. Other side effects, such as muscle fasciculations and CNS symptoms, are not controllable by the muscarinic blocking drugs and may be warning signs of an impending cholinergic crisis, which results from overdosage with the anticholinesterases. Cholinergic crisis is characterized by muscle weakness, particularly of the respiratory muscles, resulting from persistent depolarization of the neuromuscular junction.

Poisoning From Antimuscarinic Drugs

All the cholinergic drugs with muscarinic properties should theoretically be useful in antagonizing the effects of atropine, but the most effective drugs for this purpose are the anticholinesterases, and the drug of choice is physostigmine.

A number of drugs (e.g., tricyclic antidepressants, phenothiazines, and antihistamines) share to varying degrees the antimuscarinic effects of atropine. Thus, they may have an atropine-like effect and these adverse effects can be inhibited by physostigmine. Remember that physostigmine is able to enter the CNS and is able to inhibit the central effects of atropine-like drugs.

Paralytic Ileus and Bladder Atony

Neostigmine and bethanechol are used for this condition.

Senile Dementia of the Alzheimer Type

One central neurochemical affected by Alzheimer disease, especially early in the course of the illness, is ACh. Deficits in ACh and in choline acetyltransferase, the enzyme responsible for the formation of ACh from choline and acetyl coenzyme A, have been identified in the brains of Alzheimer patients. The identification of these deficiencies suggested a treatment strategy for Alzheimer disease analogous to that used in the pharmacologic therapy of Parkinson disease, namely, replacement of the missing (in this case cholinergic) agonist. In fact, early experiments with physostigmine showed some transient, if variable, improvement. The AChE inhibitors that are used to treat Alzheimer disease easily penetrate the blood–brain barrier. **Donepezil** and **rivastigmine** are two examples of AChE inhibitors used to treat Alzheimer disease. The AChE inhibitors have shown modest but significant improvement in Alzheimer patients. Their benefit seems to be in temporarily slowing memory loss and loss of function.

Antimuscarinic Drugs

Various drugs can interfere with the transmission of nerve impulses at cholinergic junctions. The drugs in this section selectively block responses at muscarinic receptors and are essentially without effect, except at inordinately high doses, at nicotinic receptors. Hence, these drugs are known as **antimuscarinic** or **muscarinic receptor–blocking drugs**; the term **anticholinergic**, although often used for this class of drugs, is somewhat inaccurate because these drugs, for the most part, are selective for muscarinic receptors, not nicotinic receptors. They are also termed **atropine-like**.

Because peripheral muscarinic receptors are the primary targets of ACh released by postganglionic cholinergic neurons, the effects achieved by the antimuscarinic drugs are chiefly on the smooth muscle, cardiac muscle, and glands that are innervated by these neurons. The prototypes of the antimuscarinics, atropine, and scopolamine, are referred to as **belladonna alkaloids** because of their plant origin.

Classification

These drugs are divided into two groups
1. Naturally occurring belladonna alkaloids—atropine and scopolamine

2. Semisynthetic and synthetic atropine-like drugs. These can be further divided into permanently charged drugs (e.g., ipratropium, tiotropium) or those that are not permanently charged (e.g., benztropine, trihexyphenidyl, tolterodine)

Mechanism of Action

The antimuscarinic drugs are **competitive antagonists of ACh at muscarinic receptors**. (Review Figs. 4.1, 4.3 and 5.3A–G for location of muscarinic receptors.) They have an affinity for muscarinic receptor sites but lack intrinsic activity. Thus, they occupy the receptor sites and prevent access of ACh, creating a blockade that is reversible. Reversible blockade means that the blockade by antimuscarinic drugs can be reversed by increasing the amount of ACh in the area of the receptor, as would occur after the administration of an anticholinesterase drug. Because atropine can antagonize the muscarinic effects of the anticholinesterases and vice versa, each drug can be used as an antidote for the other in case of poisoning. In effect, the antimuscarinic drugs are capable of blocking responses to parasympathetic nerve stimulation, to sympathetic nerve stimulation of sweat glands, to ACh protected from hydrolysis by anticholinesterases, and to directly acting muscarinic agonists.

Pharmacologic Effects

Therapeutic doses of the antimuscarinic drugs produce effects attributable to the blockade of peripheral muscarinic receptors and similar receptors in the CNS located within the medulla and higher cerebral centers.

Peripheral Nervous System Actions

The antimuscarinic drugs possess both peripheral and CNS actions. Most peripheral effects are caused by an interruption of parasympathetic impulses to a given effector tissue. This results in control of the tissue or organ by the sympathetic nervous system, which often exerts effects opposite to those of the parasympathetic nervous system. An important exception is where the sympathetic effect acts through muscarinic receptors, most notably in the sweat glands. Thus, the **sympathetic effect of sweating is inhibited by antimuscarinic drugs**. In general, atropine-like drugs block the salivation, lacrimation, urination, and defecation response to cholinergic drugs previously described and the hypotensive and bradycardic effects of muscarinic receptor stimulation. The effects of **muscarinc** stimulation are shown in Fig. 5.3A–F. The effects of **antimuscarinic** stimulation are therefore **opposite** to these effects.

Eye

Atropine-like drugs block muscarinic receptors in the sphincter of the iris and in the ciliary muscle, leading, respectively, to dilation of the pupil (mydriasis) and paralysis of accommodation (cycloplegia). Photophobia and fixation of the lens occurs for far vision, and thus vision for near objects is blurred. Intraocular pressure is not significantly affected except in the case of narrow-angle (or angle-closure) glaucoma, for which administration of these drugs may cause a dangerous rise in intraocular pressure.

Bronchi

After administration of antimuscarinic drugs, the bronchial smooth muscle is left under the sole control of the sympathetic nervous system which results in the relaxation of the bronchi. This relaxation of the smooth muscle decreases airway resistance. Secretion of all glands in the nose, mouth, pharynx, and respiratory tree is inhibited.

Salivary Glands

Parasympathetically mediated salivary secretion (and secretion of many other exocrine glands) is inhibited in a dose-dependent manner. The mouth and throat become unpleasantly dry, to the point that speech and swallowing may become difficult. Xerostomia can lead to any one of a number of adverse effects (e.g., difficulty in chewing and swallowing, increased risk for fungal infections and dental caries, etc.) on the oral cavity.

Gastrointestinal Tract

The antimuscarinic drugs are quite effective in preventing the expected motor and secretory responses of the gastrointestinal tract to administered cholinergic drugs, and to a lesser extent, vagal stimulation.

Cardiovascular System

The administration of antimuscarinic drugs, in most cases, results in an increase in heart rate. In the standing or upright patient, there is little or no change in cardiac output.

Genitourinary Tract

The ureters and the urinary bladder (detrusor muscle) are relaxed by atropine. The sphincter and trigone muscles are contracted as a result of atropine. These effects are due to muscarinic receptor blockade. Together, these changes in the bladder cause urinary retention in humans. This retention may be exacerbated in the presence of benign prostatic hyperplasia.

Effects on Body Temperature

The belladonna alkaloids suppress sweating because the sweat glands (other than the apocrine sweat glands as found on the palms of the hand) are innervated by cholinergic fibers of the sympathetic nervous system. The receptors at the neuroeffector sites in the sweat glands are therefore muscarinic. The rise in body temperature that can follow the administration of large doses of atropine or scopolamine may have a CNS component, but the primary cause is the peripheral inhibition of sweating. Hyperthermia is also the most serious and life-threatening result of an overdose of one of these drugs.

Antitremor Activity

Antimuscarinic drugs are effective in suppressing the tremor of parkinsonism due to blocking muscarinic receptors in the striatum which can compensate for a lack of dopamine.

Effect on Vestibular Function

The belladonna alkaloids have since ancient times been the basis of various remedies to treat motion sickness. Scopolamine is more effective than atropine. It acts on several areas of the brain, including the vestibular apparatus and the cerebral cortex.

Uses

The therapeutic uses of the antimuscarinic drugs are all based on the pharmacologic effects affecting peripheral organs and the CNS (Table 5.3).

Antidote to Cholinesterase Inhibitors

Toxicity from anticholinesterases may result from their use in the treatment of MG (particularly in the early phase of therapy when the patient is not as tolerant to the muscarinic effects of these drugs) or from exposure to one of the organophosphate insecticides or anticholinesterase nerve gases. These anticholinesterases typically produce a spectrum of peripheral muscarinic and nicotinic effects as well as CNS effects. Atropine is effective in **antagonizing** the **effects at muscarinic sites** and thus will relieve the hypersecretion of salivary, lacrimal, and respiratory glands; bronchoconstriction; gastrointestinal symptoms; sweating; various other manifestations of muscarinic stimulation; and some CNS actions. **Atropine does not interfere** with the desired effects of anticholinesterases at **neuromuscular junctions** when these drugs are being used for MG or to reverse

TABLE
5.3 **Effects and Indications of Antimuscarinic Drugs**

Tissue	Effect	Indication(s)	Common Drugs Used
Eye			
Sphincter of iris	Mydriasis	To dilate pupils[a]	Tropicamide[b]
Ciliary muscle	Cycloplegia		Cyclopentolate[b] Homatropine
Bronchi			
Smooth muscle	Relaxation	Asthma (certain forms)	Ipratropium[c]
Secretory cells	Reduced secretion	Bronchitis	Tiotropium[c]
Salivary glands	Reduced secretion	To reduce saliva	Glycopyrrolate
GI Tract			
Smooth muscle	Reduced peristalsis	Rarely, ulcers[d]	Glycopyrrolate
Glands	Reduced secretions	Peptic ulcer disease	Pirenzepine[e]
Heart	Tachycardia	Bradycardia[f]	Atropine
	Increased AV nodal conduction	Heart block	Atropine
Genitourinary Tract			
Bladder detrusor	Relaxation	Urinary incontinence	Oxybutynin Flavoxate
Bladder sphincter and trigone	Constriction	Overactive bladder	Darifenacin Solifenacin
CNS			
Medulla and higher centers	Sedation, euphoria, amnesia[g]	Rarely, preanesthetic medication	Scopolamine
Corpus striatum	Reduced tremor	Parkinsonian tremor	Benztropine, Trihexyphenidyl
Vestibular apparatus	Reduced activity	Motion sickness	Scopolamine

[a]The topical use of these drugs is strongly contraindicated in patients with a predisposition to narrow-angle glaucoma.
[b]Shorter duration of action than atropine.
[c]Quaternary compounds used by inhalation.
[d]Other drugs, such as proton pump inhibitors are more commonly used.
[e]Muscarinic M₁ receptor selective. Not available in the US.
[f]Also can prevent vagal reflexes in surgery.
[g]Especially scopolamine.

neuromuscular blockade induced by curare-like agents (see Chapter 6).

Antidote to Poisoning by Muscarinic Receptor Agonists

Atropine, a specific antagonist of antimuscarinic chemicals, naturally occurs in the night shade family of plants (e.g., belladonna), certain mushrooms (Inocybe lateraria), Jimson weed, and mandrake. If consumed in high quantities, these plants can produce life threatening effects.

Adverse Effects

The colloquialisms "hot as a hare, red as a beet, dry as a bone, blind as a bat, and mad as a hatter" vividly convey the symptoms of atropine intoxication, which are predictable extensions of the pharmacologic effects of this group of drugs. Present are dryness of the mouth, extreme thirst, a burning sensation in the throat, and difficulty in swallowing; dilation of the pupils and cycloplegia with severe impairment of vision and photophobia; flushing of the skin, vasodilation of skin vessels, absence of sweating, and a rise in body temperature, urinary retention; and derangements of CNS activity. Therapy for atropine poisoning involves physostigmine, which is useful in raising the amount of ACh in the vicinity of the receptors and acts rapidly to terminate the atropine blockade. The antianxiety drugs such as diazepam may be used to control CNS excitation. Therapy also includes supportive care.

Topical use of antimuscarinic drugs in the eye is absolutely contraindicated in cases of suspected or diagnosed narrow-angle glaucoma. Systemic doses of anticholinergic drugs can be used in patients with open-angle glaucoma but not in patients with narrow-angle glaucoma.

Therapeutic Uses in Dentistry

Muscarinic Receptor Agonists

All the cholinomimetic drugs that have an affinity for muscarinic sites are capable of stimulating salivation. **Xerostomia** is a common problem encountered by dentists in patients with Sjögren's syndrome, those who have had head and neck radiation, and those undergoing treatment involving drugs that produce dry mouth. Muscarinic receptor agonists may be useful in stimulating salivary flow when there is functional salivary gland tissue present and when there is no contraindication for their use. Muscarinic receptor agonists should not be administered if they will compromise other therapy that the patient is undergoing. For instance, antimuscarinic therapy for overactive bladder would tend to be compromised by the administration of a muscarinic receptor agonist. (Antimuscarinic drug therapy would also reduce the clinical efficacy of pilocarpine or cevimeline.) Muscarinic receptor agonists are contraindicated in urinary tract obstruction, hyperactive airway disease, chronic obstructive pulmonary disease, acute heart failure, gastrointestinal spasms, hyperthyroidism, and acute iritis. Pilocarpine is usually taken at doses of 5 or 10 mg three times a day, 30 minutes before each meal. Cevimeline is given at doses of 30 mg three times daily.

Antimuscarinic Drugs

The principal use of the **anticholinergic drugs** in dentistry is to **decrease the flow of saliva** during dental procedures.

Small doses given orally approximately 30 minutes to 2 hours before the procedure are effective, but the drugs may also produce side effects that may be objectionable to some patients. The same dose may also be used to diminish salivary flow in heavy metal poisoning. Atropine is often selected because it is well absorbed from the GI tract. However, because it is a quaternary amine, glycopyrrolate has fewer CNS effects than the belladonna alkaloids. Compared with atropine, it is a more selective antisialagogue and less likely to promote tachycardia in conventional doses. During general anesthesia, the anticholinergics also diminish secretions in the respiratory tract, thus lessening the likelihood of laryngospasm, and they help prevent reflex vagal slowing of the heart.

Not only do dentists occasionally have reason to use antimuscarinic drugs, but dentists often encounter patients who are taking them for any one of the reasons enumerated. Moreover, drugs of several different pharmacological classes have substantial antimuscarinic effects. The most characteristic effects of these drugs that concern dentists are xerostomia and the discomfort that this brings to the patient as well as the deterioration in oral health. In those cases in which using a muscarinic receptor agonists may antagonize therapy involving an antimuscarinic drug, patients can be advised to drink water, suck on noncariogenic lemon drops, and irrigate the mouth with saliva substitutes to alleviate xerostomia. If saliva flow is reduced, patients need to pay scrupulous attention to oral hygiene, and caries control needs to be more aggressive. If there is progressive deterioration in oral health, consultation with the patient's physician may be helpful in identifying suitable therapeutic alternatives without as much xerostomia. Finally, the contraindications of antimuscarinic drugs must be considered for a variety of adverse reactions. More specifically, the use of antimuscarinic drugs should be avoided in patients with benign prostate hypertrophy and those with atony in the urinary or gastrointestinal tract.

Suggested Readings

Barbe AG. Medication-induced xerostomia and hyposalivation in the elderly: culprits, complications, and management. *Drugs Aging*. 2018;35(10):877–885.

Tiisanoja A, Syrjälä AH, Kullaa A, Ylöstalo P. Anticholinergic burden and dry mouth in middle-aged people. *J Dent Res Clin Trans Res*. 2020;5(1):62–70.

6

Drugs Acting at Nicotinic Cholinergic Receptors or Near the Neuromuscular Junction (NMJ)

KEY POINTS

- Nicotinic cholinergic receptors respond to acetylcholine (ACh) and are located in the central nervous system, and in the peripheral nervous system, including in ganglia and at the neuromuscular junction (NMJ).
- Nicotine has complex effects on nicotinic receptors, including stimulation and inhibition.
- Skeletal NMJ blockers belong to two classes: depolarizing drugs represented by succinylcholine and nondepolarizing drugs which are curare derivatives.
- Botulinum toxin blocks the release of ACh from nerve endings.
- Dantrolene blocks the release of calcium from the inside of skeletal muscle cells.

DEFINITIONS

- Nicotinic receptors are ion channel membrane receptors that respond to acetylcholine (ACh) and nicotine.
- Nondepolarizing NMJ blockers are competitive at nicotinic binding sites.
- Depolarizing NMJ blockers are noncompetitive at nicotinic binding sites.
- Nicotine replacement agents are drugs used for smoking cessation and target nicotinic receptors in the brain.
- NMJ blocking drugs prevent the peripheral effect of ACh at skeletal NMJs.

Nicotinic Receptors

Nicotinic receptors (see Chapters 1 and 4) play a crucial role in the transmission of autonomic impulses across the ganglionic synapse. However, nicotinic drugs are rarely given for their effects on ganglia, since these drugs may have ganglionic side effects.

The pharmacology of nicotinic cholinergic receptors at the neuromuscular junction (NMJ) and in the central nervous system (CNS) has more direct clinical relevance. Fig. 6.1 is a depiction of neurotransmission at the NMJ. Remember that the neurotransmitter at the NMJ is acetylcholine (ACh) and the principle postjunctional receptors are nicotinic cholinergic. The neuronal connection to the NMJ is shown in Fig. 6.2.

Nicotinic Receptor Stimulating Drugs

Pharmacology

Nicotine is the principal psychoactive ingredient in tobacco products.

As a selective depolarizing drug at nicotinic receptors, this alkaloid stimulates transmission at autonomic ganglia and at nicotinic synapses in the CNS. It also activates various sensory fibers equipped with nicotinic receptors, including mechanoreceptors in the lung, skin, mesentery, and tongue; nociceptive nerve endings; and chemoreceptors in the carotid body and aortic arch. Stimulation of nicotinic receptors by nicotine in skeletal muscle is easily shown in the laboratory, but it is not evident normally in humans because initial stimulation is soon followed by inhibition at these nicotinic sites. Nicotine has a dual effect at nicotinic sites, which includes an initial stimulation and subsequent depression. An important feature of nicotinic receptors is their tendency to become **desensitized** (i.e., unresponsive) on continuous exposure to agonists. The actions of nicotine are highly time and concentration dependent, and complex patterns of stimulation and depression are observed.

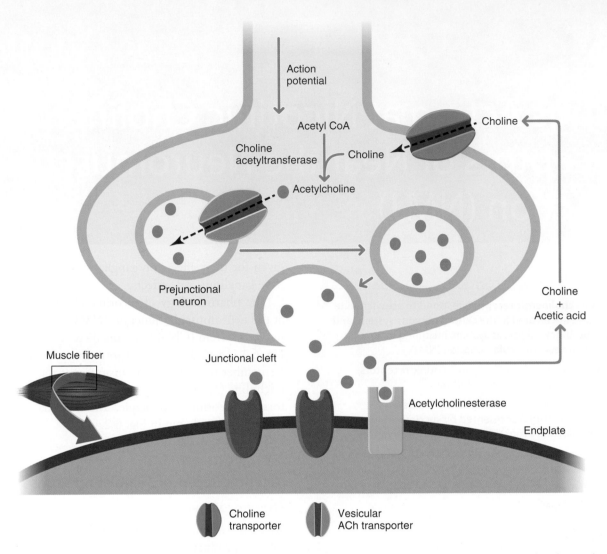

• **Fig. 6.1** Illustration of events at the neuromuscular junction. Notice the similarity with other cholinergic junctions, except that the postjunctional receptors are nicotinic and thus they are ion channel receptors. *ACh*, Acetylcholine; *CoA*, coenzyme A.

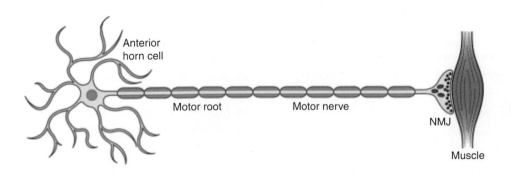

• **Fig. 6.2** Diagram of a somatic nerve and its connection to the neuromuscular junction. (Source: Preston DC, Shapiro BE. *Electromyography and Neuromuscular Disorders: Clinical-Electrophysiologic-Ultrasound Correlations*. 4th ed. Elsevier; 2021.)

Generally, usual amounts of nicotine absorbed during cigarette smoking in individuals cause mild cardiovascular stimulation, increased gastrointestinal activity, and CNS stimulation accompanied by a feeling of well-being and decreased irritability. With long-term use, tolerance and physical dependence occur. The **addictive nature of**

TABLE 6.1	Nicotine and Other Drug Products for Smoking Cessation	
Nonproprietary Product	Proprietary Name	Usual Duration of Therapy (weeks)
Nicotine transdermal patch	NicoDerm CQ	8–12[a]
Nicotine nasal spray	Nicotrol NS	≤12
Nicotine oral inhaler	Nicotrol Inhaler	≤24
Nicotine gum	Nicorette Gum	12
Nicotine lozenges	Nicorette Lozenges	12
Bupropion	Zyban	[b]
Varenicline	Chantix	[b]

[a]Patches come in three strengths designed to taper the doses.
[b]The duration depends on the patient's planned quitting date, which is set before the patient stops smoking.

nicotine is the result of its action on the reward pathway, that is, the circuitry in the brain that regulates feelings of pleasure and euphoria.

Acute overdose of nicotine causes nausea and vomiting, abdominal pain, dizziness and confusion, and muscular weakness. If untreated, death may ensue from cardiopulmonary collapse. Nevertheless, the primary health issues regarding nicotine stem from the chronic use of tobacco products. An increased incidence of cancer and cardiovascular and pulmonary disease has been well documented. In dentistry, tobacco use has been linked to oropharyngeal carcinoma, leukoplakia, periodontal disease, delayed wound healing, halitosis, and tooth staining.

Drugs Used in Smoking Cessation

The only therapeutic use of nicotine is as an adjunct in tobacco cessation programs. Nicotine is administered in multiple forms (Table 6.1) to maintain pharmacologic concentrations of the alkaloid and to prevent tobacco cessation from triggering an acute withdrawal syndrome, which includes irritability, anxiety, sleep disturbances, and cognitive impairment. The nicotine dose is reduced in a stepwise fashion over several months, during which time the patient ideally receives continued counseling and motivational assistance to remain abstinent.

Varenicline is also used for smoking cessation. It acts centrally and is a partial agonist at selective nicotinic receptors to decrease cravings for nicotine. It can cause

psychiatric side effects, such as various types of sleep disorders.

Bupropion is also a drug that acts centrally to reduce nicotine cravings (see Table 6.1). Its actions are described in Chapter 9.

Drugs That Block Nicotinic Receptors at the Neuromuscular Junction

Stimulation of the nicotinic receptors at the NMJ receptor causes opening of the ion channel and subsequent inward flow of sodium, leading to depolarization of the junctional region of the muscle fiber. This triggers an action potential in the electrically excitable muscle fiber membrane, and muscular contraction follows.

Neuromuscular blocking drugs interfere with the ability of ACh to cause muscle contraction through the nicotinic receptor. These drugs are divided into two groups based on whether the agents themselves bring about endplate depolarization in the course of their action. The depolarizing and the nondepolarizing blocking agents differ in the mechanisms through which they produce neuromuscular blockade. Their use is primarily to achieve skeletal muscle relaxation during surgery.

Nondepolarizing Drugs

Nondepolarizing, or competitive, neuromuscular blocking drugs include the prototype, tubocurarine (d-tubocurarine) (curare), and several other related drugs.

All these drugs act by occupying the endplate nicotinic receptor, blocking access of ACh to these sites. The drugs themselves do not cause endplate depolarization. Inhibition of neuromuscular transmission is essentially competitive, with the blocking agent and ACh competing for receptor sites on the muscle fiber.

Tubocurarine, was first isolated as the primary active ingredient from arrow poisons used by certain indigenous populations in South America. It is no longer used because of its tendency to evoke undesirable side effects. However, several other nondepolarizing drugs are used for skeletal muscle relaxation during surgery.

Depolarizing Drugs

Similar to most nondepolarizing blockers, succinylcholine, the major depolarizing agent, binds to the nicotinic receptor in the NMJ. However, the initial effect of the binding of this agent is a depolarization of the muscle fiber. During the early phase of its action, there is a period of excitation during which the sensitivity of the muscle to ACh is increased. It is common for the drug-induced depolarization to be great enough to trigger

TABLE 6.2	Pharmacologic Properties on Skeletal Neuromuscular Blocking Drugs	
Drug (Length of Action)	**Some Characteristics**
Ultra-short	
Succinylcholine[a]	Depolarizing, used for short procedures e.g., intubation. Metabolized by cholinesterase
Short	
Mivacurium[a]	Nondepolarizing, can be used for intubation. Metabolized by cholinesterase
Intermediate	
Atracurium[a]	Nondepolarizing, useful in renal failure patients.
Cisatracurium	Nondepolarizing
Rocuronium	Nondepolarizing, rapidly acting
Vecuronium	Nondepolarizing
Long	
Pancuronium	Nondepolarizing, vagal blockade

[a]May cause histamine release.

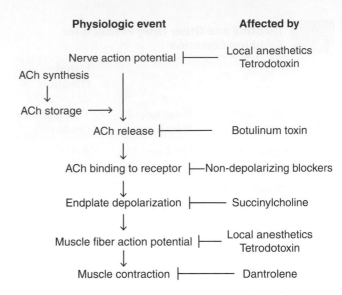

• **Fig. 6.3** Sites of action of drugs that act at the neuromuscular junction, act on peripheral nerves or directly on or in the muscle cell. *ACh*, Acetylcholine.

action potentials and fasciculations (i.e., spontaneous twitching) in the muscle fibers. What then follows is a complex inhibition of the NMJ nicotinic receptors and muscle relaxation. Succinylcholine is ultra-short acting and recovery is rapid.

Summary

Table 6.2 lists a summary of further pharmacologic characteristics and comments on several NMJ blockers.

Other Drugs That Act at or Near the Neuromuscular Junction But Do Not Act at the Nicotinic Receptors

Botulinum Toxin

Botulinum toxin is used to prevent the release of ACh from the somatic nerve at the NMJ (see Fig. 6.3). Botulinum toxin acts by binding to and inhibiting SNARE proteins. SNARE proteins are necessary for release of ACh from nerve endings. Botulinum toxin affects all peripheral

cholinergic nerves. The drug, in its various forms, is used to reduce skeletal muscle contractions in the eye, in muscles of facial expression, and elsewhere. It is also used to treat overactive bladder and in migraine prophylaxis. It has gained importance for its cosmetic effects.

Dantrolene

Dantrolene relaxes skeletal muscle by directly entering the muscle cell and blocking the release of calcium. It is used to treat malignant hyperthermia. This disorder is due to a genetic predisposition that can be triggered by the use of peripheral skeletal muscle relaxants, especially succinylcholine, and by general anesthetics. Dantrolene is also used in certain spasticity and rigidity disorders.

Summary

Several other drugs are used for muscle relaxation. Since they act in the CNS, they are discussed in later chapters. Fig. 6.3 lists some drugs that act at the NMJ, on nerves, or in the skeletal muscle.

Suggested Readings

ADA website on nicotine replacement therapy. https://www.ada.org/en/member-center/oral-health-topics/tobacco-use-and-cessation. Accessed May 2021.

Stäuble CG, Blobner M. The future of neuromuscular blocking agents. *Curr Opin Anaesthesiol.* 2020;33(4):490–498.

7

Adrenergic Receptor Agonists

KEY POINTS

- Adrenergic drugs act by stimulating a variety of adrenergic receptor types and subtypes.
- Norepinephrine and epinephrine are two important catecholamines that stimulate adrenergic receptors.
- The adrenergic receptor subtypes (α and β) and the tissues in which they are present, determine the effects of adrenergic drugs.
- The baroreceptor reflex can affect the cardiovascular effects of adrenergic drugs.
- Indirect and mixed action adrenergic agonists act by increasing the concentration of catecholamines at adrenergic nerve endings.

DEFINITIONS

- Catecholamines are aromatic amines derived from tyrosine and are monoamine neurotransmitters (e.g., norepinephrine, and dopamine). Epinephrine is a monoamine that acts pricipally as a hormone. Dopamine also acts as a hormone.
- Adrenergic receptor selectivity is the degree to which adrenergic receptor agonists can stimulate one adrenergic receptor subtype without an appreciable effect at another adrenergic receptor subtype.
  - Nonselective adrenergic agonists are drugs that can stimulate more than one type of receptor.
  - Selective adrenergic agonists are drugs that preferentially stimulate one type of receptor.
- The baroreceptor reflex is a response to a change in blood pressure, as sensed in the carotid sinus and elsewhere, which leads to a compensatory change in heart rate or blood pressure.
- Signal transduction linked to adrenergic receptor stimulation is the process by which the binding of an adrenergic receptor agonist is converted to a change in activity of a cell.

Adrenergic Receptors

Sympathetic Nerves

Adrenergic receptors are located in effector organs or tissues innervated by sympathetic nerves Fig. 7.1.

The adrenergic receptors are located at junctions of postganglionic sympathetic nerves and the organs or tissues that receive sympathetic innervation. The main exception that sympathetic nerves innervate tissues with adrenergic receptors is in the sweat glands, where the receptors are cholinergic (muscarinic).

Effects of Adrenergic Receptor Stimulation

Like the situation with cholinergic receptors, stimulation of adrenergic receptors leads to a variety of effects depending on the tissues and organs that are innervated.

Unlike the case with postganglionic cholinergic receptors, there is an important classification system for postganglionic adrenergic receptors. The following list summarizes the complexity of the adrenergic receptors and their pharmacology:

- Adrenergic receptors are divided into alpha (α) and beta (β) with further subdivisions as shown in Fig. 7.2.
- Each receptor subtype has its own effects.
- Each receptor subtype has a distinct distribution throughout the body.
- Often the effect of one adrenergic receptor subtype is opposite to, or at least distinct from, those of other adrenergic receptor subtypes.
- Adrenergic drugs can be selective or nonselective depending on the drug.

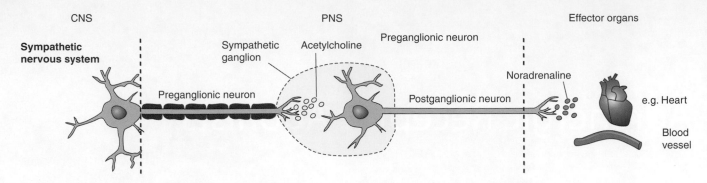

• **Fig. 7.1** A two neuron chain from central nervous system (CNS) to peripheral nervous system, to effector organs. *NE*, Norepinephrine. (From: Craft J. et al.: Structure and function of the neurologic system, *Understanding pathophysiology,* ed. 7, Australian adaptation, ed 2, Marrickville, Australia, Elsevier Australia, 2015.)

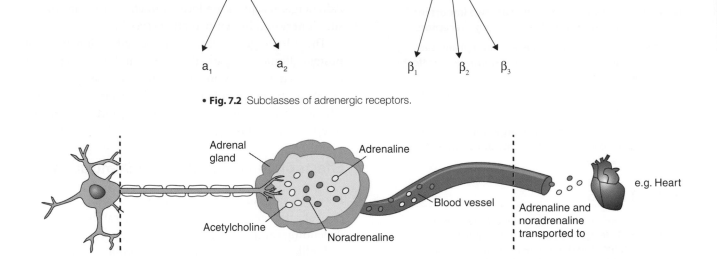

• **Fig. 7.2** Subclasses of adrenergic receptors.

• **Fig. 7.3** Release of epinephrine from the adrenal medulla into the blood. *ACh*, Acetylcholine. (From: Craft J. et al.: Structure and function of the neurologic system, *Understanding pathophysiology,* ed. 7, Australian adaptation, ed 2, Marrickville, Australia, Elsevier Australia, 2015.)

• Knowledge of the pharmacology of adrenergic drugs and the sympathetic system requires understanding the receptor preference(s) of each drug, the location of various adrenergic receptors, and the effect of stimulation of each adrenergic receptor in tissues and organs.

Adrenergic Receptor Agonists

Catecholamines

Two endogenous compounds, **epinephrine (adrenaline) norepinephrine** and **norepinephrine(noradrenaline)norepinephrine**, are agonists at adrenergic receptors. Epinephrine is released from the adrenal medulla into the blood and therefore acts as a hormone (Fig. 7.3).

Norepinephrine is released primarily from adrenergic nerve endings (see Fig. 7.1). Some is released from the adrenal medulla. In Fig. 7.3, notice that acetylcholine is released from the nerve, which then stimulates the release of epinephrine and some norepinephrine from the adrenal gland. The structures of epinephrine and norepinephrine are shown in Fig. 7.4. Notice that they contain a benzene ring with two attached hydroxyl groups. In this configuration, this part of the structure is referred to as a catechol. The ring structure is separated from an amino group by two carbons. The entire structure is referred to as a catecholamine.

Several other adrenergic receptor agonists share this catecholamine structure or are a modified form of the catecholamine structure.

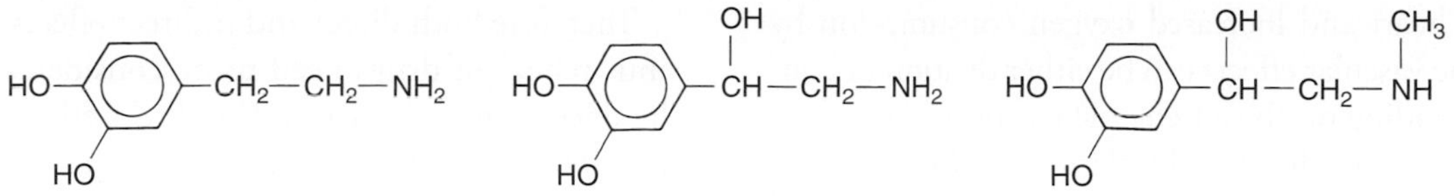

Dopamine Norepinephrine Epinephrine

• **Fig. 7.4** Structures of norepinephrine and epinephrine.

TABLE 71 **Tissue Responses and the Adrenergic Receptors Involved (exception sweat glands)**

Tissue	Response	Receptor(s)	Clinical Use
Eye			
Radial muscle	Contraction (mydriasis)	α_1	Dilation of pupil
Ciliary body	Decreased AQ[a] production (also increased outflow)	α_2 and β	Treat glaucoma
Heart			
Sinoatrial node	Increased rate	β_1, β_2	Cardiac stimulation
Atria	Increased rate and contractility	β_1, β_2	
AV node	Increased automaticity and conduction velocity	β_1, β_2	
Ventricles	Increased contractility, conduction velocity, and automaticity	β_1, β_2	
Blood vessels			
Most blood vessels	Vasoconstriction	α_1, α_2	Constrict blood vessels in hypotension and other situations
Blood vessels to skeletal muscle	Vasodilation	β_2	
Lungs, bronchial smooth muscle	Bronchodilation	β_2	Treat asthma and COPD[b]
Urinary bladder			
Detrussor muscle	Relaxation	β_2, β_3	Treat overactive bladder
Trigone and sphincter	Contraction	α_1	
Uterus	Relaxation	β_2	Inhibit premature contractions
Pilomotor muscle	Contraction	α_1	
Sweat glands	Secretion	Muscarinic	
Liver	Glycogenolysis, gluconeogenesis	α_1, β_2	
Adipose tissue	Lipolysis	α_1, β_1, β_3	

[a]Aqueous humor.
[b]Chronic obstructive pulmonary disease.
AV, Atrioventricular.

Tissue Responses

Tissue responses to adrenergic receptor agonists are shown in Table 7.1.

Highlights From Table 7.1

The cardiovascular effects of adrenergic receptor agonists are among the most important. As indicated in Table 7.1, they include cardiac stimulatory effects, leading to increased work of the heart and increased oxygen consumption by the heart. The vascular effects can be either dilation or constriction depending on the adrenergic receptor.

Bronchodilation, due to stimulation of the β_2 adrenergic receptor, is useful in the treatment of asthma and chronic obstructive pulmonary disease (COPD).

Receptor Selectivity

Notice the varied tissue selectivity among those adrenergic receptor agonists shown in Table 7.2.

Table 7.2 lists the receptors stimulated by various adrenergic receptor agonists. The drugs listed in Table 7.2 vary in their degree of selectivity. (Notice that epinephrine stimulates all four receptors.) We can determine the effect, and possible clinical use, by matching the receptor stimulation by a drug in Table 7.2, with the receptor effect(s) listed in **selective** Table 7.1.

Cardiovascular Effects of Adrenergic Receptor Agonists

Now let us look more closely at the effects of three adrenergic receptor agonists on blood pressure and heart rate. It should be remembered that, due to the baroreceptor reflex, a drug that directly causes vasodilation will indirectly cause a increase in heart rate. Likewise, a drug that directly causes vasoconstriction will indirectly cause a decrease in heart rate, as mechanistically shown in Fig. 7.5.

In the example shown in Fig. 7.5, the afferent nerves from the carotid sinus and aortic baroreceptors send signals (blue arrows) to a cardiac control center. Efferent nerves, both parasympathetic and sympathetic, are linked to the cardiac control center, and conduct signals to the heart and blood vessels (red arrows). Thus, an increase in blood pressure activates stretch receptors in the carotid sinus, which increases stimulation to the cardiac control center, resulting in a decrease in sympathetic outflow and an increase in parasympathetic outflow. The opposite happens if blood pressure falls.

Therefore both direct and indirect effects (e.g., carotid sinus reflex) of drugs need to be considered to interpret the effects on end organs. The direct effect of a drug on heart rate may be opposed by its indirect effect. On the other hand, the effect of a direct effect may be amplified by its indirect effect.

Based on receptor preference, and the effects of the drug on heart rate and arterial blood pressure, one can predict the actions of drugs as shown in Fig. 7.6.

Adrenergic Receptor Agonists and Indications

A list of several adrenergic receptor agonists, their receptor preferences, and clinical indications is given in Table 7.3.

Signal Transduction of Adrenergic Receptors

The signal transduction pathways for the adrenergic receptors are shown in Fig. 7.7. The G protein is identified as well as the effect on either calcium or cyclic adenosine monophosphate (AMP). These pathways are dependent on receptor subtype. (Chapter 1 has more information regarding signal transduction.)

Indirect Agonists and Mixed-Acting Agonists

An indirect adrenergic agonist is a drug that stimulates adrenergic receptors by increasing the level of norepinephrine at adrenergic nerve terminals or increases the release of catecholamines. **Amphetamine** and amphetamine-like drugs as well as **tyramine** enter the nerve terminal to cause this release.

Mixed-acting drugs cause the release of catecholamines but also are direct agonists at adrenergic receptors. **Ephedrine**, in addition to its indirect effect of releasing catecholamines, it also directly stimulates α and β adrenergic receptors.

TABLE 7.2	Receptor Selectivity of Adrenergic Receptor Agonists		
Epinephrine	Epinephrine	Epinephrine	Epinephrine
Levonordefrin	Levonordefrin	Levonordefrin	
Norepinephrine	Norepinephrine	Norepinephrine	
		Isoproterenol	Isoproterenol
α_1	α_2	β_1	β_2
Phenylephrine	Oxymetazoline	Dobutamine	Salmeterol
Methoxamine	Tetrahydrolozine		Bitolterol
	Clonidine		Albuterol

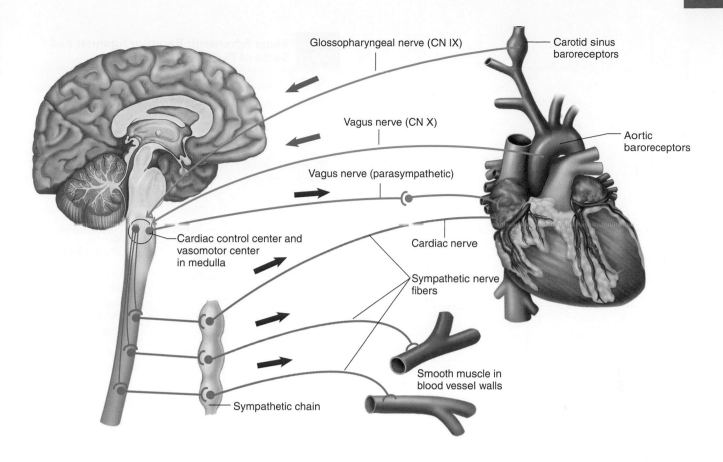

• **Fig. 7.5** Simple scheme for the baroreceptor (carotid sinus) reflex. (From: Patton KT et al: *Anatomy and physiology*, ed 11, ch 30, Elsevier, 2022.)

Metabolism of Catecholamines

Two major pathways are involved in the metabolism and inactivation of catecholamines. Monoamine oxidase (MAO) is an enzyme that oxidizes catecholamines and is present in adrenergic nerve terminals. The enzyme is important in controlling cytoplasmic concentrations of catecholamines.

In regard to the type of drug inhibitor, there is a spectrum of actions by MAO inhibitors. Nonselective MAO inhibitors are associated with important drug-drug interactions. More selective MAO inhibitors, such as those used to treat Parkinson disease, have fewer such interactions.

Catechol-O-methyl transferase (COMT) also participates in metabolism of catecholamines. This metabolism takes place largely outside of nerves. Inhibitors of this enzyme are also used in the treatment of Parkinson disease.

Adverse Effects of Adrenergic Agonists

The adverse effects are generally extensions of their receptor effects. These include vascular and cardiac effects.

Those drugs that have **β-adrenergic** effects can cause tachycardia and arrhythmias. This can lead to myocardial ischemia. Hypertension can result from over aggressive IV use of **α-receptor** agonists. Adverse central nervous system (CNS) effects, such as sedation, can result from $\alpha\alpha_2$-**adrenergic** receptor agonists like **clonidine**. In addition, clonidine can cause xerostomia. It can also lead to rebound hypertension if withdrawn abruptly. Installation of an $\alpha\alpha_1$-**adrenergic** receptor agonist in the eye can lead to a dangerous increase in intraocular pressure in a patient with narrow angle glaucoma.

Dopamine

Dopamine is the third major endogenous catecholamine. It has important cardiovascular effects as well as effects in the CNS, including hormonal effects. Its role in the CNS will be discussed in later chapters. Dopamine is also used to treat certain types of shock.

In dentistry, adrenergic agonists are important drugs that are commonly used in patient management. For instance, some benefits of epinephrine in the treatment of dental patients include its use in prolonging the action of local anesthesia and reducing gingiva bleeding during

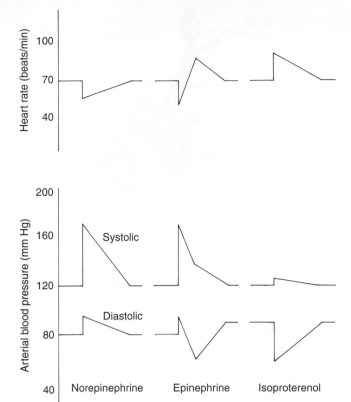

• **Fig. 7.6** Schematic representation of the effects of three catecholamines on heart rate and arterial blood pressure in the dog. The drugs were administered intravenously by bolus injection at a dose of 1 μg/kg. Note the biphasic effect of epinephrine. Initially, the drug resembles norepinephrine by causing an increase in blood pressure and reduction in heart rate. As the concentration of epinephrine falls into the physiologic range, however, β-adrenergic receptor activation predominates. Diastolic pressure decreases, and direct cardiac effects are unmasked. The decreased heart rates seen with norepinephrine and at the beginning of the epinephrine response are produced indirectly by the baroreceptor reflex. The drug effects shown here last for approximately 5 minutes. Isoproterenol causes vasodilation via **β**$_2$ adrenergic receptor stimulation. The drug's indirect effect on the heart amplifies its direct effect of increasing heart rate. The drug's indirect effect on the heart amplifies its direct effect of increasing heart rate.

TABLE 7.3	Some Adrenergic Receptor Agonists and Some of Their Uses	
Drug	**Receptor(s)**	**Use**
Phenylephrine	α$_1$	Nasal vasoconstriction. Treatment of hypotension.
Oxymetazoline, Tetrahydrolozine	α$_2$	Nasal vasoconstriction.
Dobutamine	β$_1$	Cardiogenic shock.
Levonordefrin	α$_1$, α$_2$	Local vasoconstriction.
Epinephrine	α$_1$, α$_2$, β$_1$, β$_2$	Vasoconstriction. Treatment of acute allergic reactions.[a] Cardiac stimulation.
Clonidine	α$_2$	Treatment of hypertension.[b]
Apraclonidine, Brimonidine	α$_2$	Treatment of glaucoma.[c]
Albuterol, Bitolterol, Salmeterol	β$_2$	Treatment of asthma and COPD.[d]

[a]In addition to vasoconstriction, epinephrine has several mechanisms that aid in the treatment of anaphylactic shock and other acute allergic reactions.
[b]α$_2$ adrenergic receptor agonists lower blood pressure by action in the central nervous system which results in a decrease of sympathetic outflow.
[c]Drugs that stimulate α$_2$-adrenergic receptors reduce the production of aqueous humor in the eye.
[d]Adrenergic drugs that are β$_2$-adrenergic receptor agonists, relax bronchial smooth muscle resulting in opening of the airway.
COPD, Chronic obstructive pulmonary disease.

restorative treatment. Epinephrine is the drug of choice in treating acute anaphylaxis.

Suggested Reading

Bylund DB. Alpha- and beta-adrenergic receptors: Ahlquist's landmark hypothesis of a single mediator with two receptors. *Am J Physiol Endocrinol Metab.* 2007;293:E1479–E1481.

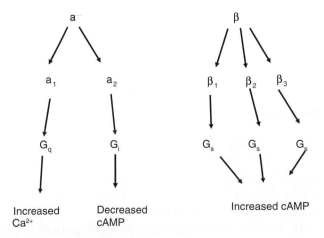

• **Fig. 7.7** Signal transduction pathways for the adrenergic receptors. *cAMP,* Cyclic adenosine monophosphate.

8
Adrenergic Receptor Antagonists

KEY POINTS

- Adrenergic receptor antagonists block the effect of endogenous and exogenous adrenergic receptor agonists.

- Both α- and β-adrenergic receptor blockers vary in their degree of selectivity and therefore can be classified as either selective or nonselective antagonists.

- α-Adrenergic blockers are used to lower blood pressure and to reduce prostate hypertrophy.

- β-Adrenergic blockers are widely used for a variety of indications including hypertension, ischemic heart disease, myocardial infarction, heart failure, arrhythmias, performance anxiety, etc.

DEFINITIONS

- **Sympatholytic** is a general term used to describe a drug that inhibits sympathetic effects.
- **Adrenergic receptor antagonists** are also called adrenergic receptor blockers, such as α-blocker or β-blocker depending on their selectively.
- **Suffixes of nonproprietary names** for adrenergic receptor blockers that help in drug identification include the following:
  ○ … osin for an α_1-adrenergic receptor blocker.
  ○ … olol for a β-adrenergic receptor blocker.
  ○ … ilol or … alol that pertain to carvedilol and labetalol, respectively. They are β-blockers with added properties.

Mechanism of Action

Most adrenergic receptor antagonists (i.e., sympatholytics) are competitive antagonists at either α- or β-adrenergic receptors. A few are antagonists at both. A thorough knowledge of the effects of stimulation of the various adrenergic receptors provides insight into the effects of drugs that block those receptors. It is important to remember that the effects of norepinephrine and epinephrine are antagonized by the appropriate adrenergic blocking drugs. Therefore adrenergic blocking drugs have important effects without an adrenergic receptor agonist being administered.

Fig. 8.1 shows a functional schematic diagram of adrenergic nerve endings and location of adrenergic receptors.

Selectivity of Adrenergic Receptor Antagonists and Clinical Characteristics

Table 8.1 shows the receptor preferences for representative antagonists. Individual drugs are listed as either, alpha antagonists, beta antagonists, or mixed antagonists. The ability of each drug to block receptors (α_1, α_2, β_1, β_2) is listed.

Selective α_1-Adrenergic Receptor Antagonists

The most important α_1-adrenergic receptors are located **on smooth muscle**. The vasoconstrictor effects of norepinephrine and other α_1-adrenergic receptor agonists are blocked by α_1-adrenergic receptor antagonists. The primary indication for these drugs is **hypertension**. Prazosin, terazosin, and doxazosin are the ones used for this purpose.

Alpha$_1$-adrenergic receptor antagonists are also effective in treating **benign prostatic hyperplasia**, since, by their action, they inhibit smooth muscle contraction in the bladder neck and the prostate. Two drugs, alfuzosin and tamsulosin, are the most often used for this purpose because they have a degree of selectivity for the prostate. These actions are shown in Fig. 8.2.

Adverse Effect of α_1-Adrenergic Receptor Blockers

In some cases adverse events are due to effects of these drugs at their adrenergic receptors. Blocking α_1-adrenergic receptors in blood vessels can lead to

hypotension and notably, orthostatic hypotension. This is particularly the case when the drugs are first administered, known as the **first dose effect**. This necessitates careful initial dosing and a gradual build-up of doses until the therapeutic dose is reached. Another example

of the adverse effects is **intraoperative floppy iris syndrome** that can occur during cataract surgery.

Nonselective α-Adrenergic Receptor Blockers

Phenoxybenzamine and phentolamine block both α_1- and α_2-adrenergic receptors. Phenoxybenzamine is an irreversible antagonist, whereas phentolamine is a competitive reversible antagonist. They are occasionally used to treat pheochromocytoma.

Phentolamine, however, is used in dentistry to attain more rapid reversal of soft tissue anesthesia. Its mechanism is most likely to block sympathetic tone allowing the more rapid removal of local anesthesia from the injection

Sites of action for sympatholytic drugs

MAO inhibitors

DOPGAL MAO

NE

NE

NE

NE transporter (NET)

NE NE NE

Competitive antagonists at alpha or beta adrenergic receptors

Alpha or beta adrenergic receptors

• **Fig. 8.1** Potential sites of action for sympatholytic drugs. *DOPGAL*, 3,4 dihydroxyphenylglycolaldehyde; *MAO*, Monoamine oxidase; *NET*, norepinephrine transporter Table 8.1.

TABLE 8.1	Receptor selectivity of adrenergic receptor antagonists			
Drug	**Receptor blocked**			
	α_1	α_2	β_1	β_2
Alpha Antagonists				
Phentolamine, phenoxybenzamine	√	√		
Prazosin, terazosin, doxazocin	√			
Beta Antagonists				
Propranolol, pindolol			√	√
Metoprolol, atenolol			√	
Mixed Antagonists				
Labetalol, carvedilol	√		√	√

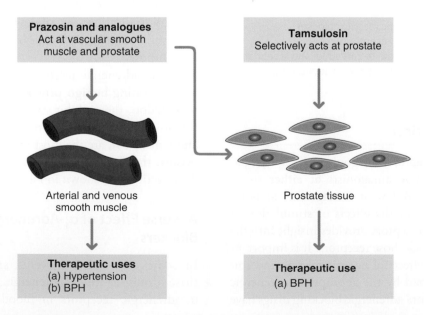

Prazosin and analogues
Act at vascular smooth muscle and prostate

Tamsulosin
Selectively acts at prostate

Arterial and venous smooth muscle

Prostate tissue

Therapeutic uses
(a) Hypertension
(b) BPH

Therapeutic use
(a) BPH

• **Fig. 8.2** Sites of action and therapeutic uses of selective α_1-adrenergic receptor antagonists. *BPN*, Benign prostatic hyperplasia.

site. Phentolamine mesylate is available in 1.7 mL dental cartridges containing 0.4 mg of the drug.

β-Adrenergic Receptor Blockers

Beta-adrenergic receptor blockers, often referred to as **beta-blockers**, are a large class of drugs that are widely used in therapy. They have important cardiovascular indications as well as a number of other indications.

The first important consideration in classification of β-blockers is whether or not the drug is selective for β_1-adrenergic receptors. (Drugs that selectively block β_2-adrenergic receptors are not useful clinically). A major advantage of selective β_1-adrenergic receptor antagonists is that they are less likely to cause bronchoconstriction in patients with asthma or chronic obstructive pulmonary disease (COPD).

A second consideration is whether the drug also blocks α_1-adrenergic receptors as do two drugs listed below.

Additional actions of some β-blockers include generation of nitric oxide and reducing reactive oxygen species. These effects may contribute to the therapeutic effect of the drug.

Table 8.1 lists several β-blockers and their level of selectivity. Additional effects of some β-blockers are shown in Table 8.2.

Comments on Table 8.2.

Blockade of α_1-adrenergic receptors contributes to the antihypertensive effects of labetalol and carvedilol. The antioxidant properties of carvedilol are also beneficial in treating heart failure. The ability of nebivolol to generate nitric oxide likely contributes to its antihypertensive properties.

Cardiovascular Indications for β-Blockers

- **Hypertension**
  Blockade of β_1-adrenergic receptors leads to a decrease in cardiac rate and force of contraction. **Renin release is also decreased**. Eventually peripheral resistance decreases. Relief of hypertension is therefore the result of several factors.
- **Heart failure**
  The reduction in force of contraction appears counterintuitive when treating heart failure and it can be harmful if the dose is not regulated carefully. However, the excessive adrenergic stimulation seen in heart failure is controlled by β-blockers. In addition, the reduction in peripheral resistance reduces the load on the heart. Carvedilol and metoprolol succinate (in an extended-release preparation) have been shown to be beneficial.
- **Ischemic heart disease**
  Beta-blockers reduce the work of the heart and therefore improve the balance between oxygen demand and oxygen delivery to the myocardium.
- **Myocardial infarction**
  Beta-blockers reduced the risk of infarction and reinfarction in patients with acute coronary syndrome. The ability of these drugs to reduce the work of the heart and their ability to reduce arrhythmias contribute to the cardiac benefits.

TABLE 8.2	Some Properties of β-Adrenergic Receptor Antagonists				
Drug	RECEPTOR BLOCKED			Generates Nitric Oxide	Antioxidant Properties
	β_1	β_2	α_1		
Nonselective (First Generation)					
Propranolol	Yes	Yes	No	No	No
Nadolol	Yes	Yes	No	No	No
Selective (Second Generation)					
Metoprolol	Yes	No	No	No	No
Atenolol	Yes	No	No	No	No
Esmolol	Yes	No	No	No	No
β-Blockers With Additional Properties (Third Generation)					
Labetalol	Yes	Yes	Yes	No	No
Carvedilol	Yes	Yes	Yes	No	Yes
Nebivolol	Yes	No	No	Yes	No

- **Arrhythmias**

  Sympathetic stimulation of the heart is inhibited by β-blockers. This results in the slowing of the heart rate and a reduction in atrioventricular (AV nodal) conduction velocity. In addition, β-blockers reduce automaticity in regions such as the Purkinje fibers in the heart.

Other Indications for β-Blockers

- **Hyperthyroidism**

  Hyperthyroidism occurs when excess amounts of thyroid hormone are secreted from the thyroid gland. The increase in thyroid hormones can cause a rapid or irregular heartbeat as well as other cardiovascular problems. This excessive cardiac stimulation in hyperthyroidism can be reduced using β-blockers.

- **Pheochromocytoma**

  Beta-blockers reduced the cardiac stimulation due to excessive release of catecholamines from the adrenal medulla. An α-adrenergic receptor antagonist is also required in this situation.

- **Glaucoma**

  β-Blockers are among the drugs used to treat open-angle glaucoma because they reduce intraocular pressure by reducing the production of aqueous humor.

- **Migraine**

  β-Blockers are used to prevent migraine headache attacks. The mechanism is not established.

- **Performance anxiety (stage fright); essential tremors**

  Excessive skeletal muscle tremors due to anxiety and other causes accompanied by excessive sympathetic activity can be relieved by β-blockers.

- **Variceal bleeding prophylaxis**

  A relevant clinical condition causing this disorder is portal hypertension in a patient with cirrhosis of the liver.

Adverse Effects of β-Blockers

Important adverse effects are listed in Table 8.3.

TABLE 8.3 Adverse Effects of β-Blockers

Organ or Tissue	Effect
Heart	Bradycardia
	Heart block
	Excessive decrease in cardiac output—heart failure.
Bronchus	Bronchoconstriction in sensitive patients especially with nonselective β-blockers.
Central nervous system	Sleep disturbances
Blood	Hypoglycemia may be prolonged in patients treated with hypoglycemic drugs.
Liver and elsewhere	May often involve the effect of other drugs on the metabolism of the β-blocker.

These effects are dose-related and careful consideration should be given to drug dosage and contraindications to β-blockers.

An important consideration of a **drug-drug interaction in dentistry** involves the use of a vasoconstrictor, epinephrine as a main example, in patients taking a nonselective β-blocker. Given higher doses of the vasoconstrictor, hypertension and bradycardia can ensue after inadvertent intravascular injection. This could be a risk in patients with underlying cardiovascular disorders.

Suggested Readings

Dowd FJ, Mariotti AJ, eds *Adrenergic Antagonists. Pharmacology and Therapeutics for Dentistry*. St Louis: Elsevier; 2017:2024.

Hersh EV, Giannakopoulos H. Beta-adrenergic blocking agents and dental vasoconstrictors. *Dent Clin North Am*. 2010;54(4):687–696.

9

Central Nervous System Drugs

KEY POINTS

- Sedative hypnotics
  - Sedatives of the benzodiazepine class, like drugs, enhance the effect of gamma aminobutyric acid (GABA) at GABA$_A$ receptors, thereby increasing chloride conductance.
  - The elimination half-times of benzodiazepines depends on their routes of metabolism.
  - The "Z" drugs act in a similar manner as the benzodiazepines.
  - Additional sedatives include the barbiturates, antihistamines, dexmedetomidine, and melatonin receptor agonists.
  - The sedative properties of select drugs are used for muscle relaxation.

- Antipsychotic drugs
  - Antipsychotic drugs (i.e., neuroleptics) are generally dopamine (D$_2$) receptor blockers and/or blockers of serotonin (5-HT$_2$) receptors.
  - Newer atypical antipsychotic drugs have a different mechanism of action compared to the older (i.e., typical) drugs.
  - Adverse effects vary depending on the drug but often include motor side effects.

- Mood stabilizers
  - Mood stabilizer drugs are used to treat large emotional swings in affective disorders.
  - The mechanism of action of mood stabilizer drugs, lithium, carbamazepine, and valproic acid, varies depending on the agent.

- Antidepressants
  - Most antidepressants inhibit the reuptake of norepinephrine and serotonin with different degrees of selectivity.
  - The adverse effects vary greatly between groups of antidepressants.

DEFINITIONS

- Sedative hypnotics are drugs that depress the central nervous system (CNS) and are used to relieve anxiety or to induce sleep.
- Antipsychotic drugs are agents used to treat changes in personality, impaired mental functioning, or a distorted sense of objective reality (typical characteristics of schizophrenia).
- Mood stabilizers are drugs that prevent or relieve extensive fluctuations in emotional range (e.g., bipolar disorders).
- Antidepressants are drugs used to treat mood disorders related to depression.
- Serotonin syndrome occurs when an excessive accumulation of serotonin in the body causes changes in mental status, motor abnormalities, cardiovascular changes, and gastrointestinal (GI) problems.
- Gamma aminobutyric acid (GABA) is an amino acid neurotransmitter that primarily causes inhibitory actions in the brain and spinal cord (i.e., blocks brain signals or decreases nervous system activity). GABA$_A$ and GABA$_B$ receptors are the two receptor types activated by GABA.
- Melatonin is a hormone released from a small mass of tissue behind the third ventricle of the brain, which is called the pineal gland.
- Ion channels are pathways through the lipid cell membrane for the passage of charged ions.
- G protein-coupled receptors are proteins in the cell membrane. When activated, the receptors transmit signals within the cell via an intracellular G-protein molecule.
- Monoamine oxidases (MAOs) are enzymes that metabolize catecholamines and serotonin. Inhibitors of MAO (MAOI) increase the concentration of these neurotransmitters in the cytosol of nerve endings.

Sedative Hypnotics

A drug class of central nervous system (CNS) depressants, which cause drowsiness, sleep, and reduction in anxiety, are known as sedative hypnotics. The different classes of these drugs vary in their magnitude and quality of CNS depression. The mechanisms of action by which sedative hypnotics cause CNS depression vary; however, a key mechanism is the ability of many of these drugs to enhance the activity (conductance) of the chloride ion channel in brain neurons.

Benzodiazepines

This is a major class of sedatives represented by **diazepam (Valium)**. A list of some members of this group is given in Table 9.1.

The elimination half-lives of these drugs can be influenced by the concurrent administration of drugs that either induce or inhibit drug metabolism. For instance, rifampin, by inducing liver enzymes, can greatly reduce the effect of triazolam. Nonetheless, not all benzodiazepines are similarly affected by inducers or inhibitors of liver enzymes.

Mechanism of Action

The action of benzodiazepines is linked to the **increase in conductance of the chloride ion channel**, resulting in an increase in chloride ion influx into nerve cells in the brain. This leads to hyperpolarization and reduced activity of nerve cells with major effects in the limbic system and other regions of the brain.

Since the **benzodiazepine receptors** are located on an ion (i.e., chloride) channel, other drugs can also bind and influence the chloride channel. The chloride channels are composed of five subunits as shown in Fig. 9.1. Notice that the subunits are surrounding the channel.

Gamma aminobutyric acid (GABA) is a neurotransmitter that opens the chloride channel and the effects of benzodiazepines depend on the presence of GABA. These drugs and others that stimulate the benzodiazepine receptors increase the frequency of channel opening as long as GABA is present. The chloride channel that contains a GABA receptor is termed the **GABA$_A$** receptor.

TABLE 9.1	Representative Benzodiazepines
Drug	Elimination Half-Life (h)
Triazolam	1.5–5
Midazolam	2–5
Oxazepam	5–15
Lorazepam	10–18
Alprazolam	12–15
Chlordiazepoxide	5–30
Diazepam	30–60
Flurazepam	50–100

Another complexity to the chloride channel and benzodiazepine receptors is that the subunits of the channel can vary, leading to two different types of benzodiazepine receptors. Drugs other that benzodiazepines can also bind to the chloride channel as shown in Figs. 9.1 and 9.2.

Effects of Benzodiazepines

There is a dose-dependent increase in CNS depression that is produced by benzodiazepines (Table 9.2). Certain benzodiazepines are also used as anticonvulsants. Benzodiazepines typically cause amnesia during moderate to deep sedation procedures, resulting in the patient not remembering events during the sedation.

Biotransformation

Although benzodiazepines are metabolized by a variety of metabolic pathways, which vary according to the drug, all of them are eventually converted to the glucuronide.

Adverse Effects

Most adverse events are extensions of the therapeutic effects. Benzodiazepines are relatively safe drugs with a high

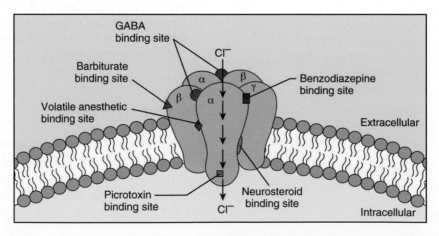

• **Fig. 9.1** Structural model of the γ-aminobutyric acid (GABA)- benzodiazepine (BZ) receptor complex. The arrangement of the subunits (α, β, γ) forms the Cl– channel. GABA-binding sites are illustrated at the two analogous interfaces between the α and β subunits. The BZ-binding site is associated with the interface of the α and γ subunits. (Reproduced with permission from Wecker Lynn, Sanchez Deborah L., Currier Glenn W. Brody's Human Pharmacology. Published January 1, 2019. Pages 143-156. © Elsevier 2019.)

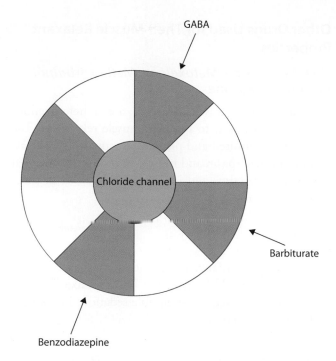

• **Fig. 9.2** Arrangement of allosteric-binding domains on the γ-aminobutyric acid (GABA)$_A$ receptor complex. The complex is composed of five subunits. Multiple receptor subtypes are possible on the basis of different combinations of the subunits. Binding sites for picrotoxin (a convulsant), barbiturates, GABA, and benzodiazepines are presented for illustrative purposes. In addition, distinct binding sites for other chemical agents have been identified (shown as blank areas). The figure does not identify which receptor subunits are involved in the binding of each drug. (Adapted from Sieghart W. GABAA receptors: ligand-gated Cl− ion channels modulated by multiple drug-binding sites. *Trends Pharmacol Sci*. 1992;13:446–450.)

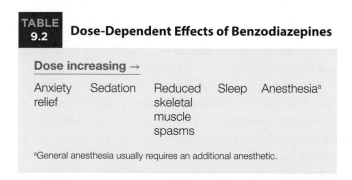

TABLE 9.2 Dose-Dependent Effects of Benzodiazepines

Dose increasing →				
Anxiety relief	Sedation	Reduced skeletal muscle spasms	Sleep	Anesthesia[a]

[a]General anesthesia usually requires an additional anesthetic.

therapeutic index because their toxicity is controlled by the limited presence of GABA. Nevertheless, serious respiratory depression can result when benzodiazepines are combined with ethanol or opioids. Although benzodiazepines can induce sleep, they can also change, to some degree, sleep architecture. With chronic use, the benzodiazepines can cause dependence and they do have abuse potential leading to addiction. **Flumazenil** is an **antagonist** at the benzodiazepine receptors and can be used in cases of overdose.

Other Sedatives

The "Z" Drugs

The "Z" term refers to a class of benzodiazepine-like sedative-hypnotics (e.g., **zolpidem**, **zaleplon**, and **eszopiclone**) that have similar pharmacologic profiles to the benzodiazepines. Their similarities to benzodiazepines include the following:
- bind to benzodiazepine receptors;
- inhibited by flumazenil;
- cause sedation;
- enhance the effect of GABA at the GABA$_A$ receptors (chloride channel); and
- have abuse potential.
  Unlike the benzodiazepines, "Z" drugs are
- more selective for a subgroup of benzodiazepine receptors;
- less effective as muscle relaxers;
- less effective as anticonvulsants;
- metabolized and eliminated more rapidly (i.e., shorter half-lives); and
- used primarily to reduce the time to sleep onset in patients with insomnia.

The "Z" drugs are commonly used today and compare favorably with the benzodiazepines.

Barbiturates

The mechanism by which the barbiturates exert their CNS depressant effects bears a striking similarity to the effects of benzodiazepines. Barbiturates **enhance GABA-activated chloride channel opening** by acting at specific barbiturate-binding sites on the GABA$_A$ receptor complex (see Fig. 9.2). In addition, at high concentrations, barbiturates also act directly on the chloride channel, not requiring the presence of GABA. It is this latter action that accounts for the **lower margin of safety** of the barbiturates. This is one reason why the use of these drugs has greatly declined. **Pentobarbital and phenobarbital** are two examples of these drugs. Adverse effects include the following:
- Severe CNS depression and death due to respiratory arrest in overdose.
- Significant changes in sleep patterns e.g., reduced time spent in rapid eye movement (REM) sleep.
- Drug-drug interactions due to induction of liver enzymes by barbiturates.

Antihistamines

Hydroxyzine and **diphenhydramine** are earlier antihistamines (histamine (H$_1$) receptor antagonists) that are noted to cause considerable sedation. Diphenhydramine is an over-the-counter drug. Hydroxyzine is useful for sedation in a number of clinical settings.

Later H$_1$ receptor antagonists do not cause significant sedation. These drugs and drugs that block histamine H$_2$ receptors are discussed further in Appendix 3.

Alpha$_2$-adrenergic Receptor Agonists

Alpha$_2$-adrenergic receptors (see Chapter 7) are proteins in cell membranes and are responsive to alpha$_2$-adrenergic agonists that generally produce inhibitory responses. **Tizanidine** increases presynaptic inhibition of motor neurons and is useful in treating disorders involving excessive muscle tone, such as amyotrophic lateral sclerosis and multiple sclerosis. The mechanism of action of **dexmedetomidine** is similar to tizanidine and is useful in treating critical care patients when sedation is needed. Both of these drugs do not cause respiratory depression, however they can lower blood pressure.

Melatonin Receptor Agonists

Melatonin, which is secreted by the pineal gland, follows a circadian pattern that is synchronized to the light/dark cycle. Melatonin rises as daylight diminishes and helps to prepare the body for sleep. Melatonin receptor subtypes, which are members of the G protein-coupled receptor (GPCR) family, are located in many areas of the brain as well as a variety of peripheral tissues. Melatonin receptor ligands have been used to treat sleep and circadian dysfunction. **Ramelteon**, an agonist at melatonin receptors, is used to treat insomnia and jet lag. **Tasimelteon** is used primarily to treat non-24-hour sleep/wake disorder.

Suvorexant

Orexin, which is a neuropeptide produced by hypothalamic neurons, promotes the awake state. Suvorexant is an antagonist at orexin receptors in the hypothalamus and the blocking of orexin receptors promotes sleep. Suvorexant is used to treat insomnia.

Baclofen

Baclofen is a drug that stimulates another GABA receptor, the **GABA$_B$** receptor. This receptor is a G protein-coupled receptor (GPCR) which, when stimulated, reduces calcium conductance and increases potassium conductance. The net effect is to reduce nerve activity, in part by reducing neurotransmitter release and effect. It is used to reduce muscle spasticity in disorders such as **multiple sclerosis**. It also may be helpful in managing trigeminal neuralgia, although it is not usually as effective as other drugs (e.g., carbamazepine) for this indication. Baclofen has sedative properties as well.

Other Drugs Used for Their Muscle Relaxant Properties

Cyclobenzaprine, Metaxalone, Methocarbamol, and Chlorzoxazone

Centrally acting muscle relaxants are a heterogenous group of drugs used to produce muscle relaxation. The clinical use is limited and primarily focused in the treatment of muscle spasm and muscle immobility associated with strains, sprains, and injuries. A side effect of these agents is sedation.

Buspirone

Buspirone is an antianxiety agent that is a partial agonist at the serotonin 5-HT$_{1A}$ receptor. The antianxiety effects are not accompanied by noticeable sedation, in contrast with other antianxiety drugs.

Antipsychotic Drugs (Neuroleptics)

Mechanisms of Action

Antipsychotic drugs, also called neuroleptics, are used to treat schizophrenia and other psychoses.

In treating psychotic disorders, these drugs act by **blocking dopamine (D$_2$) receptors** and **serotonin (5-HT$_2$) receptors**. However, depending on the drug class, they also block muscarinic, alpha$_1$-adrenergic, and other receptors, in addition to other subtypes of dopamine receptors. The earlier conventional antipsychotic drugs are characterized by their major antipsychotic action on the D$_2$ receptor, whereas newer drugs generally achieve antipsychotic effects by blocking both 5-HT$_{2A}$ and D$_2$ receptors.

Schizophrenia is characterized by a variety of symptoms that can be classified as either positive symptoms or negative symptoms (Table 9.3). The mechanisms of the antipsychotic drugs, determine the relative effect on adverse symptoms.

Fig. 9.3 portrays the ability of antipsychotic drugs to block postsynaptic dopamine receptors.

Examining the regions of the brain that contain dopamine receptors helps explain the therapeutic effects as well as adverse effects of dopamine receptor antagonism. Fig. 9.4 shows four dopaminergic pathways. The **mesocortical/mesolimbic pathway**, involving the D$_2$ receptors, is linked to the **antipsychotic effect**.

Fig. 9.4 shows the mesocortical/mesolimbic pathway starting from the ventral tegmentum, as well as other dopaminergic pathways that are associated with other effects of the antipsychotic drugs. Adverse motor effects are linked to blocking dopamine receptors in the nigrostriatal pathway (substantia nigra to basal ganglia). Reduction in nausea and vomiting occurs from blocking dopamine receptors in the chemoreceptor trigger zone CTZ). Hyperprolactinemia is due to dopamine receptor blockade in the hypothalamus (tubero-infundibular system).

What is the role of the 5-HT$_{2A}$ receptor compared to the D$_2$ receptor in alleviating the symptoms of schizophrenia? Whereas excessive dopamine in the mesolimbic pathway is linked to positive symptoms of schizophrenia, negative symptoms result from a deficiency of dopamine in the cortex (i.e., mesocortical pathway) (Fig. 9.5). Serotonin 5-HT$_{2A}$ receptor antagonists selectively increase dopamine release in the cortex. Thus they have a more selective action in reducing negative symptoms. Moreover, 5-HT$_{2A}$ receptor antagonists cause fewer motor adverse effects because these drugs have less effect of dopamine receptors in the basal ganglia.

Types of Drugs

Based primarily on the different mechanisms of action, antipsychotic drugs can be classified as either typical (older) or atypical (newer) drugs (Table 9.4). Generally, the atypical drugs show more blocking ability on 5-HT$_{2A}$ receptors than do the typical drugs. This is a major, but not the only, difference between the two groups.

Adverse Effects

Motor adverse effects (Table 9.5) are seen more often with the typical drugs. Other adverse effects, depending on the drug, include weight gain, sedation, and anticholinergic effects.

Mood-Stabilizing Drugs

The term *mood stabilizer* can have a variety of different meanings. For pharmacology, mood-stabilizing drugs are a class of medications that treat mania or manic depressive-illness (bipolar disease). The following are three important drug groups that act as mood stabilizes:
- Lithium, which inhibits turnover of inositol phosphates in the brain.
- Carbamazepine, which blocks sodium channels.
- Valproic acid, which blocks both sodium channels and calcium channels.

Lithium is removed largely by renal excretion. Sodium and lithium compete with each other for tubular

TABLE 9.3	Clinical Efficacy and Antipsychotic Mechanisms	
	ANTIPSYCHOTIC MECHANISM	
Symptoms	D$_2$ Receptor Blockade	5HT$_{2A}$ Receptor Blockade
Positive (hallucinations, disorganized speech, abnormal thought processes)	+++	++
Negative (lack of emotion, withdrawal, hesitant speech)	+	+++

The number of "+" signs indicates the relative effectiveness.

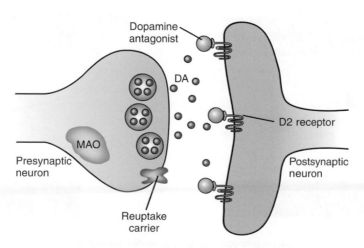

• **Fig. 9.3** Dopamine blockade by antipsychotic drugs. *DA*, Dopamine (released from presynaptic neuron). (Taken from: Holliday C. In: Banasik J., ed, et al. *Neurobiology of Psychotic Illnesses in Pathophysiology*. St. Louis: Elsevier; 2022. 7th ed. pii:B9780323761550000481/f48-05-9780323761550.)

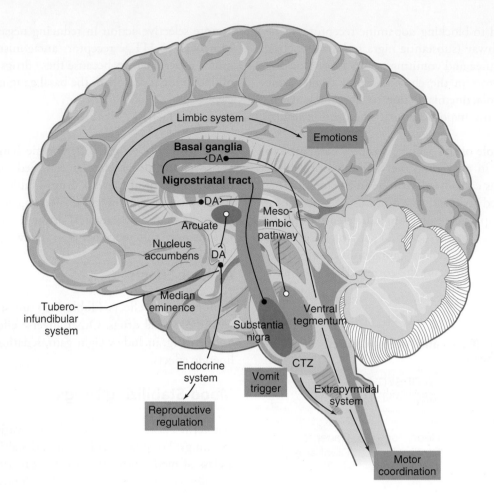

• **Fig. 9.4** Dopaminergic pathways in the brain. The mesolimbic system (shown from the ventral tegmentum through the meso-limbic pathway to the limbic system) is linked to the antipsychotic mechanism of antipsychotic drugs. *CTZ*, Chemoreceptor trigger zone; *DA*, dopamine. (Modified from Kester M. et al. *Elsevier's Integrated Pharmacology*, Philadelphia: Mosby; 2012. 2nd ed.)

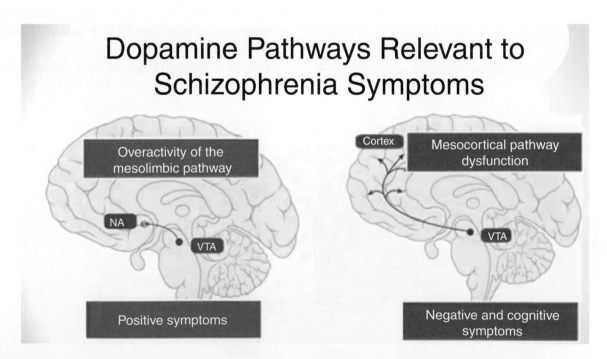

• **Fig. 9.5** Location of two pathways that are involved in schizophrenia symptoms. *NA*, nucleus accumbens; *VTA*, ventral tegmental area. (Taken from Flavio Guzman, ed. *The Four Dopamine Pathways Relevant to Antipsychotics Pharmacology*, [Open access article]. Psychopharmacology Institute. 2016.)

reabsorption. Therefore a significant decrease of sodium in the diet can increase lithium in the plasma. Ibuprofen and similar drugs may also increase plasma levels of lithium. These interactions are important because lithium has a narrow margin of safety.

Toxicity due to lithium includes diuresis and thirst due to inhibition of antidiuretic hormone effects on the kidney, as well as tremors, weight gain, and fatigue.

Carbamazepine and valproic acid are discussed further under antiepileptic drugs (Appendix 2). Carbamazepine is also mentioned in Chapter 14. Antipsychotic drugs are also useful in disorders such as acute mania.

TABLE 9.4	Examples of Antipsychotic Drugs	
Typical (Older) Drugs	**Atypical (Newer) Drugs**	
Chlorpromazine	Olanzapine	
Thioridazine	Risperidone	
Haloperidol	Quetiapine	

TABLE 9.5	Some Motor Adverse Effects (Extrapyramidal Effects) from Antipsychotic Drugs	
Adverse Effect	**Description**
Parkinsonism	Bradykinesia, rigidity, tremor
Akathisia	Motor restlessness
Acute dystonia	Spasms of face, tongue, and back
Tardive dyskinesia	Abnormal muscle activity of the face and mouth and other muscles

Antidepressant Drugs

Mechanism of Action

Unlike the antipsychotic drugs, most of which are receptor blockers, most antidepressant drugs act by **blocking the reuptake** of norepinephrine and serotonin.

The classification of antidepressant drugs depends on their relative effect on norepinephrine and serotonin, and in a few cases, whether they have other mechanisms.

The major classes of drugs used to treat depression block the reuptake of norepinephrine (noradrenaline) and serotonin (5-HT), as shown in Fig. 9.6. This takes place in CNS synapses after these neurotransmitters are released from the presynaptic neurons. The reuptake mechanism, through the reuptake transporter, maintains the level of neurotransmitter in the synapse at low levels.

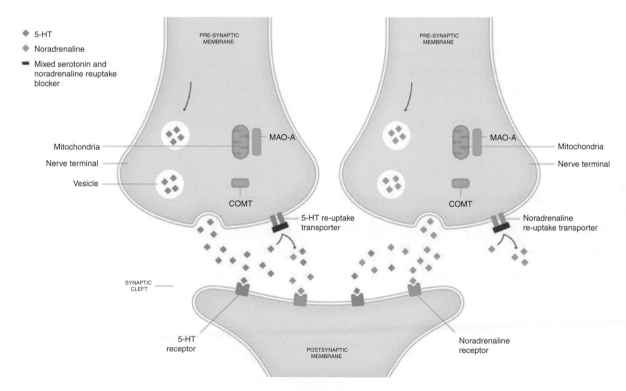

• **Fig. 9.6** Action of antidepressants (reuptake inhibitors). *MAO-A*, Monoamine oxidase-A; *COMT*, catechol-O-methyltransferase; *5HT*, 5-hydroxytryptamine (serotonin). (Image from an image bank at © 2020 H. Lundbeck Institute Campus A/S. All rights reserved. Website: institute.progress.im.)

The action of antidepressants leads to:

(1) An acute increase of the neurotransmitter in the synapse.

(2) A long-term effect, in which the postsynaptic receptors are changed. These changes include a disproportionate increase (up-regulation) in certain receptors more than other receptors.

(3) An alleviation of symptoms of depression beginning weeks after initiation of therapy.

Ultimately, the actions of antidepressants lead to changes in transmission in **noradrenergic** and **serotonergic pathways** in the limbic system and cerebral cortex.

It is important to remember that antidepressants have other actions that can lead to adverse effects (see Table 9.8).

Classification

The classes of antidepressant drugs and examples of each are listed in Tables 9.6 and 9.7.

Not mentioned in this chapter are other drugs within each of the above classes that have antidepressant actions.

Adverse Effects

Most antidepressant drugs have effects other than to inhibit neurotransmitter reuptake. An example is the antimuscarinic effects of the tricyclic drugs. Dry mouth is a common occurrence with these drugs. Tricyclic antidepressant drugs cause sedation, which is not as likely with the newer drugs. Table 9.8 shows the relative risk of certain adverse effects of the antidepressant drugs.

Other adverse effects may include the following:

- convulsions and insomnia with bupropion,
- GI upset and insomnia with the selective serotonin reuptake inhibitors (SSRIs),
- agitation and confusion with the tricyclics.

Furthermore, combinations of antidepressant drugs may lead to serotonin syndrome. Other antidepressant drugs should not be combined with monoamine oxidase inhibitors. A number of **drug-drug interactions** may occur with the antidepressant drugs and other drugs based on the ability of other drugs to either increase or decrease the metabolism of antidepressants.

Monoamine oxidase inhibitors (MAOIs) pose a significant risk if taken with foods that contain tyramine or drugs that can cause the release of catecholamines from nerve endings.

TABLE 9.7	List of Some Major Drugs by Class
Class	**Drugs**
Tricyclics	Amitriptyline Imipramine Protriptyline
SSRIs	Fluoxetine Paroxetine Citalopram Escitalopram Sertraline
SNRIs	Duloxetine Venlafaxine
Atypical drug	Bupropion[a]
MAOI	Phenelzine Tranylcypromine

MAOI, Monoamine oxidase inhibitor; *SNRIs*, serotonin-norepinephrine reuptake inhibitors; *SSRIs*, selective serotonin reuptake inhibitors.
[a]Bupropion is also used for smoking cessation. When used as an antidepressant it is marketed under the proprietary name of **Wellbutrin**, whereas when used for smoking cessation, it is marketed as **Zyban**.

TABLE 9.6	Classification of Antidepressants Drugs and Their Specific Mechanisms
Drug Class	**Mechanism**
Tricyclic antidepressants	Block reuptake of norepinephrine and serotonin
Selective serotonin reuptake Inhibitors (SSRI's)	Block reuptake of serotonin with greater potency than reuptake of norepinephrine
Serotonin-norepinephrine reuptake inhibitors (SNRI's)	Block reuptake of serotonin and norepinephrine but have fewer effects as blockers of various receptors
Atypical drug (Bupropion)	Has some inhibitory effect on dopamine reuptake and causes release of serotonin and nor epinephrine from nerve endings
Monoamine oxidase inhibitor (MAOI)	Increases norepinephrine and serotonin by blocking MAO

TABLE 9.8	**Adverse Effects of Antidepressant Drugs**				
Class	Antimuscarinic Action	Sedation	Orthostatic Hypotension (α_1-Adenergic Receptor Blockade)	Sexual Dysfunction	Weight Gain
Tricyclics	+++	+++	+++	+	++
SSRI's	−−	−−	−−	++	+
SNRI's	−−	−−	−−	+	+
Bupropion	++	−−	−−	+	+
MAOI	+	+	+	−−	I

The number of "+" signs is the relative degree to which the drug or drug class is likely to cause the effect. The sign "−−" indicates no or little effect. Relative differences in effects can vary within each class. *MAOI*, Monoamine oxidase inhibitors; *SNRI's*, serotonin-norepinephrine reuptake inhibitors; *SSRI's*, selective serotonin reuptake inhibitors.

Suggested Readings

Drugs for anxiety disorders. *Med Lett Drugs Ther*. 2019;61: 121–126.

Ramsford N, Marnell B, Randall C, et al. Systemic medicines taken by adult special care dental patients and implications for the management of their care. *Br Dent J*. 2021;231:33–42.

10
General Anesthetics

The histories of dentistry and anesthesia intersect.

- The mechanism(s) of action of general anesthetics are not well understood.
- The options for general anesthesia are classified as either inhalation and/or intravenous.
- Balanced anesthesia, using multiple drugs, is the common technique.
- Inhalational anesthetics (e.g., nitrous oxide, isoflurane, desflurane, and sevoflurane) are used primarily for maintenance of anesthesia.
- Intravenous anesthetics (e.g., propofol, methohexital, ketamine, midazolam) are used for induction of anesthesia.
- Adjuvant drugs (e.g., skeletal neuromuscular blockers, analgesics, sedatives, antihistamines, antimuscarinics) are also added to contribute to balanced anesthesia.

DEFINITIONS

- **Minimal sedation** or anxiolysis is a state in which the patient is relaxed and awake and can respond to verbal commands. An example is the oral administration of a low dose of midazolam.
- **Moderate sedation** was formally known as conscious sedation. It is a drug-induced depression of consciousness while the patient can respond to verbal commands. An example is the intravenous administration of midazolam and meperidine.
- **Deep sedation** is a drug-induced depression of consciousness during which the patient cannot be easily aroused. In this level of sedation, the patient can respond to purposefully repeated verbal commands. This level of sedation is usually approved for trained personnel for short procedures (i.e., 10 minutes or less).
- **General anesthesia** is a drug-induced loss of consciousness.

History

Although the effects of ethyl alcohol, opiates, and some other agents had been known for centuries, early experimental use of drugs for anesthesia date from the 1840s. Two dentists were among those early experimenters. With varying degrees of success, Horace Wells utilized nitrous oxide and William Morton used diethyl ether. Further intriguing information on early events in the development of general anesthetics can be found in the textbook, *Pharmacology and Therapeutics for Dentistry*.

Today we have several anesthetics, administered both by inhalation and intravenously, that provide effective general anesthesia for a variety of clinical situations.

Mechanisms of Action for General Anesthesia

An early theory stated that general anesthetics act nonselectively on neurons as a function of their lipid solubility. This characteristic of the drugs would allow them to dissolve into neurons and disrupt neuronal activity.

The latest information indicates that anesthetics have more selective actions aimed at the synapses in the brain and multiple mechanisms of action of anesthetic agents may include:

- inhibiting stimulatory receptors, such as receptors for glutamate (i.e., N-methyl D-aspartate [NMDA] receptors), and acetylcholine
- stimulating the inhibitory circuitry via action on glycine and $GABA_A$ receptors
- activating potassium channels causing hyperpolarization of neurons.

Among the important regions of the brain accounting for the effects of general anesthetics are the:

- relay circuits between the thalamus and the cerebral cortex
- hippocampus
- reticular activating system.

Factors Affecting the Rate of Onset of Anesthesia

The rate of onset of anesthesia depends on several factors including the cardiac output, the concentration of inhaled drug, as well as the depth and rate of inhalation. One important characteristic of the drug itself is the **blood/gas partition coefficient**. If the ratio of the drug in the blood/inspired air is very low, the rate of onset or induction of anesthesia is high. Although this may seem counterintuitive, drugs with a low blood/gas partition coefficients allow rapid equilibrium of drugs between blood and gas. This correlates with a rapid onset of anesthesia, which is a desirable trait in an inhaled anesthetic. Thus, for inhaled anesthetics in which blood/gas partition coefficients are low, recovery from anesthesia is also rapid.

Stages of Depth of Anesthesia

The classical stages were developed from observations of diethyl ether. They are listed as a progression in depth of anesthesia. That progression is listed in Table 10.1. Two points should be made.

1. The information is derived from the use of diethyl ether and does not closely parallel the characteristics of modern-day anesthetics.
2. Modern-day general anesthesia is attained rapidly with very few adverse effects seen in stage II. A combination of drugs is usually given resulting in **balanced anesthesia.**

Nitrous Oxide (N$_2$O)

Uses

Nitrous oxide is a drug that is sometimes used for induction of general anesthesia. It has major application in dentistry for conscious sedation (stage I anesthesia). In its use in conscious sedation, it is often started at 20% nitrous oxide and 80% oxygen. Greater sedative effects can be achieved by increasing the ratio of N$_2$O to O$_2$.

Mechanism of Action

Nitrous oxide inhibits NMDA receptors. The inhibition of these glutamate stimulatory receptors likely contributes to its anesthetic action. Other mechanisms are likely involved.

Central Nervous System Effects of Nitrous Oxide

Nitrous oxide causes a dose-dependent depression of the central nervous system (CNS). In dentistry its purpose is to achieve conscious sedation at various levels. This is associated with a **reduced anxiety** while still allowing the dentist and patient to communicate. The drug is an effective **analgesic**.

Advantages to Using Nitrous Oxide

The **rapid onset and recovery** are ideal characteristics for dental procedures, especially in the apprehensive patient. The rapid onset and recovery are due to its low blood/gas partition coefficient. Nitrous oxide does not significantly depress the cardiovascular system. The drug is **pleasant** and is not associated with nausea (Table 10.2).

The drug is stored in cylinders under pressure (750 PSI). Therefore, upon opening the valve of the cylinder, nitrous oxide is released as a gas, thus not requiring a vaporizer prior to inhalation, since the drug vaporizes when released from its cylinder. (The anesthetic equipment includes a cylinder for N$_2$O and one for O$_2$. The gas released from each cylinder is controlled by regulator valves, allowing mixing of the two gases at varying proportions.)

The drug is inert, but an extremely small amount is metabolized. It is nonflammable, although, similar to oxygen, it will support combustion (see Table 10.2).

Disadvantages of Nitrous Oxide and Precautions

The rate of recovery from nitrous oxide is rapid. When delivery of the drug is terminated, the drug exits the blood back into the alveoli of the lungs with the tendency to severely reduce the oxygen level. This phenomenon is called **diffusion hypoxia** (see Table 10.2). To avoid this, 100% oxygen should be inhaled for 3 to 5 minutes after the nitrous oxide is terminated.

Nitrous oxide penetrates into **closed air spaces** in the body. This can lead to expansion of these spaces, with

TABLE 10.1	Stages of Anesthesia
Stage	**Characteristics**
I	Analgesia, patient is conscious. Amnesia may occur. Conscious sedation from such drugs as nitrous oxide is in this stage.
II	Loss of consciousness, delirium, hyperreflexia, hypertension. (Overall an undesirable stage)
III	Surgical anesthesia, progressive loss of reflexes and progressive loss of spontaneous ventilation mechanisms.
IV	Respiratory paralysis and circulatory collapse.

TABLE 10.2 Characteristics of Nitrous Oxide		
Physical Properties	Advantages	Disadvantages
Stored in cylinders at 750 PSI	Analgesic	Without precautions can cause diffusion hypoxia
Released as a gas	Rapid onset and termination	Diffuses into closed air spaces in the body
Odorless, colorless	Pleasant and well tolerated	Potential for chronic abuse
Inert, nonflammable	Not associated with nausea unless hypoxia exists	At high doses can cause bone marrow suppression
1.5 times heavier that air	Does not require a vaporizer	Potential reproductive toxicity
	Only minor effects on respiratory and cardiovascular function	

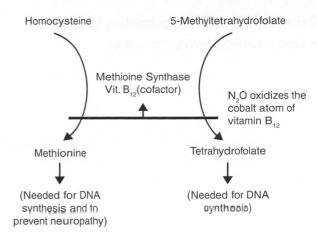

• **Fig. 10.1** Effect of nitrous oxide on DNA synthesis *(red arrow)*. Nitrous oxide inhibits methionine synthase, resulting in reduced production of methionine and tetrahydrofolate. Both are required for DNA synthesis.

• BOX 10.1 Steps to Reduce Nitrous Oxide Exposure

Facility and Equipment Preparation

- Purchase scavenging nitrous oxide delivery systems with air sweeper capabilities
- Check plumbing for leaks by pressure retention of closed system
- Check all fittings for leaks with disclosing solution or nitrous oxide analyzer
- Ensure exhaust system vents to the outside away from air intake
- Maximize room air circulation
- Consider use of a local exhaust system

Daily Use

- Adjust vacuum setting to manufacturer 's maximum recommended value
- Place hood on nose before administering nitrous oxide
- Adjust flow to patient 's minute respiratory volume
- Instruct patient to exhale through nose
- Instruct patient not to talk
- Use rubber dam whenever possible
- Use high-vacuum suction when mouth is open
- Administer 100% oxygen for 3–5 min before removing hood

Monitoring

- Inspect delivery apparatus each day of use, particularly the reservoir bag
- Periodically monitor exposure by passive dosimetry or nitrous oxide analyzer
- Record monitoring results

---

damage, sometimes severe, to tissues. Relevant situations include chronic lung disease and pneumothorax, a bowel obstruction, and eustachian tube obstruction. In circumstances where a gas, such as perfluoropropane, was instilled into the eye, to treat a detached retina, administration of nitrous oxide can lead to nitrous oxide diffusing into the eye and expanding the gas space, resulting in changes in the central retinal artery leading to retinal ischemia and infarction. Nitrous oxide should be avoided for at least 3 months in these patients. Furthermore, nitrous oxide can cause dilation of cerebral blood vessels leading to an increase in intracranial pressure in patients with head injuries.

Nitrous oxide has been used as a recreational drug (whippits) and is subject to **chronic abuse**. This is more likely to be seen in those, such as dentists, who have ready access to nitrous oxide. Abuse can lead to neurologic changes such as paresthesias and shooting pains.

Continuous exposure (several hours) to nitrous oxide can lead to **suppression of DNA synthesis** followed by pernicious anemia and infertility in both men and women. The relevant mechanisms involved are shown in Fig. 10.1. It has been shown that nitrous oxide blocks methionine and tetrahydrofolate synthesis, both of which are needed for DNA synthesis.

The risk to dental personnel from exposure to nitrous oxide has been a concern because of potential reproductive risks such as infertility and miscarriage. As a result of these concerns, steps must be taken to limit exposure to health care workers. Box 10.1 lists steps used to reduce such exposure.

Other Inhalation Anesthetics (Volatile Halogenated Hydrocarbons)

The three agents discussed below have several traits in common. Among them is their high potency, which provides for complete surgical anesthesia in stage III. Furthermore, they are nonflammable and are generally given with an intravenous anesthetic for rapid induction. These drugs depress cardiovascular function and respiration. Unlike earlier drugs, they do not significantly sensitize the heart to the effects of epinephrine and other catecholamines. These drugs may be associated with malignant hyperthermia, especially in the presence of peripheral skeletal muscle relaxants. Therefore they are contraindicated in patients with a history of this disorder. Some properties of these anesthetics and nitrous oxide are given in Table 10.3.

Isoflurane

Isoflurane is a commonly used anesthetic. Very little gets metabolized. It is combined with other drugs because of its slower onset. Isoflurane may have irritating effects on the patient during induction.

Desflurane

Desflurane has a fast onset of action, based on its low blood/gas partition coefficient. It nonetheless irritates the respiratory tract.

Sevoflurane

Sevoflurane is nonirritating. It undergoes some metabolism, although this does not typically cause toxicity.

Table 10.3 compares some characteristics of general anesthetics.

Intravenous Anesthetics

Propofol

Propofol is commonly used for induction of general anesthesia. It has a rapid onset and a rapid recovery. It has no analgesic effect and is not characterized by postoperative nausea. It tends to cause pain during the injection. Propofol is an agonist at $GABA_A$ receptors. Without adequate precautions, apnea may occur after induction.

Ketamine

Ketamine is noted for causing dissociative anesthesia. Analgesia and amnesia are present in addition to a trance-like state and unconsciousness. The drug is an NMDA receptor antagonist. It is sometimes used alone for very short procedures. Ketamine stimulates the cardiovascular system and can provide a benefit for patients with hypotension. The delirium and hallucinations that often occur during emergence can be prevented with the use of a benzodiazepine.

Benzodiazepines

The drugs in this class are used in several settings for induction and sedation. The principal benzodiazepine used in this setting is midazolam, although lorazepam can also be used for sedation. The short half-life and short duration of action of midazolam make it particularly desirable for short procedures.

Dexmedetomidine

Dexmedetomidine is an alpha$_2$-adrenergic receptor agonist. Its actions in the central nervous system results in sedation and analgesia. Its role related to anesthetics

TABLE 10.3	Properties of Inhalation Anesthetics		
Anesthetic	Blood/Gas Partition Coefficient[a]	Physical State (at Standard Temperature and Pressure)	Metabolism (%)
Nitrous oxide	0.47	Gas	0.004
Isoflurane	1.4	Liquid	< 0.2
Desflurane	0.42	Liquid	< 0.02
Sevoflurane	0.65	Liquid	3–5

[a]All coefficients are taken at 37°C.

centers around its analgesic effect and its sedative effects in the intensive care unit and before surgery. At sedative doses, it has little effect on the cardiovascular system and on respiration.

Other Drugs

Opioids such as morphine and fentanyl as well as non-opioids can be useful perioperative analgesics. Recent practice has focused on the use of nonopioids and reducing opioids in perioperative analgesia. Peripherally acting skeletal muscle relaxants (curare-type) provide useful muscle relaxation and also reduce, in some cases, the need for higher doses of anesthetics to provide adequate muscle relaxation, particularly surgeries of the chest and abdomen.

Suggested Readings

Dowd FJ, Mariotti AJ, eds *General Anesthesia: Pharmacology and Therapeutics for Dentistry*. St Louis: Elsevier; 2017:2024.

Hemmings HC, Riegelhaupy PM, Kelz MB, et al. Towards a comprehensive understanding of anesthetic mechanisms of action: a decade of discovery. *Trends Pharmacol Sci.* 2019;40:464 181.

11

Local Anesthetics

KEY POINTS

All local anesthetics in use today share similar chemical structures and can be categorized as being either esters or amides.

Their mechanism of action is by blockade of the propagation of peripheral nerve impulses through binding to their receptor within sodium channels.

Their duration of anesthetic action is determined by redistribution away from the site of action, not metabolism.

Most local anesthetics cause vasodilation, necessitating addition of a vasoconstrictor to provide appropriate duration of action for use in dentistry.

The most common adverse reaction is psychogenic in nature, manifested as syncope.

DEFINITIONS

- Many drugs used in therapy are either weak acids or weak bases. Local anesthetics are weak bases and as such are subject to changes in the ratio of their charged form to their noncharged form (BH^+/B). This ratio is determined by the pH of the solution and the pK_a of the drug.
- Nerve fiber myelination is categorized into heavily myelinated (group A fibers), moderately myelinated (group B fibers), and unmyelinated (group C fibers).
- Methemoglobinemia is a blood disorder when a significant amount of methemoglobin is produced resulting in reduced release of oxygen to tissues.

Background

Local anesthetics are one of the most important drug groups in dentistry. These agents reversibly block nerve conduction when applied to a circumscribed area of the body. Although numerous substances of diverse chemical structure are capable of producing local anesthesia, most drugs of proven clinical usefulness share a fundamental configuration with the first true local anesthetic, cocaine.

The abuse liability of cocaine led to a chemical search for safer, nonaddicting local anesthetics leading to the synthesis of procaine. Since then, numerous improvements in the manufacture of local anesthetic solutions have been made, and many useful agents have been introduced into clinical practice.

Chemistry and Classification

Certain physicochemical characteristics are required of a drug intended for clinical use as a local anesthetic. One prerequisite is that the agent **must depress nerve conduction**. Because an axon whose cytoplasmic contents have been completely removed can still transmit action potentials, a drug must be able to interact directly with the axolemma to exert local anesthetic activity. A second important consideration is that the agent **must have both lipophilic and hydrophilic properties** to be effective by parenteral injection. Lipid solubility is essential for penetration of the various anatomic barriers existing between an administered drug and its site of action, including the nerve sheath. Water solubility ensures that the drug can be dissolved in an aqueous medium, and when injected in an effective concentration, the drug does not precipitate on exposure to interstitial fluid. These requirements have placed important structural limitations on the clinically useful local anesthetics.

The typical **local anesthetic molecule can be divided into three parts**: (1) an aromatic group, (2) an intermediate chain, and (3) a secondary or tertiary amino terminus (Fig. 11.1). All three components are important determinants of a drug's local anesthetic activity. The aromatic residue confers lipophilic properties on the molecule, whereas the amino group furnishes water solubility. The intermediate portion is significant in two respects. First, it provides the necessary spatial separation between the lipophilic and hydrophilic ends of the local anesthetic, which is important for binding to its receptor. Second, the chemical link between the central hydrocarbon chain

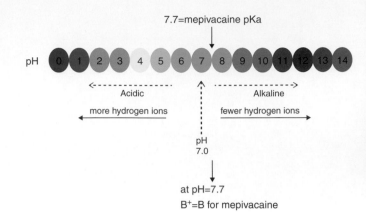

• **Fig. 11.1** Chemical structure of lidocaine.

• **Fig. 11.2** The effect of pH on the ionization of mepivacaine. The scale shows the relative ratios of mepivacaine in the ionized form (BH+) to the nonionized form (B) as a function of pH. The ionized form results from association of mepivacaine with a hydrogen ion as pH is lowered. As pH drops (more acidic) a greater and greater percentage of the anesthetic is in the ionized form. The opposite happens as the pH rises and becomes more basic. "B" in this figure refers specifically to mepivacaine.

and the aromatic moiety serves as a suitable basis for classification of most local anesthetics into two groups: the esters (—COO—) and the amides (—NHCO—). This distinction is useful because there are marked differences in allergenicity and metabolism between these two local anesthetic groups.

Influence of pH

Local anesthetics exist as either nonionized (uncharged) or ionized (charged) forms of the molecule. The ionized form is more water soluble and can pass through the aqueous environment, but it is the nonionized form that is able to diffuse rapidly into the nerve (Fig. 11.2). As a result, both the pH of the tissue and the pK_a of the drug determine the degree of ionization of the drug in the tissue and the onset of action. The pK_a of a weak acid or weak base is the pH at which the drug is half in the ionized form and half in the nonionized form. Therefore, when the tissue pH is lower, there is reduced diffusion of local anesthetic into the nerve membrane because there is a greater percentage of the ionized form of the drug. Moreover, local anesthetics with a higher pK_a tend to be slower in onset of action than similar agents with more favorable dissociation constants (i.e., lower pK_a).

Mechanism of Action

Local anesthetics block the sensation of pain by interfering with the propagation of peripheral nerve impulses. Therefore, the generation and the conduction of action potentials are inhibited. Local anesthetics do not significantly alter the normal resting potential of the nerve membrane but instead impair certain dynamic responses to nerve stimulation. More specifically, local anesthetics block Na^+ channels, thereby blocking nerve conductance. A developing local anesthetic block is characterized by inhibiting the voltage-gated Na^+ channels on the nerve membrane. This leads to a progressive reduction in the rate and degree of depolarization as well as slowing of conduction. Conventional **local anesthetics generally inhibit high-frequency trains of impulses more readily than they do single action potentials.**

Local anesthetics block nerve conduction by (1) impeding the **gating mechanisms** that underlie cycling of the Na^+ channel (Fig. 11.3), (2) physical occlusion of the Na^+ channel, (3) an allosterically mediated change in channel conformation, and/or (4) a distortion of the local electrical field.

Clinically, neurons vary according to fiber size and type in their susceptibility to local anesthetics (Fig. 11.4). In myelinated nerves, action potentials are propagated from one node of Ranvier to the next in a saltatory fashion, with a safety factor sufficient to require **at least three consecutive nodes to be completely blocked before impulse transmission is interrupted.** Because internodal distance is directly related to fiber diameter, small neurons tend to be more sensitive clinically than large fibers to conduction block. As a local anesthetic diffuses into the nerve trunk, it reaches an effective concentration over a length required to inhibit small axons before it spreads sufficiently to block large fibers. Differences in modes of impulse transmission preclude direct comparisons based on fiber size between myelinated and unmyelinated axons. Smaller in diameter, C fibers (unmyelinated) nevertheless have approximately the same apparent critical length as small, myelinated axons. Generally, the more susceptible a fiber is to a local anesthetic agent, the faster it is blocked, and the longer it takes to recover. **Modalities listed in increasing order of resistance to conduction block include the sensations of pain, cold, warmth, touch, and deep pressure.**

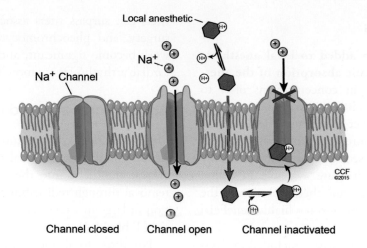

• **Fig. 11.3** The interaction of local anesthetics with the Na$^+$ channel. Figure illustration by Department of Medical Art and Photography—Cleveland Clinic and Mr. Dave Schumick, image (pii:B9780323757898001572/f157-04-9780323757898)

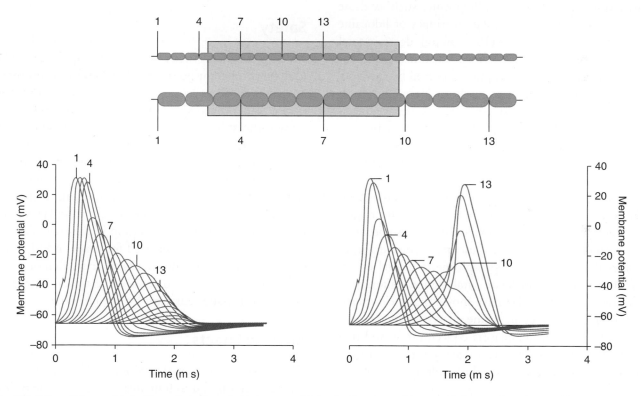

• **Fig. 11.4** Differential nerve block. Two adjacent myelinated axons, differing in diameter and internodal distance by a factor of 2, are exposed to a local anesthetic *(gray zone)*. Impulses arising from successive nodes of the small axon are plotted on the left. Exposure of 14 nodes to a specific concentration of local anesthetic causes conduction to fail. Identical exposure of the larger axon (right) results in seven nodes being affected, an insufficient number to prevent conduction at this local anesthetic concentration.

Pharmacologic Effects

Although primarily used to depress peripheral nerve conduction, **local anesthetics are not selective and may interfere with impulse transmission in any excitable tissue.** Most prominent of the systemic effects of local anesthetics are effects related to the cardiovascular system and the central nervous system (CNS), but virtually any organ with dependence on nervous or muscular activity may be affected. Local anesthetics may also influence various tissues through actions unrelated to specific disturbances in Na$^+$ conductance. In the peripheral vasculature, **local anesthetics reduce vascular tone** related to autonomic function by diminishing neurotransmitter release and smooth muscle responsiveness. Local anesthetics administered submucosally inhibit myogenic activity and autonomic tone clinically and cause vasodilation in the area of injection.

Vasoconstrictor Effects

Vasoconstrictors are often added to local anesthetic solutions to impede systemic absorption of the anesthetic agent. Epinephrine in concentrations of 5 to 20 μg/mL (1:200,000 to 1:50,000) is most commonly used for this purpose, but other sympathomimetic amines, including levonordefrin, norepinephrine, and phenylephrine, are or have been used. In North America, only epinephrine and levonordefrin are available in dental cartridges. Localization of the anesthetic solution in the area of injection by epinephrine is often highly beneficial (Table 11.1).

Normally, sympathomimetic drugs included in anesthetic formulations produce no pharmacologic effects of clinical consequence other than **localized** arteriolar constriction. Low doses of epinephrine, such as those contained in one or two dental cartridges of lidocaine with 1:100,000 epinephrine (18 to 36 μg), decrease total peripheral resistance by 20% to 30%, but a commensurate increase in cardiac output supported by increases in stroke volume, heart rate, or both leaves the mean blood pressure unchanged. Injudicious dosage, accidental intravascular injection, or adverse drug interactions may promote clinically noticeable effects on the CNS and sympathetic nervous system. Heart rate and systolic blood pressure may be elevated by epinephrine, causing uncomfortable palpitation and pain in the chest. Restlessness and apprehension similar to the effects produced by local anesthetics in overdose may also occur.

As a guideline for cardiac patients, current evidence indicates that minimizing epinephrine to a level of less than 40 μg with appropriate vital sign monitoring is appropriate. Several studies have shown that the intraoral injection of 20 μg of epinephrine effectively doubles the preoperative epinephrine plasma concentration and that higher doses produce proportionately greater elevations. At doses approaching 200 μg, the resulting epinephrine titers can surpass titers associated with heavy exercise, surgery, and pheochromocytoma. Increases in cardiac work become significant, and myocardial ischemia and cardiac arrhythmias are more likely to occur.

Absorption, Fate, and Excretion

Pharmacokinetic considerations regarding local anesthetics are vital because the balance between the uptake of a local anesthetic into the systemic circulation and its removal through redistribution, metabolism, and excretion in large measure determines the drug's toxic potential (Table 11.2).

For those local anesthetics used in dentistry (Table 11.3), the onsets of action and the durations of the effect are shown in Table 11.4.

Safety

Modern local anesthetic solutions are quite safe when used by competent personnel. Further, local anesthetics are generally regarded as safe for use throughout pregnancy. When needed, a reversal agent may be used to reverse the soft tissue anesthetic effect. Phentolamine mesylate (OraVerse) is a medication that is indicated for the "reversal" of soft tissue anesthesia. It is marketed to shorten the duration of action of local anesthetics containing a vasoconstrictor. Phentolamine mesylate produces α-adrenergic blockade of vascular smooth muscle, resulting in vasodilatation in the area of administration. OraVerse is approved for usage in individuals 6 years of age and older. Clinical trials demonstrated that OraVerse is able to reduce the time to return to normal soft tissue sensation by 50% to 60%.

Adverse Effects

Given the common use of local anesthetics, adverse events can be categorized into four areas: systemic toxicity, local tissue responses, psychogenic/idiosyncratic reactions, and allergic reactions.

Systemic Toxicity

Most serious systemic toxic effects are related to excessive blood concentrations caused by inadvertent intravascular injection or the administration of large quantities of drug. Such reactions can usually be prevented by observing three precautions: **(1) administer the smallest dose that provides effective anesthesia; (2) use proper injection techniques, including aspiration; and (3) use a vasoconstrictor-containing solution when not contraindicated by patient history or operative need.**

TABLE 11.1	Benefits of Vasoconstrictors Added to Local Anesthetics
Prolonged duration of action
Improved success rate of nerve block
Enhanced intensity of nerve block
Reduction in toxicity of the anesthetic
Less anesthetic required for nerve block
Anesthetic metabolism is more likely to keep pace with drug absorption
Less bleeding

TABLE 11.2	Pharmacokinetic Properties and Their Effects on Local Anesthetics	
Pharmacokinetic Property	**Effect**	
Absorption	Absorption depends on dosage and pharmacologic profile of the drug used, the presence of a vasoconstrictor agent, and the nature of the administration site. Topically applied local anesthetics are readily absorbed from most mucosal surfaces.	
Distribution	It is important to note that the duration of action of local anesthetics is dependent on its absorption into the bloodstream and distribution away from the site of injection. Distribution to peripheral tissues is a major means for the removal of amide and slowly metabolized ester local anesthetics from the bloodstream and for keeping their plasma concentrations below the toxic range.	
Metabolism	The metabolic fate of a particular agent largely depends on the chemical linkage between the aromatic residue and the rest of the molecule.	
	Esters: Ester drugs are inactivated by hydrolysis. Derivatives of *p*-aminobenzoic acid (PABA), such as procaine and tetracaine, are preferentially metabolized in the plasma by pseudocholinesterase; the ratio between plasma and tissue hydrolysis with other esters is variable.	
	Amides: Metabolism of amide drugs primarily occurs in the liver. Hepatic blood flow is often the rate-limiting factor governing metabolism of many amides.	
Excretion	Esters: Products of hydrolytic cleavage undergo further biotransformation in the liver before being eliminated in the urine. The half-life for the hydrolysis of procaine is normally less than 1 min and less than 2% of the drug is excreted unchanged by the kidneys.	
	Amides: As with the ester compounds, small amounts (1%–20%) of administered amides appear in the urine as unmetabolized compounds.	

TABLE 11.3	A Summary of the Local Anesthetics and Related Drugs Available for Dentistry	
Nonproprietary (Generic) Name	**Proprietary (Trade) Names**	
Agents for Parenteral Administration		
Articaine	Articadent, Orabloc, Posicaine, Septocaine, Zorcaine	
Bupivacaine	Marcaine, Sensorcaine, Surgicaine, Vivacaine	
Lidocaine	Xylocaine, Lignospan, Lignospan Forte, Octocaine	
Mepivacaine	Carbocaine, Isocaine, Polocaine, Scandonest	
Prilocaine	Citanest, Citanest Forte	
Procaine	Novocain (brand discontinued in United States)	
Ropivacaine	Naropin	
Tetracaine	Pontocaine	
Agents Limited to Surface Application		
Benzocaine	Americaine, Gingicaine, Hurricaine, Topicale, in Cetacaine	
Butamben	Butesin Picrate, in Cetacaine	
Dibucaine	Nupercainal	
Lidocaine/ prilocaine	EMLA, Oraqix	
Other Related Drugs		
Sodium bicarbonate injection	OnPharma, Anutra	
Phentolamine mesylate	OraVerse	

The first five are the ones prepared in dental cartridges and most commonly used. *EMLA,* Eutectic mixture of local anesthetics.

Regarding excessive doses, in general, there is a correlation between potency and toxicity. The rate of injection can be a factor, since the faster the rate, the more likely the toxicity. Toxicity manifests primarily in the CNS, with the cardiovascular system the next most susceptible.

This has led to recommended maximum doses, as seen in Table 11.5. It is apparent that overdose should be a rare event in healthy adult patients. Toxicity has been a more common issue in pediatrics, simply because of the greater likelihood of an inadvertent overdose.

In Table 11.6 the maximum doses recommended for adults are used to calculate the values for the local anesthetics for children weighing 14, 18, and 23 kg. These

TABLE 11.4 Physicochemical Correlates of Local Anesthetic Activity

Drug	Octanol/Buffer Distribution Coefficient[a]	Anesthetic Potency (Tonic Block)	Duration of Anesthesia (half-life in minutes)	pK_a[a]	Rate of Onset (in minutes)
Procaine	3	Low	30–60	8.9	5–10
Articaine	17	Moderate	30–146	7.8	2–3
Mepivacaine	42	Moderate	114	7.7	1.5–2.0
Prilocaine	55	Moderate	93–96	7.8	2–4
Lidocaine	110	Moderate	80–96	7.8	2–3
Bupivacaine	560	High	162–210	8.1	6–10

[a]Measurements made at 36°C except for prilocaine, which is extrapolated from the value taken at 25°C. (Data from Strichartz GR, Sanchez V, Arthur GR, et al. Fundamental properties of local anesthetics, II: measured octanol/buffer partition coefficients and pK$_a$ values of clinically used drugs. Anesth Analg. 1990;71:158–170.) Data also from; Martin, E., Nimmo, A., Lee, A. et al. Articaine in dentistry: an overview of the evidence and meta-analysis of the latest randomised controlled trials on articaine safety and efficacy compared to lidocaine for routine dental treatment. BDJ Open 7, 27 (2021).

TABLE 11.5 Comparisons of Local Anessthetics Used in Dentistry

Preparation Contents	Proprietary (Trade) Name	MAXIMUM DOSE[a] (mg/kg)	(mg) (adult)	DURATION OF ANESTHESIA (SOFT TISSUE) Maxillary Infiltration (min)	Inferior Alveolar Block (min)
2% lidocaine hydrochloride; 1:100,000 epinephrine	Xylocaine with epinephrine, 1:100,000	7	500	170	190
2% lidocaine hydrochloride; 1:50,000 epinephrine	Xylocaine with epinephrine, 1:50,000	3.5[b]	250[b]	170	190
2% lidocaine	Xylocaine	4.5	300	40[c]	100[c]
2% mepivacaine hydrochloride; 1:20,000 levonordefrin	Carbocaine 2% with Neo-Cobefrin	5.7	400	150	190
3% mepivacaine hydrochloride	Carbocaine	5.7	400	90	165
4% prilocaine hydrochloride; 1:200,000 epinephrine	Citanest Forte	8	600	140	205
4% prilocaine hydrochloride	Citanest	8	600	105	175
0.5% bupivacaine hydrochloride; 1:200,000 epinephrine	Marcaine with epinephrine	1.3	90	340	440
4% articaine hydrochloride; 1:100,000 epinephrine	Septocaine with epinephrine, 1:100,000	7		200	230
4% articaine hydrochloride, 1:200,000 epinephrine	Septocaine with epinephrine, 1:200,000	7		180	200

[a]The maximum dose is the smaller of the two values (e.g., 7 mg/kg lidocaine up to a maximum dose of 500 mg).
[b]Lower doses than those approved by the U.S. Food and Drug Administration are recommended on the basis of the high epinephrine content.
[c]Lidocaine without epinephrine produces unreliable pulpal anesthesia, especially of the maxilla.

TABLE 11.6	Maximum Number of Dental Anesthetic Cartridges for Children		
Child's Age	3-Year-Old	5-Year-Old	7-Year-Old
Weight at 50th percentile for that age	14 kg	18 kg	23 kg
Maximum Number of Cartridges[a]			
Articaine (4%) with epinephrine (1:100,000)	1.4	1.8	2.2
Lidocaine (2%) with epinephrine (1:100,000)	2.7	3.5	4.5
Mepivacaine (3%) plain	1.5	2.0	2.4
Mepivacaine (2%) with levonordefrin (1:20,000)	2.2	2.9	3.6
Prilocaine (4%) with epinephrine (1:200,000)	1.6	2	2.6

[a]Using the 50th percentile weight for age. Calculations should be based on the child's body weight and not his or her age.

weights correspond to the 50th percentile weight for a 3-, 5-, and 7-year-old child, respectively. Bupivacaine is not listed, as it is not a preferred agent in the young child.

Methemoglobinemia is a subcategory of toxicity found with certain agents. It is most common with prilocaine or benzocaine overdose, although it can occur with any local anesthetic in susceptible individuals. For instance, prilocaine, by being metabolized to o-toluidine, can increase the risk of methemoglobinemia especially in susceptible individuals (Fig. 11.5). For individuals susceptible to methemoglobinemia, bupivacaine should be considered for administration when a local anesthetic is needed, since it is least likely to induce a response. When methemoglobinemia occurs, it should be considered a medical emergency, and treatment includes intravenous administration of methylene blue (Fig. 11.5).

Local Tissue Responses

Commercially available local anesthetics are relatively non-irritating to tissues. Local anesthetic concentrations necessary to damage peripheral nerves usually far exceed the concentrations required for transmission blockade. Accidental intraneural injection may lead to nerve damage, however, from the combination of undiluted local anesthetic, strong hydrostatic pressure, and direct physical injury.

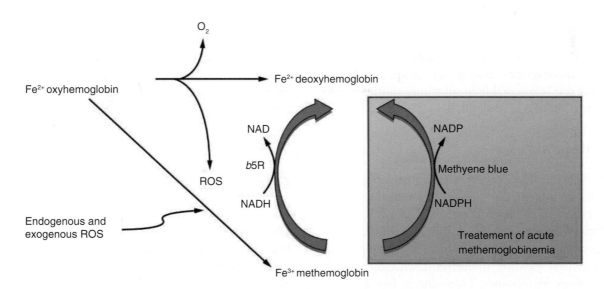

• **Fig. 11.5** Methemoglobinemia and the effect of a prilocaine metabolite. Formation of methemoglobin and its physiologic *(open space)* and therapeutic reductions *(shaded space)* are shown. Iron is in the ferrous state (Fe^{2+}) in oxygenated and deoxyhemoglobin (deoxyHb). When oxygen is released to the tissues, a small proportion of oxygen-bound hemoglobin iron is then converted by ROS to the ferric state (Fe^{3+}); i.e., methemoglobin. Methemoglobin can result from an exogenous source such as o-toluidine, a metabolite of prilocaine. NADH, is a cofactor for methemoglobin reduction mediated by cytochrome b5 reductase (b5R), keeping methemoglobin at low levels (approximately 1%). **O-toluidine** is one of the chemicals that can inhibit cytochrome b5 reductase (b5R), (methemoglobin reductase). When this physiologic reduction of NADH-dependent methemoglobin reduction is either insufficient because of excessive ROS or decreased b5R activity, methemoglobinemia can occur. Exogenously administered methylene blue utilizing NADPH can nonenzymatically convert methemoglobin to Fe^{2+} hemoglobin *(shaded space)*. *b5R*, Cytochrome b5 reductase; *NAD*, nicotinamide adenine dinucleotide phosphate; *NADH*, the reduced form of NAD; *NADP*, oxidized form of nicotinamide adenine dinucleotide phosphate; *NADPH*, reduced form of NADP; *ROS*, reactive oxygen species. (From: Gregg XT, Prchal JT, in Hematology: Basic Principles and Practice, ed 7, pp 616–625, 2018. [image identfier] pii:B9780323357623000445/f044-003-9780323357623.)

Adverse tissue responses to injected local anesthetic preparations are usually caused or augmented by vasoconstrictor additives. Epinephrine can create tissue hypoxia by reducing local blood flow while increasing oxygen consumption.

Psychogenic Reactions

A psychogenic reaction is the most common adverse event from the injection of local anesthetic in dental practice. It must be made clear that these reactions are not due to the local anesthetic drug but to the insertion of the needle. The most common manifestation of this is syncope, very often vasovagal in nature. Another common manifestation of a psychogenic reaction to the injection of local anesthetic is hyperventilation.

Allergic Phenomena

Local anesthetics rarely cause allergic reactions; however, when one does occur, an ester derivative of *p*-aminobenzoic acid (PABA) is usually involved. PABA is a breakdown product of the ester local anesthetics, and it is the most likely antigen when an allergy occurs after its administration. Since procaine and similar ester local anesthetics produce PABA, an allergy to one ester local anesthetic rules out the use of all esters. Although articaine has an ester in its structure, it does not produce PABA.

A confirmed allergy in a patient to an amide anesthetic is rare. In the event that this does occur, there is no evidence of cross-reactivity among the amide anesthetics, meaning that it is acceptable to substitute another amide when a local anesthetic is required.

Drug Interactions

Because of their influences on excitable membranes, local anesthetics are potentially capable of interacting with a wide spectrum of therapeutic agents. The CNS depressant effects of local anesthetics summate with the effects of the general anesthetics, barbiturates, opioid analgesics and others, yielding interactions with therapeutic and toxicologic significance. Lidocaine in blood stream combined with another antiarrhythmic drug may generate disturbances in cardiac automaticity and conduction, in excess of what either compound would have caused if given alone.

A unique interaction may occur between certain esters and the sulfonamides. As mentioned earlier, procaine and several other local anesthetics (benzocaine, tetracaine) are metabolized to yield *PABA*. The antibacterial

action of sulfonamides is competitively antagonized by this metabolite. This interaction is not relevant for amide dental anesthetics; however, it is a likely interaction with the use of high levels of PABA in certain "health food supplements."

Although the potential for interactions involving local anesthetics is great, clinical manifestations appear infrequently outside the hospital and more often when very large doses are used or when unusual patient factors are present. Much more likely to occur are interactions between various drugs and the vasoconstrictors used during local anesthesia. Epinephrine may generate ventricular arrhythmias during general anesthesia given by some inhaled agents. Similarly, catecholamines can induce undesirable changes in cardiac action and blood pressure in patients taking tricyclic antidepressants and related norepinephrine transporter inhibitors, cocaine, nonselective β-adrenergic blockers, digoxin, inhibitors of catechol-O-methyltransferase, or adrenergic neuron–blocking drugs (e.g., guanethidine). Compounds with prominent α-adrenoceptor-blocking activity, such as the phenothiazine and butyrophenone antipsychotics, may lead to hypotension if coadministered in large doses with epinephrine.

Despite statements to the contrary in local anesthetic product information approved by the US Food and Drug Administration (FDA), local anesthetics containing epinephrine may be used without special reservation in patients taking monoamine oxidase (MAO) inhibitors. Exogenous catecholamines are mostly degraded by the enzyme catechol-O-methyltransferase; inhibition of MAO has little impact on their respective metabolic fates or cardiovascular actions. Moreover, the effect of injected catecholamines is not appreciably affected by MAO inhibitors because these injected catecholamines do not release endogenous prejunctional catecholamines.

General Therapeutic Uses

Local anesthetics are widely used for pain relief. By obviating the necessity of general anesthesia, these drugs have been instrumental in reducing the mortality and morbidity associated with various operative procedures. They also render valuable service by obtunding the pain of sunburn, toothache, and other ailments.

The onset, quality, extent, and duration of local anesthesia vary markedly with the technique of administration used. As might be expected, no single agent is optimal for all purposes. There are a variety of anesthesia techniques that include surface application, infiltration, field block, nerve block, spinal anesthesia, epidural block, and intravascular injection (Fig. 11.6).

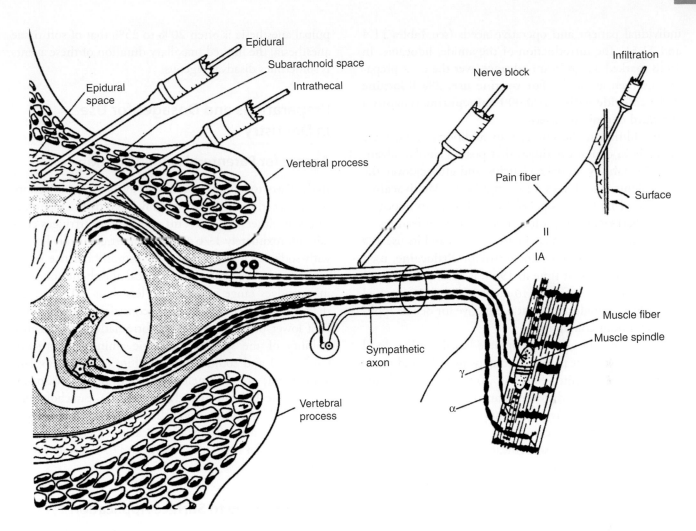

• **Fig. 11.6** Anatomic location of four different types of injection of local anesthetics.

Uses in Dentistry

By eliminating nociceptive sensations associated with dental care, local anesthetics improve patient acceptance of dental treatment and thereby contribute significantly to oral health. Because local anesthetics are so frequently used, the toxicity and efficacy of these agents are of particular interest and concern.

Safety in Dentistry

General Considerations

Because most, but not all, of the complications observed with local anesthetic (i.e., pallor, unrest, sweating, fatigue, palpitation, nausea, and fainting) are common manifestations of acute anxiety, it is evident that many adverse effects ascribed to local anesthesia are actually generated by the process of injection and not by the drugs themselves.

Safety in Pediatric Patients

The use of local anesthetics without vasoconstrictors in pediatric dentistry warrants special comment. Consideration of systemic toxicity should limit the pediatric dental use of local anesthetics without vasoconstrictors. **Because the safety margin of local anesthetics is quite low in small children, it is advisable to use a preparation containing a vasoconstrictor, if not doing so would result in more total drug being administered.** After termination of the dental procedure, injection of phentolamine (OraVerse) will reduce the duration of soft tissue anesthesia and thereby likely reduce the incidence of accidental soft tissue injury, such as that caused by the patient.

Drug Selection

Selection of a local anesthetic for dental application must include considerations of efficiency, safety, and individual patient and operative needs (see Tables 11.4 and 11.5). The introduction of the amide, lidocaine, in 1948 marked a significant advance over the ester preparations then available. **For routine use, 2% lidocaine hydrochloride with 1:100,000 epinephrine remains a standard dental anesthetic**.

In addition to lidocaine, four additional amides are available in dental cartridges that possess similar advantages in stability, nonallergenicity, and efficacy over the ester agents (see Tables 11.4 and 11.5). **Mepivacaine**, introduced in 1957, is generally equivalent to lidocaine in its pharmacologic profile. Two distinctive features of mepivacaine are its topical ineffectiveness and its use as a 3% solution without a vasoconstrictor. **Prilocaine**, used clinically for the first time in 1960, is a less potent alternative to lidocaine. Similar to mepivacaine, it is not used topically as a single agent but is effective for dental application without epinephrine.

Articaine, the only thiophene-based amide local anesthetic, was first tested in humans in 1970 and made available in the United States in 2000. An issue of current interest is whether the marketed formulations of 4% articaine are equivalent or superior to other amide preparations. Properly controlled clinical trials have not generally shown increased efficacy with standard mandibular block injections. Several studies have indicated clinical superiority of articaine over lidocaine (both with epinephrine) when injected supraperiosteally for mandibular anesthesia.

Bupivacaine was used initially in 1963 but not marketed in a dental cartridge until 1983. It exhibits a slightly slower onset time than the other amides but is similarly efficacious after nerve block and has a much longer duration of action, making it well suited for providing postoperative pain relief. Given its slow onset and yet prolonged duration of action, consideration can be given to administering this at the end of the dental procedure before the duration of action of the initial local anesthetic has worn off and to provide more prolonged postoperative pain control. The bupivacaine preparation intended for dental use is a 0.5% solution with 1:200,000 epinephrine.

A significant dissimilarity among the amide preparations concerns the presence or absence of a vasoconstrictor additive. Local anesthetic formulations without epinephrine-like drugs are particularly useful when sympathomimetic amines are contraindicated. Plain solutions are additionally promoted on the basis of a shorter duration of action. Although soft tissue anesthesia is comparatively brief after maxillary injection with 3% mepivacaine or 4% prilocaine (both without vasoconstrictor), differences in duration after mandibular nerve block are trivial (see Table 11.5). Because the period of

pulpal anesthesia is often 20% to 25% that of soft tissue anesthesia, the limited maxillary duration of these agents is sometimes disadvantageous.

Preparations and Dosages for Use in Dentistry

Agents for Parenteral Administration

In dentistry today, only amides are available for injection. As stated earlier, although variably listed by the manufacturers as either 1.8 or 1.7 mL, all dental cartridges contain approximately 1.76 mL. Pyrogen-free distilled water with sodium chloride added for osmotic balance serves as the local anesthetic vehicle. Local anesthetic solutions in cartridges range in pH from less than 3.0 to greater than 6.0; preparations with vasoconstrictors are adjusted to a lower pH than are plain formulations to enhance stability of the sympathomimetic amine constituents. Citric acid and sodium metabisulfite (or an equivalent antioxidant) are also included to help prevent vasoconstrictor breakdown. (Oxidation of the catecholamine compounds produces acids that tend to lower the pH over time.) Currently available local anesthetics marketed for dentistry in the United States and Canada are shown in Table 11.3.

Agents Limited to Surface Application

Topical anesthetics are used in the oral cavity for various purposes. Formulations marketed as pressurized sprays produce widespread surface anesthesia appropriate for making impressions or intraoral radiographs. Such preparations are potentially hazardous, however, and only products with metered valve dispensers to help prevent inadvertent overdose should be used. Topical liquids, which avoid the possibility of aerosol inspiration, may also be used for anesthetic coverage of large surface areas. Nonaqueous topical preparations are suitable for most other procedures. Common local anesthetic vehicles include lanolin, petrolatum, sodium carboxymethylcellulose, and polyethylene glycol.

Benzocaine

Benzocaine is a derivative of procaine in which the amino terminus is lacking. Poorly soluble in aqueous fluid, benzocaine tends to remain at the site of application and is not readily absorbed into the systemic circulation. Because of its low toxic potential, benzocaine is especially useful for anesthesia of large surface areas within the oral cavity. Benzocaine is not totally innocuous, however; cases of methemoglobinemia have been reported after the administration of very large doses, especially in unmetered spray form. Benzocaine is available in a variety of preparations; a 20% concentration in the form of an aerosol spray, gel, ointment, paste is available. A mucosal gel patch, containing 18% benzocaine, is also available.

Tetracaine Hydrochloride

Tetracaine is an ester derivative of PABA in which a butyl chain replaces one of the hydrogens on the *p*-amino group. The drug has approximately 10 times the toxicity and potency of procaine. It is no longer available for injection in dentistry; for surface application, it is most commonly marketed as a 2% hydrochloride salt in combination with 14% benzocaine and 2% butamben, a PABA derivative, in an aerosol spray, solution, gel, and ointment under the proprietary name Cetacaine. Tetracaine is one of the most effective topical anesthetics, but the drug's toxic potential after surface application should dictate caution in its use.

Lidocaine/Prilocaine

This is marketed under the acronym of Eutectic Mixture of Local Anesthetics (EMLA). In this case, a eutectic mixture of 2.5% lidocaine and 2.5% prilocaine is available in the form of a cream for topical anesthesia of the skin. When placed under an occlusive dressing for 1 hour, EMLA obtunds the pain of venipuncture and is useful in young children and other patients intolerant of needle insertion. Although this formulation is not intended for topical anesthesia of the oral cavity (it has a poor taste and unfavorable physical characteristics for intraoral use), several investigations have proved its superiority over other topical anesthetics in relieving pain associated with manipulation of oral tissues. EMLA has significantly relieved the discomfort of palatal injections after a 5-minute application and allowed deeper probing of the gingival sulcus without discomfort compared to 5% topical lidocaine.

An intraoral preparation with the same active ingredients of EMLA has been marketed with the trade name of Oraqix. A low-viscosity fluid at room temperature, the anesthetic mixture becomes an elastic gel after being applied to the gingival sulcus to provide local anesthesia for periodontal scaling and root planing. The packaging of Oraqix is intended to avoid the possibility of administering the drug by parenteral injection. The overall effect is approximately a 50% reduction of treatment pain.

Suggested Readings

Daublander M, Liebaug F, Niedeggen G, et al. Effectiveness and safety of phentolamine mesylate in routine dental care. *J Amer Dent Assoc*. 2017;148(3):149–156.

Gamal El-Din TM, Lenaeus MJ, Zheng N, et al. Fenestrations control resting-state block of a voltage-gated sodium channel. *Proc Natl Acad Sci USA*. 2018;115:13111–13116.

Saraghi M, Moore PA, Hersh EV. Local anesthetic calculations: avoiding trouble with pediatric patients. *Gen Dent*. 2015;63:48–52.

Strichartz GR, Sanchez V, Arthur GR, et al. Fundamental properties of local anesthetics, II: measured octanol/buffer partition coefficients and pKa values of clinically used drugs. *Anesth Analg*. 1990;71:158–170.

12

Principles of Antimicrobial Therapy

Antibacterial Drugs

Mechanisms and Sites of Action

The targets of antibacterial drugs' actions are on various sites of the bacteria cell (Fig. 12.1).

Inhibition of Cell Wall Synthesis

The bacterial cell wall is not found in mammalian cells. This fact provides selectivity to the drug. Many important antibacterial drugs inhibit bacterial cell wall synthesis.

Inhibition of Ribosomal Protein Synthesis

Although mammalian cells contain ribosomes, they differ from those of bacteria, resulting in selective inhibition of bacterial protein synthesis by many antibacterial drugs.

Inhibition of Folate Metabolism

Selectivity of the antibacterial effect is a result of the fact that, for certain antibacterial drugs, the corresponding enzymes in bacteria are orders of magnitude more sensitive than those in mammalian cells.

Inhibition of Cell Membrane Function

Select bacteria offer targets in their cell membranes that are unique to those organisms and can be inhibited by some antibacterial drugs.

Inhibition of Nucleic Acid Function and Metabolism

Enzyme targets associated with nucleic acids are sufficiently different from those in mammalian cells so as to be selective targets of some antibacterial drugs.

Mechanisms of Resistance (Each Can Lead to a Lack of Effect of the Drug) (Fig. 12.1)

- Alteration of the drug target site reduces or removes the effectiveness of the drug.

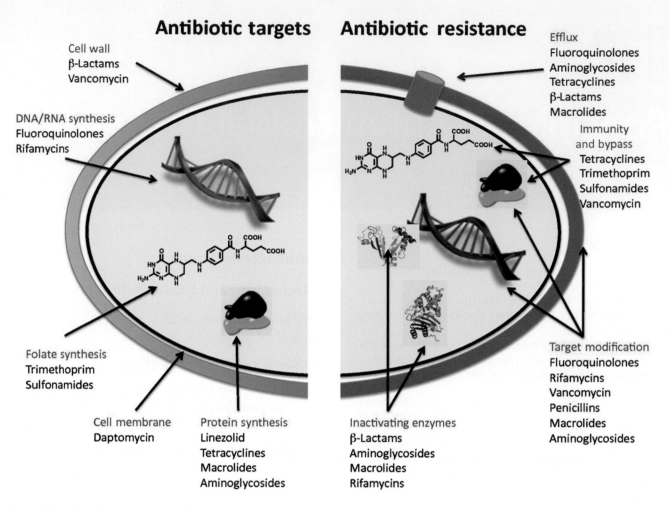

• **Fig. 12.1** Examples of various antibacterial drugs and their sites of action as well as mechanisms of antibiotic resistance by bacteria. (Taken from Sen S, and Sarkar K: Molecular Techniques for the Study of Microbial Diversity with Special Emphasis on Drug Resistant Microbes" in Microbial Diversity in the Genomic Era, Das S, and Dash HR editors, 2019, Elsevier, India.)

- Development of an efflux pump removes the drug from the microbe.
- Development of reduced permeability of the organism to the drug reduces access of the drug.
- Enzymatic breakdown. This occurs when the organism produces an enzyme that can metabolize the drug.
- Growth requirement changes. The organism may develop alternative growth pathways, bypassing the inhibition of growth by the drug.
- Overproduction of target sites. The organism produces an excess of ineffective target sites for the drug, reducing or eliminating the effect of the drug.

How to Avoid or Reduce the Likelihood of Developing Microbial Resistance

- Use an appropriate drug for the infection.
- Use the appropriate dose as well as the appropriate duration of therapy.
- Use drug combinations, **when indicated**. Certain drug combinations will reduce the risk of developing resistance. Further, drug combinations may enhance

the antimicrobial effect compared to a single drug effect.

Adverse Effects

- Allergies: Similar to other drug classes, antimicrobial agents can cause a damaging immune response by the body. Penicillin allergies are a prime example.
- Superinfections: Organisms that are insensitive to an antimicrobial drug are allowed to multiply when sensitive organisms are greatly reduced by the drug.
- Direct organ toxicity: Harmful and unpleasant effects on organs can occur due to actions of certain drugs. Nephrotoxicity and ototoxicity are two relevant examples with specific antimicrobial drugs.
- Photosensitivity is the added sensitivity to sunlight caused by certain drugs or their metabolites.
- Long QT syndrome: Specific antimicrobial drugs may cause an abnormal cardiac rhythm.
- Drug-drug interactions: Certain antimicrobial drugs enhance or inhibit the effect of other antimicrobial drugs as well as other drug classes.

Antifungal Drugs

Types of Infections

- Fungal disease can occur from a number of fungi.
- Systemic disease is the most serious form, although a number of topical infections may occur.
- Fungal infections are more likely to occur in patients with a compromised immune system.
- Certain geographical areas are more likely to harbor a specific fungal pathogen.

Mechanisms of Action Drugs (Either Fungicidal or Fungistatic)

These mechanisms of action on the fungal cell are:
1. Disruption of ergosterol function in the membrane.
2. Inhibition of ergosterol synthesis for the membrane.
3. Inhibition of glucan synthesis for the membrane.
4. Inhibition of deoxyribonucleic acid (DNA) and ribonucleic acid (RNA) synthesis.
5. Inhibition of microtubule function.

Mechanisms or Resistance by Fungi

1. Decrease in or alteration of the membrane target site.
2. Change in the enzyme target site.
3. Increased metabolism of the drug.

Antiviral Drugs

Viral Characteristics

- Viruses are composed of DNA or RNA enclosed in a capsid.
- Some viruses are also enclosed in an envelope
- Viruses enter host cells where they cause disease.

- Drugs can be classified according to the viruses they are used to treat. Examples of viral targets are listed below.
  Herpes and varicella viruses
  Cytomegalovirus
  Human immunodeficiency virus (HIV)
  Hepatitis viruses
  Influenza viruses

Major Mechanisms of Action of Antiviral Drugs Include

- Inhibition of viral attachment to the host cell.
- Inhibition of viral penetration into the host cell.
- Prevention of uncoating of the virus.
- Blockade of viral nucleic acid synthesis.
- Inhibition of integration of viral DNA into host DNA.
- Inhibition of viral protein synthesis.
- Inhibition of the release of the virus from the host cell.

Resistance to Antiviral Drugs

Acquired resistance to the above mechanisms do occur. Using HIV as an example, mutations in the virus can reduce the effect of antiviral drugs. An important strategy to deal with this is to use combinations of drugs that attack different targets in the virus.

Suggested Reading

Bennet JE, Dolin R, Blaser MJ. *Mandell, Douglas and Bennett's Principles and Practice of Infectious Disease.* 9th ed. New York: Saunders; Elsevier; 2019.

13

Antimicrobial Drugs

KEY POINTS

- Antibacterial drugs are based on classification according to structural class and mechanism of action. The mechanism of antibiotic drugs include:
  - Inhibition of cell wall synthesis
  - Alteration of cell membrane function
  - Inhibition of ribosomal protein synthesis
  - Inhibition of DNA or RNA synthesis and function
  - Inhibition of folic acid synthesis
- Antifungal drugs are classified according to their site of action in the fungal cell.
- Antiviral drugs are classified according to viral diseases and by mechanism.

DEFINITIONS

- An antibiotic is a chemical substance, often produced by another microorganism, that can kill bacteria or arrest the multiplication of bacteria.
- An antifungal drug is a chemical that kills or inhibits the multiplication of fungal organisms.
- An antiviral drug is a chemical that kills or inhibits the multiplication of viral organisms.
- β-lactam refers to a key part of the chemical structure of penicillins and related drugs.
- β-lactamases are enzymes that disrupt the β-lactam ring of penicillins and related compounds and destroys their antimicrobial activity.
- First-line therapy refers to drugs used most commonly. Second-line therapy refers to drug alternatives in case of resistant bacterial strains.
- MRSA is an acronym for methicillin-resistant *Staphylococcus aureus*.
- Nosocomial infection refers to a hospital-acquired infection.
- The spectrum of bacterial action can either be narrow spectrum (effective against a limited number of bacteria), extended spectrum (a penicillin that is effective against a larger number of bacteria), or broad spectrum (an antibiotic that inhibits a wider range of organisms such as both gram-positive and gram-negative bacteria). The distinction between extended spectrum and broad spectrum is sometimes blurred.

Antibacterial Drugs

Antibacterial drugs are primarily classified according to their chemical class and mechanism of action. They also can be distinguished based on spectrum and adverse effects.

Penicillins

Penicillins belong to the β-lactam family of antibiotics, which remain the most widely used antibiotics in the world. **β-lactams** are composed of five different groups of antibiotics, with the β-lactam nucleus as the common feature. Examples of β-lactam antibiotics include **penicillins, cephalosporins, carbapenems, and monobactams**. Penicillins and cephalosporins are most commonly used, with carbapenems (imipenem, meropenem, ertapenem), and monobactams (aztreonam), reserved for infections such as nosocomial infections. β-Lactams vary greatly from one another in their spectrum of antimicrobial activity, ranging from an extremely narrow spectrum to a very wide spectrum.

Fig. 13.1 shows the chemistry of penicillins. Notice the β-lactam (four-member ring) structure and the substitutions that render different drugs.

Penicillin is a generic term for a group of β-lactam antibiotics that have similar adverse drug reactions, and similar mechanism of action, but differ in their antibacterial spectrum, pharmacokinetics, and resistance to β-lactamase enzymes.

On the basis of the substitutions (R- Groups) shown in Fig. 13.1, penicillins can be divided into four groups: **(1) penicillin G and penicillin V, (2) anti-staphylococcal penicillins (e.g., dicloxacillin) that are resistant to β-lactamase produced by staphylococci, (3) aminopenicillins with an extended-spectrum (e.g. amoxicillin), and (4) extended-spectrum penicillins with added activity against gram-negative organisms, such as *Pseudomonas aeruginosa*** (Table 13.1).

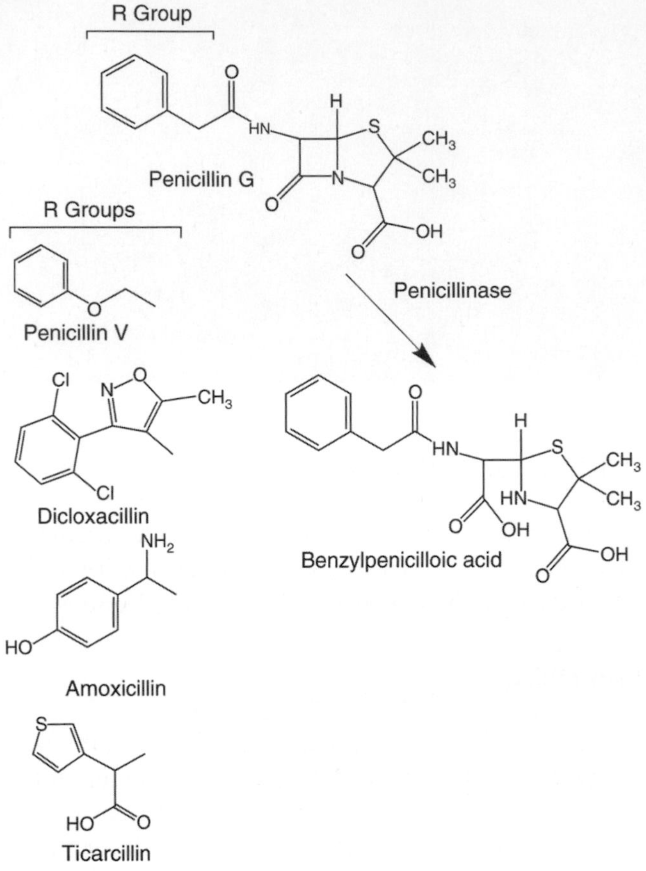

• **Fig. 13.1** Structure of penicillin G and structures of penicillin V, dicloxacillin, amoxicillin, and ticarcillin, as shown by replacement of the R group of penicilloic G. Also shown is the effect of penicillinase in producing the penicilloic acid metabolite, which is inactive as an antimicrobial drug.

Acid-stable penicillins are resistant to breakdown in stomach acid, indicating their usefulness as oral drugs. Penicillin V and amoxicillin are examples. Penicillin G is not acid stable and is not often used orally. Penicillinase-resistant penicillins are resistant to some β-lactamases, particularly those produced by staphylococci. Staphylococci develop resistance to penicillins chiefly through the elaboration of β-lactamase, enzymes (e.g., penicillinases) that inactivate the penicillins by cleavage of their structure to yield penicilloic acid derivatives.

Extended-spectrum penicillins are represented by two groups of penicillin derivatives. One group is the aminopenicillin group (ampicillin and amoxicillin), and the second group is represented by ticarcillin and piperacillin that exhibit activity against *Pseudomonas* and indole-positive *Proteus* species.

Mechanism of Action

Penicillins are structural analogs of an amino acid, D-alanine, which occupies a key site in the final step in the formation of the bacterial rigid cell wall. This **transpeptidation** reaction involves the enzymatic removal of a terminal D-alanine in cell wall proteins to allow for the formation of the cross-linked **peptidoglycan cell wall** (Fig. 13.2). **β-Lactams are competitive inhibitors** of various enzymes, (transpeptidases, carboxypeptidases), collectively termed penicillin-binding proteins (PBPs). β-Lactams promote the formation of cell wall–deficient microorganisms of different shapes (oval, oblong, spherical) depending on the particular PBP affected. As a result,

TABLE 13.1	Penicillin Groups			
Group	**Examples**	**Acid Stable**	**Spectrum**	**Penicillinase Resistant**
Penicillin G and congener	Penicillin G	No	Narrow	No
	Penicillin V	Yes	Narrow	No
Anti-staphylococcal	Methicillin[a]	No	Narrow	Yes[b]
	Nafcillin	Somewhat[c]	Narrow[d]	Yes[b]
	Oxacillin	Yes	Narrow[d]	Yes[b]
	Cloxacillin	Yes	Narrow[d]	Yes[b]
	Dicloxacillin	Yes	Narrow[d]	Yes[b]
Amino-penicillins, extended-spectrum	Ampicillin	Yes	Extended	No
	Amoxicillin	Yes	Extended	No
Extended-spectrum[e]	Ticarcillin[a]	No	Extended[e]	No
	Piperacillin	No	Extended[e]	No

[a]No longer used clinically.
[b]Resistant to penicillinase from *Staphylococcus aureus*.
[c]Although nafcillin is somewhat acid stable, it is used parenterally.
[d]Limited to use against staphylococcal organisms.
[e]Spectrum includes other gram-negative bacteria (e.g., *Pseudomonas aeruginosa* and indole-positive *Proteus*).

the organisms cannot maintain their internal osmotic pressure and will eventually burst.

In Fig. 13.3, a simplified view of the action of penicillins and other β-lactams is depicted. The absence of crosslinking results in a "leaky" cell wall which is lethal to sensitive bacteria.

Penicillins and other β-lactam antibiotics are bactericidal drugs. In other words, they kill the organisms that are inhibited by these drugs. Nonetheless, the effect of these drugs requires that the organisms are actively

reproducing because penicillins, and other β-lactam antibiotics, only inhibit new cell wall production.

Antibacterial Spectrum

The spectrum of penicillin G and penicillin V is narrow. These drugs are effective against several gram-positive cocci, gram-negative cocci, some gram-positive rods, and some gram-negative oral bacteria (Table 13.2). Despite the narrow spectrum, penicillin V is effective against many oral bacteria. Penicillin V is a useful drug for oral

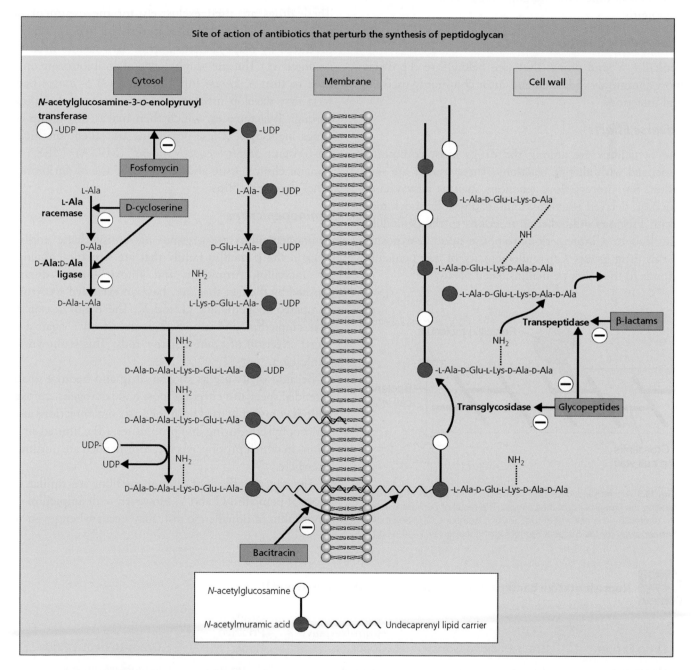

• **Fig. 13.2** The sites of action of several antibiotic drugs are shown. On the right side of the figure, the action of penicillins and other β-lactams is shown, namely, the inhibition of transpeptidase. The action of the β-lactams results in the the failure of the bacterium to form the crosslinking which is necessary for a stable cell wall. *UDP*, uridine diphosphate.

infections because of its spectrum and administration by the oral route.

Pharmacokinetics

Orally useful drugs (those that are acid stable) are shown in Table 13.1. Most penicillins are removed from the body by renal excretion. For example, penicillins G and V are rapidly eliminated with terminal half-lives of 20 to 30 minutes. The short half-life is due to the active renal tubular secretion of these penicillins.

Penicillins do not effectively pass through the blood-brain barrier unless the meninges are inflamed, such as in meningitis.

Therapeutic Uses

Penicillin V and amoxicillin (see below) are the drugs most commonly indicated and most commonly used for oral infections.

Adverse Effects

The penicillins are among the drugs most commonly associated with allergic reactions. These usually are skin rashes, but more serious reactions such as airway constriction, delayed reactions, and anaphylactic shock may occur. Previous mild allergic reactions to the penicillins may lead to a more serious response upon re-exposure to this drug group. Cross allergenicity of one penicillin extends to the other penicillins listed below.

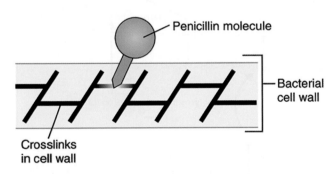

• **Fig. 13.3** A simplified depiction of effect of the action of penicillin inhibiting the crosslinking of the cell wall. The result of penicillin's action is to destabilize the cell wall. (From Snyder, Katherine C., Keegan, C., *Pharmacology for the Surgical Technologist*. Elsevier; 2017. 4th ed.)

Very large doses of a penicillin can cause seizures, especially in patients with compromised renal function.

Drug-Drug Interactions

Bacteriostatic drugs block the growth of bacteria and therefore may inhibit the therapeutic effect of the penicillins, which require proliferation of the bacteria to be effective.

Other Groups of Penicillins

Anti-Staphylococcal Penicillins

These drugs are used exclusively for the treatment of Staphylococcal infections that are resistant to β-lactamases produced by *Staphylococcus aureus*. Two factors need to be noted: (1) The anti-staphylococcal antibiotics are only used to treat *S. aureus* infections and (2) *S. aureus* bacteria may develop mechanisms of resistance other than through β-lactamases, which then makes this group of drugs ineffective. These organisms are called "methicillin-resistant *Staphylococcus aureus*" (MRSA). MRSA is a major clinical issue and requires the use of antibiotics other than penicillins.

Aminopenicillins

Aminopenicillins are a group of semisynthetic antibiotics in the penicillin family that are structural analogs of ampicillin. Ampicillin and amoxicillin are distinguished by the fact that they have an extended spectrum compared to penicillin G and V. The major reason is that ampicillin and amoxicillin are effective against a larger selection of gram-negative rods. This is shown in Table 13.3.

Because of its use as an oral drug and because of its extended spectrum covering most oral pathogens, amoxicillin is commonly used both for acute oral infections and for prophylaxis during oral procedures. (The limited situations in which prophylaxis is recommended are outlined elsewhere.)

The adverse effects of aminopenicillins are similar to those of penicillin G and V. However, with ampicillin or amoxicillin, a nonallergic rash may occur when given to

TABLE 13.2	Representative Bacteria That Are Sensitive to Penicillin G and V			
Drug Group	Gram-Positive Cocci	Gram-Negative Cocci	Gram-Positive Rods	Gram-Negative Rods
Penicillin G, penicillin V (narrow spectrum)	Viridans group streptococci, *Streptococcus pyogenes*, Peptostreptococci	*Neisseria meningitidis*	*Clostridium perfringens*	*Leptotrichia buccalis*, oral bacteroides, fusobacterium species

TABLE 13.3	Representative Bacteria That Are Sensitive to Ampicillin or Amoxicillin[a,b]				
Drug Group	Gram-Positive Cocci	Gram-Negative Cocci	Gram-Positive Rods	Gram-Negative Rods
Ampicillin, amoxicillin	Viridans group streptococci, *Streptococcus pneumoniae*, *Enterococcus faecalis*	*Moraxella catarrhalis*	*Bacillus anthracis*	Oral *Bacteroides*, *Haemophilus influenzae*, *Salmonella typhi*

[a]Therapy may also require a β-lactamase inhibitor.
[b]Either ampicillin or amoxicillin is preferred for treating many of the above infections.

TABLE 13.4	Some Organisms Sensitive to Piperacillin	
Drugs	Sensitive Gram-Negative Organisms
Piperacillin/ tazobactam	*Pseudomonas aeruginosa, Proteus mirabilis, Klebsiella pneumoniae, Escherichia coli*

a patient with cytomegalovirus infection/mononucleosis or a patient taking allopurinol.

Extended-spectrum penicillins with added activity against gram-negative organism (e.g., Pseudomonas

The drug listed in this class has utility against several gram-negative organisms including *Pseudomonas aeruginosa*. Piperacillin is administered with a β-lactamase inhibitor as indicated in Table 13.4. It is administered parenterally.

β-Lactamase inhibitors are often used with extended spectrum penicillins to protect these penicillins from inactivation by β-lactamase-producing bacteria. The β-lactamase inhibitors are clavulanate, sulbactam, tazobactam (see Table 13.4), and avibactam.

Cephalosporins

The cephalosporins are another class of β-lactams derived from the mold *Acremonium*.

Mechanism of Action

Besides being structurally related to the penicillins, cephalosporins have a mechanism of antimicrobial action that is very similar to that of penicillins. Cephalosporins vary in their sensitivity to β-lactamases but are generally more resistant to these enzymes than are the penicillins.

Spectrum

The antibacterial spectrum of cephalosporins is broad, but the classification of cephalosporins is by generations based on antimicrobial activity. Cephalosporins' main use in dentistry is as an alternative to penicillin for prophylactic treatment. However, cephalosporins are useful for a wide variety of serious infections and this depends on susceptibility based on the different generations of cephalosporins. Table 13.5 lists representative drugs and some important properties.

Pharmacokinetics

Only some cephalosporins are well absorbed orally (see Table 13.5). These include cephalexin, cefadroxil, and cefaclor. Renal excretion plays a major role in elimination of the cephalosporins. The half-lives are longer than those of penicillin V and penicillin G but vary among the drugs.

Adverse Effects

The cephalosporins may produce allergies and show some cross-allergenicity with the penicillins. Patients with a history of anaphylactic shock to penicillins should not receive cephalosporins. Superinfections can occur due in part to their broad spectrum.

Drug-Drug Interactions

Cephalosporins are bactericidal and, like penicillins, the bactericidal effect can be compromised by administration of bacteriostatic antibiotics.

Other β-Lactam Antibiotics

Carbapenems have a similar structure to the other β-lactam antibiotics. The drugs are useful for treating resistant organisms over a wide spectrum and are resistant to many β-lactamases. Table 13.6 summarizes some key information about these drugs.

Mechanism of Action

These drugs inhibit cell wall synthesis similar to other β-lactam antibiotics.

TABLE 13.5	Representative Cephalosporins and Their Characteristics	
	Spectrum[a]	
Drugs (Route of Administration)	Gram Positive	Gram Negative
First generation Cephalexin (O) Cefazolin (IV) Cefadroxil (O)	Streptococci, *Staphylococcus aureus*	*Klebsiella pneumoniae, Escherichia coli*
Second generation[b] Cefuroxime (O/IV) Cefoxitin (IV)[c] Cefaclor (O)	Streptococci, *S. aureus*	*E. coli, K. pneumoniae, Haemophilus influenzae*
Third generation Ceftriaxone (IV) Cefotaxime (IV)	Streptococci	*E. coli, K. pneumoniae, H. influenzae, Serratia marcescens, Neisseria gonorrorheae*
Antipseudomonal drugs Ceftazidime (IV) Cefepine (IV)	(Cefepine has activity vs. some gram-positive organisms)	*Pseudomonas aeruginosa,* other gram-negative organisms similar to third generation
Anti-MRSA drug Ceftaroline (IV)	MRSA, streptococci	Similar to 3rd generation

[a]Partial list.
[b]Less active against gram-positive organisms compared to first generation.
[c]Cefoxitin is more active against anaerobes (e.g., *Bacteroides fragilis*) than others listed in 2nd generation.
IV, Intravenous; *MRSA*, methicillin-resistant Staphylococcus aureus; *O*, oral.

Spectrum

Some sensitive organisms are shown in Table 13.6. Carbapenems are broad-spectrum antibiotics. Aztronam's spectrum is limited to aerobic gram-negative species.

Pharmacokinetics

The carbapenems and aztreonam are administered parenterally. Renal excretion occurs. Imipenem requires cilastatin to protect it from renal dehydropeptidase (dipeptidase).

Adverse Effects

Nausea and vomiting may occur. The carbapenems, in a few cases, may show cross-allergenicity with penicillins. Aztreonam lacks cross-allergenicity with most other β-lactams.

Drug-Drug Interactions

Carbapenems may reduce the level of valproic acid.

Macrolides

Mechanism of Action

Macrolides are bacteriostatic agents that inhibit the translocation step in protein synthesis. Macrolides prevent elongation of the polypeptide chain via reversible binding to the P site of the 50 S ribosomal subunit (Fig. 13.4).

Spectrum

Table 13.7 summarizes their spectrum, which is considered to be narrow.

Some macrolides are used in dentistry as alternatives to penicillin V or amoxicillin for acute oral infections and for prophylaxis. **They are effective in treating infections from many oral pathogens**.

TABLE 13.6	The Antibiotic Spectrum of Carbapenems and Aztreonam	
	Spectrum	
Drug Class and Drugs	Gram Positive	Gram Negative
Carbapenems Imipenem Meropenem Doripenem Ertapenem	Streptococci, Methicillin- sensitive staphylococci	*Haemophilus influenzae, Klebsiella, Serratia, Escherichia coli, Pseudomonas aeruginosa, Bacteriodes* species
Monobactam Aztreonam	None	*H. influenzae, Klebsiella, Serratia, E. coli, Pseudomonas aeruginosa*

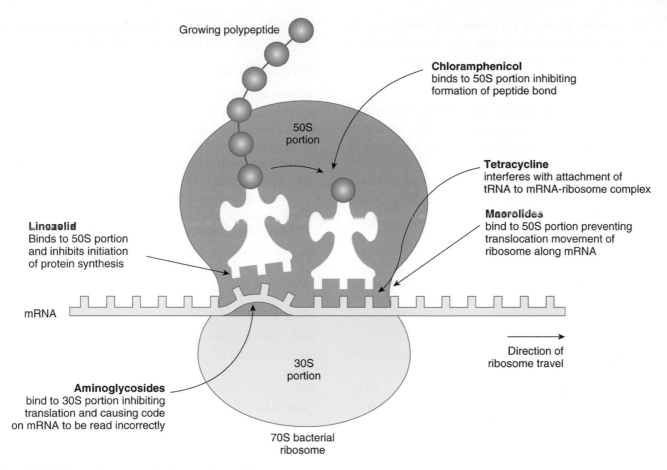

• **Fig. 13.4** Inhibition of protein synthesis by antimicrobial drugs.

TABLE 13.7	The Antibiotic Spectrum of the Macrolides			
	Spectrum			**Half-Life (Hours)**
Drug	**Gram Positive**	**Gram Negative**	**Other**	
Erythromycin	Streptococci, Pneumococci,	*Legionella pneumophila*, *Corynebacterium diphtheriae*	*Mycoplasma pneumoniae, Clamydia trachomatis*	1–2
Clarithromycin	Similar but not identical spectrum to erythromycin			3–7
Azithromycin	Similar but not identical spectrum to erythromycin			40–68
Fidaxomicin	Used to treat *Clostridioides difficile* infections			

Pharmacokinetics

The macrolides can be given orally. Erythromycin and azithromycin can also be given intravenously (IV).

Fidaxomicin is used orally for its local effect on the gastrointestinal (GI) tract, which is the location of the *Clostridioides difficile* infection. Very little of the drug gets into the systemic circulation.

The half-lives of the macrolides are listed in Table 13.7.

Adverse Effects

Gastric pain may occur with the macrolides. Erythromycin is used less often than clarithromycin or azithromycin. One reason is that **erythromycin is most likely to cause nausea and vomiting** because of its action in stimulating the motilin receptor in the GI tract. Erythromycin is not a part of the prophylactic protocol during oral procedures and is not often used for treating active oral infections.

The **estolate form of erythromycin** should not be used because **cholestatic jaundice** may result. Macrolides are contraindicated in previous allergic hepatitis.

Drug-Drug Interactions

Erythromycin and clarithromycin inhibit liver microsomal enzymes and can increase the effect of several other drugs because of this effect. Azithromycin has little effect on these enzymes.

Macrolides are contraindicated in patients taking medications that are a risk of lengthening the QT interval of the heart.

Tetracyclines

Tetracyclines are derived from *Streptomyces* bacteria or are semisynthetically produced.

Mechanism of Action

Tetracyclines inhibit protein synthesis by binding to the 30 S ribosomal subunit, inhibiting the binding of aminoacyl-tRNA to the mRNA translation complex (see Fig. 13.4). Tetracyclines also inhibit metalloproteinases, accounting for benefits in the periodontium.

Spectrum

Tetracyclines are considered broad-spectrum antibiotics but may have limited use because many bacteria are resistant. However, this drug class has found a use in the **treatment of periodontal diseases** in high-dose (500 mg) and low-dose (50 mg) formulations (Table 13.8).

Pharmacokinetics

Tetracycline and especially doxycycline are well absorbed after oral use. The half-life of tetracycline is approximately 15 hours, whereas that of doxycycline is about 20 hours, and tigecyline's half-life is over 27 hours. Tigecycline is only administered parenterally. Tetracycline is eliminated mainly by renal excretion. Doxycycline and tigecycline are eliminated both by the liver and kidney.

Adverse Effects

Adverse effects of the tetracyclines include GI upset, liver toxicity during pregnancy, permanent tooth staining if given during tooth development during pregnancy or in children less than 8 years of age.

Superinfections may be an issue given the broad spectrum of these drugs. Phototoxicity is a risk.

Outdated tetracyclines can cause a Fanconi-like syndrome resulting in kidney damage.

Polyvalent cations (e.g., calcium in cheese, milk, etc.) can decrease the absorption of tetracyclines from the GI tract and therefore should not be administered concurrently.

Drug-Drug Interactions

Barbiturates, carbamazepine, and hydantoins can increase the metabolism of tetracyclines and decrease their effect. Tetracyclines can increase the effect of warfarin because tetracyclines tend to reduce intestinal flora that produce vitamin K.

Metronidazole

Mechanism of Action

Metronidazole is of the nitroimidazole class and functions by inhibiting nucleic acid synthesis by forming free radicals to disrupt bacterial deoxyribonucleic acid (DNA). This unique mechanism of action is shown in Fig. 13.5.

Spectrum

Metronidazole's antibacterial effect is only useful against **obligate anaerobes**, making it useful in treating anaerobic bacterial infections. It is also useful in treating some protozoal infections.

TABLE 13.8   Summary of Three Tetracyclines and Some Important Clinical Uses Based on Organisms

	Spectrum		
Drug	Gram Positive	Gram Negative	Other
Tetracycline		*Helicobacter pylori*, *Legionella pneumophila*	*Chlamydia* species, Richettsiae, *Nocardia asteroides*,
Doxycycline	Similar to above, more effective in some cases. Effective against *Hemophilus influenzae*, *Moraxella catarrhalis*, and others, and more commonly used than tetracycline.		
Tigecycline	Effective against methicillin-resistant *Staphylococcus aureus* and some enterococci.		

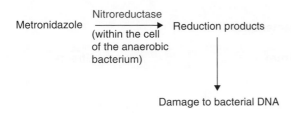

• **Fig. 13.5** Mechanism of action of metronidazole.

TABLE 13.9	Some Characteristics of Clindamycin	
	Examples of Spectrum	Adverse Effects
Clindamycin	Bacteroides species, some staphylococci, streptococci, fusobacterium species	Mostly GI effects, **Clindamycin-induced colitis**

Dental applications for metronidazole are anaerobic infections including **treatment of periodontitis**.

Organisms that are sensitive include Fusobacterium species, Bacterioides species, and Clostridioides species. The drug is bactericidal.

Pharmacokinetics

Metronidazole is well absorbed by the oral route. It has a half-life of about 8 hours.

Adverse Effects

The adverse effects include a disulfiram-like effect if taken with ethanol, a metallic taste, discoloration of the urine, and peripheral neuropathy.

Drug-Drug Interactions

The drug should not be given with alcohol because of the disulfiram-like effect.

Clindamycin

Mechanism of Action

Clindamycin is a bacteriostatic drug that blocks protein synthesis by inhibiting ribosomal translocation in a manner similar to that of the macrolides (see Fig. 13.4).

Spectrum

The spectrum of clindamycin is narrow but includes some anaerobes.

The drug has the ability to penetrate into bone and may be useful for infections in bone. Clindamycin is sometimes used in dentistry for oral infections.

Examples of sensitive organisms and adverse effects are listed in Table 13.9.

Pharmacokinetics

Clindamycin is well absorbed by the oral route. The drug is highly metabolized with metabolites eliminated in urine and the bile. The elimination half-time is about 3 hours.

Adverse Effects

Clindamycin may induce **colitis**, which is associated with an overgrowth of *Clostridioides* (formerly *Clostridium*) *difficile* in the colon. Patients who have had a recent *C. difficile* infection should not receive clindamycin.

Clindamycin can also cause GI symptoms (which may include diarrhea) that are not associated with *C. difficile*.

Drug-Drug Interactions

Clindamycin tends to increase the effect of peripherally acting skeletal muscle relaxers. This combination may pose a risk.

Clindamycin and erythromycin antagonize each other; clindamycin should not be given concurrently with a macrolide antibiotic.

Other antibacterial drugs that are not commonly used or are rarely used in dentistry.

See Table 13.10 for classes, action mechanism, spectrums, and adverse effects of such drugs.

Prophylactic Use of Antibiotics in Dentistry

A course of antibiotics to prevent systemic diseases prior to dental treatment has evolved significantly in the past years. Originally, the administration of an antibiotic prior to dental treatment was thought necessary to prevent problems in patients with prosthetic joint replacements or heart murmurs due to the bacteremia caused by a dental procedure. The deleterious risk of a dentally induced bacteremia continues to be re-evaluated. The previous recommendations for prophylactic antibiotic use have changed except in a relatively limited number of patients. It must be noted that the unnecessary use of antibiotics increases the risk of antibiotic resistance, allergic reactions, and other side effects. In essence, the risk for adverse reactions to antibiotic use often outweighs the benefits for prophylactic antibiotic administration.

Prosthetic Joint Replacement

The prophylactic use of antibiotics in patients with replaced joints is generally no longer recommended to prevent prosthetic joint infection. The new guidelines

TABLE 13.10   Summary of Some Antibacterial Drugs and Their Characteristics

Drug (Class)	Mechanism of Action	Spectrum	Adverse Effects
Vancomycin (Glycopeptide)	Bactericidal, inhibition of cell wall synthesis by binding to the D alanine-D alanine peptide and inhibiting the trans glycosylase reaction (see Fig. 13.2)	Gram-positive (e.g., methicillin-resistant *Staphylococcus aureus* [MRSA], Staphylococcus endocarditis, Streptococci, some enterococci)	Flushing with histamine release, kidney toxicity, ototoxicity
Gentamicin, Streptomycin, Amikacin (Neomycin topical only, has broader spectrum) (Aminoglycosides)	Bactericidal, inhibition of protein synthesis by binding to the 30 S ribosome and blocking initiation of protein synthesis, and causing misreading of mRNA (see Fig. 13.4)	Only aerobic bacteria, gram-negative bacteria, *Pseudomonas, Klebsiella, Escherichia coli, Proteus mirabilis* (often combined with another antibiotic)	Ototoxicity, kidney toxicity, skeletal neuromuscular blockade
Ciprofloxacin, levofloxacin, moxifloxacin (Fluoroquinolones)	Bactericidal, disrupt deoxyribonucleic acid (DNA) by inhibiting DNA gyrase and topoisomerase	Both gram-negative and gram-positive This varies depending on the drug, *Neisseria meningitides, Bacillus anthracis, E. coli, Haemophilus, Klebsiella, Pseudomonas aeruginosa,* some Staphylococci and Streptococci	Gastrointestinal (GI) effects, neuropathy, dermatitis, joint swelling, may prolong cardiac QT interval, Colitis, phototoxicity
Sulfisoxazole, Trimethoprim-sulfamethoxazole, Silver sulfadiazine, mafenide (last two for topical burn therapy) (Sulfonamides)	Usually bacteriostatic, They inhibit folic acid synthesis (Trimethoprim is not a sulfonamide but inhibits folic acid synthesis at a site distinct from the sulfonamides.)	*E. coli, Nocardia* Trimethoprim-sulfamethoxazole is more widely used: Staph. and Strept., *E. coli, Proteus, Klebsiella, Serratia, Nocardia*	Skin eruptions and allergies, GI reactions, blood dyscrasias
Chloramphenicol (rarely used)	Bacteriostatic, it inhibits protein synthesis by binding to the 50 S ribosomal subunit and inhibits transpeptidation. (see Fig. 13.4)	Broad spectrum, *Salmonella* species, *S. pneumoniae, Haemophilus influenzae, N. meningitides,* Rickettsiae	Anemia including **Aplastic anemia**, Gray baby syndrome, It must be used with **extreme caution**. There is no use in dentistry, and rarely used in medicine.
Telavancin, Dalbavancin, (Lipoglycopeptides)	Bactericidal, inhibit cell wall synthesis similar to vancomycin	MRSA, Streptococci,	Hepatoxicity, nephrotoxicity
Linezolid (Oxazolidinone)	Bacteriostatic/bactericidal, Inhibits protein synthesis by binding to P site of the 50 S subunit. It prevents initiation of protein synthesis (see Fig. 13.4)	MRSA, Streptococci	Myelosuppression, tongue discoloration, GI effects
Daptomycin (Lipopeptide)	Bactericidal, damages membranes leading to depolarization	Gram positive both aerobic and anaerobic	Myopathy, pneumonitis
Quinupristin-dalfopristan (Streptogramins)	Bactericidal, inhibit protein synthesis similar to macrolides	*Enterococcus faecium,* Strept. and Staph.	Arthralgias, myalgias,

Continued

TABLE 13.10 Summary of Some Antibacterial Drugs and Their Characteristics—cont'd

Drug (Class)	Mechanism of Action	Spectrum	Adverse Effects
Fosfomycin	Bactericidal, inhibits initial transferase step in cell wall synthesis (see Fig. 13.2)	Broad spectrum, (urinary antiseptic)	Headache, GI effects, vaginitis
Bacitracin (Topical only) (Peptide)	Inhibits cell wall synthesis by preventing transfer of peptidoglycan subunits (see Fig. 13.2).	Narrow spectrum, gram-positive, Strept., Staph.	
Polymyxin B (Topical use) (Peptide)	Makes the cell membrane permeable by disrupting phospholipids in the membrane.	Narrow spectrum, Gram-negative, P. aeruginosa	

take into account the possible need for prophylactic antibiotics in limited patient populations. For example, it may be necessary to prescribe antibiotics prior to dental treatment for patients with a previous history of prosthetic joint infection, patients with immunocompromising diseases or conditions, as well as the patients with uncontrolled diabetes mellitus. Consultation with the patient's orthopedic surgeon is recommended.

Endocarditis

The prophylactic use of antibiotics in patients to prevent bacterial infection of the cardiac endocardium is no longer recommended except for a few patients. For infective endocarditis prophylaxis, only a small subset of patients will require premedication. The recommendation for prophylactic antibiotics prior to dental procedures to prevent infective endocarditis should be for patients with underlying cardiac conditions associated with the highest risk for adverse outcomes to the endocardium. Consultation with the patient's cardiologist is recommended.

Patients with artificial heart valves

Patients with artificial heart valves are at greater risk of developing infective endocarditis from a dental procedure. The need to use antibiotic prophyllaxis before a dental procedure should be discussed with the patient's cardiologist before a dental procedure, especially one in which bleeding is likely.

Antituberculosis Drugs

For active infection, these drugs are given in combination to avoid resistance in the *Mycobacterium tuberculosis*

organism. The mechanisms of action are different from the drugs above because, for the most part, the targets in *M. tuberculosis* are different (Table 13.11).

Successful therapy against this disease requires a minimum of several weeks.

Antifungal Drugs

Fungal pathogens present unique targets for drugs. Oral infections with *Candida albicans* are common and therefore this organism is a target for many antifungal drugs. Topical application to treat Candida albicans is the usual route of administration, but sometimes systemic administration is appropriate. Fig. 13.6 depicts the target sites unique to the fungal organisms and the sites of action of several classes of antifungal drugs. Table 13.12 lists drug examples for the antifungal drug classes as well as indications for use and some adverse reactions. A summary of the mechanisms of action, spectrum, pharmacokinetics, therapeutic uses, adverse reactions, and drug interactions for five classes of antifungal drugs are described below.

Polyenes

Polyenes are natural products of *Streptomyces nodosus*. A single agent, amphotericin B, is available for systemic fungal infections. This drug is often used for life-threatening fungal infections. **Nystatin is commonly used topically for the treatment of Nystatin is commonly used topically for the treatment of** *Candida albicans*.

Mechanism of Action

Polyenes bind to ergosterol in the cell membrane, causing hydrophobic interactions, thereby allowing the efflux of potassium resulting in cell death.

TABLE 13.11	Antituberculosis Drugs	
Only First Line Therapy Is Listed		
Drug	**Mechanism of Action**	**Adverse Effects**
Isoniazid	Inhibition of cell wall synthesis by inhibition of mycolic acid synthesis	Hepatitis, peripheral neuropathy,
Rifampin	Inhibition of DNA-dependent RNA polymerase	Thrombocytopenia, nephritis, cholestatic jaundice, flu-like syndrome when given less that twice a week. (It is an important inducer of liver microsomal enzymes.)
Ethambutol	Inhibition of cell wall synthesis by inhibition of arabinosyl transferases	Optic neuritis with vision changes and red–green color blindness, GI effects, hyperuricemia
Pyrazinamide	Inhibits cell membrane function, stimulates protease activity	Hepatotoxicity, photosensitivity, hyperuricemia, GI adverse effects

DNA, Deoxyribonucleic acid; *GI*, gastrointestinal; *RNA*, ribonucleic acid.

Antifungal Spectrum

Amphotericin B is one of the most potent antifungals with activity against a variety of yeasts and filamentous fungal pathogens.

Pharmacokinetics

Amphotericin B is poorly absorbed enterally and must be administered parentally. It is widely distributed and exhibits a long half-life (15 days).

Therapeutic Uses

Amphotericin B is used to treat many invasive fungal infections including candidiasis, aspergillosis, cryptococcosis, blastomycosis, histoplasmosis, mucomycosis, and sporotrichosis. Nystatin is used mainly to treat *Candida* species and is only used topically.

Adverse Effects

Amphotericin B has significant toxicities, especially adverse effects on the kidney.

Drug-Drug Interactions

Amphotericin B has limited drug interactions. Most concern must be focused on drugs that also reduce renal function.

Pyrimidine

Flucytosine is a pyrimidine analogue used in a limited number of fungal infections.

Mechanism of Action

Flucytosine is converted in the fungal cell to 5-fluoro-uracil by the enzyme cytosine deaminase. Resulting

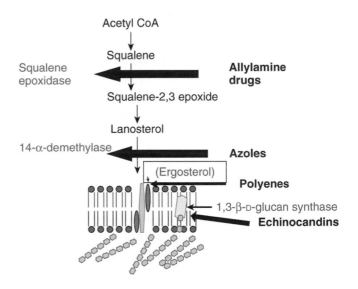

• **Fig. 13.6** Mechanism of action of four classes of antifungal drugs. Allylamines, such as terbinafine, block the synthesis of squalene-2,3 epoxide by inhibiting squalene epoxidase. Azoles, such as itraconazole, block the synthesis of ergosterol by inhibiting 14-α-demethylase. Polyenes, such as amphotericin B, bind to ergosterol and form pores in the membrane. Echinocandins, such as caspofungin, block the synthesis of β (1-3) glucan for insertion into the cell wall by inhibiting 1,3-β-D-glucan synthase. Note that synthesis begins in the membrane to form 1,3-β-D-glucan polymers (bottom), which are crucial components of the cell wall. Other elements of the cell membrane and cell wall are not pictured.

metabolism in the fungal cell leads to inhibition of thymidylate synthetase and impaired DNA synthesis.

Antifungal Spectrum

The use of flucytosine is limited to common pathogenic yeasts, such as many *Candida* species.

TABLE 13.12   Major Antifungal Drugs by Class

Class	Drug Examples	Indications	Adverse Effects
Polyene	Amphotericin B	Most systemic fungi	Chills and fever with infusion, renal toxicity which limits maximum dose
	Nystatin (topical only)	*Candida* species	Bitter taste
Pyrimidine	Flucytosine	Cryptococcal meningitis	Bone marrow toxicity
Azoles	**Clotrimazole** topical	Oral candidiasis, Oral troche available	Altered taste, oral burning, dry mouth
	Miconazole topical	Oral candidiasis, Oral (buccal) tablet available	Altered taste, oral burning, dry mouth
	Itraconazole	*Candida* species, *Cryptococcus* and many other systemic fungal infections	Liver dysfunction, hypokalemia
	Fluconazole	Cryptococcal meningitis, *Candida* species	Liver dysfunction, hypokalemia, cardiac QT elongation
	Voriconazole	*Candida* species, *Aspergillus*	Rash, headache, visual effects, liver dysfunction
	Posaconazole	*Candida* species, *Aspergillus, mucormycosis*	GI effects, Liver dysfunction, cardiac QT elongation
	Isavuconazole	*Candida* species, *Aspergillus, mucormycosis*	GI effects, hypokalemia, liver dysfunction
Echinocandins	Caspofungin	*Candida* species, *Aspergillus*	Liver dysfunction, hypokalemia
	Micafungin	*Candida* species, *Aspergillus*	Histamine release
	Anidulafungin	*Candida* species, *Aspergillus*	GI effects
Allylamine	Terbinafine	Dermatophytes in skin	GI effects, rash

Amphotericin is associated with the most serious adverse effects.
GI, Gastrointestinal.

Pharmacokinetics

Flucytosine is easily absorbed by the gastrointestinal tract and due to the short half-life must be given four times daily. The drug is not normally metabolized in humans and is excreted unchanged by the kidneys.

Therapeutic Uses

Flucytosine, along with amphotericin B, is the first-line therapy for treatment of cryptococcal meningitis. Due to the concentration of this drug in the kidney, flucytosine can be used to treat fungal infections that primarily affect renal tissue.

Adverse Effects

Flucytosine is primarily associated with bone marrow suppression and liver toxicity and GI side effects. If these toxic effects occur, they may result from the release of 5-fluorouracil form fungi and intestinal microbes.

Drug-Drug Interactions

Drugs that reduce kidney function may increase the level of flucytosine.

Azoles

The azole drug class is composed of imidazoles (clotrimazole, ketoconazole, miconazole) and triazoles (fluconazole, itraconazole, voriconazole, posaconazole, isavuconazole). Certain drugs in this class are used to treat dental fungal infections.

Mechanism of Action

Azoles inhibit 14-α-demethylase, causing impaired ergosterol synthesis leading to cell membrane disruption.

Antifungal Spectrum

Azoles are active against many *Candida* spp. Newer triazoles have an extended spectrum of activity which includes *Aspergillus* and *Cryptococcus*.

Pharmacokinetics

Azoles are primarily available for topical or oral use, and fluconazole, voriconazole, posaconazole, and isavuconazole can also be administered intravenously. Many triazoles are metabolized by hepatic CYP 450 enzymes. Depending on the azole drug, the half-life varies between 1.5 and 30 hours.

Therapeutic Uses

Azole antifungal agents can be used to treat internal fungal infections. Skin infections include onychomycosis, ringworm, and tinea pedis (athlete's foot). Azoles are also effective against oral and vaginal candidiasis.

Adverse Effects

The imidazole, ketoconazole, exhibits significant toxicity due in part to ability to alter sex hormone levels. Ketoconazole is rarely used. The newer triazoles have improved safety parameters but can cause hypokalemia and liver dysfunction. Azoles used by topical oral application can cause altered taste and can cause dry and burning mouth.

Drug-Drug Interactions

Ketoconazole can increase the toxicity of several other drugs because it is an inhibitor of liver metabolism of those drugs. Other azoles have less or very little effect on drug metabolism.

Echinocandins

The echinocandins are unique semisynthetic molecules that consist of a lipid connected to a peptide (i.e., lipopeptide). Antifungals in this drug class include micafungin, anidulafungin, and caspofungin.

Mechanism of Action

Echinocandins reduce production of glucan by inhibiting synthesis of (1,3) β-glucan, causing damage to the fungal cell wall (Fig. 13.6).

Antifungal Spectrum

Echinocandins exhibit potent activity against many *Candida* species and *Aspergillus*.

Pharmacokinetics

Echinocandins are poorly absorbed through the gastrointestinal tract and are administered in parenteral formulations. These drugs are given once a day and have 10- to 26-hour half-lives. Echinocandins are not metabolized.

Therapeutic Uses

Echinocandins are used for the prevention of invasive fungal infections, treatment of candidiasis, and empiric treatment of fungal infections.

Adverse Effects

Echinocandins are well tolerated with few side effects. Some of the most commonly reported side effects include headache and gastrointestinal upset.

Drug-Drug Interactions

There are relatively few drug interactions with echinocandins.

Allylamines

Allylamines are synthetic molecules represented by naftifine and terbinafine.

Mechanism of Action

Allylamines work in a similar fashion to azole antifungals by inhibiting the synthesis of ergosterol and causing membrane disruption. Unlike azoles, allylamines act at an earlier step in the ergosterol synthesis pathway by inhibiting the enzyme squalene epoxidase (Fig. 13.6).

Antifungal Spectrum

Allylamines are fungicidal against dermatophyte organisms (e.g., *Trichophyton* spp., *Microsporum* spp., and *Epidermophyton floccosum*) as well as many *Candida* species.

Pharmacokinetics

Naftifine can cause serious health issues if taken orally and should only be used topically. Terbinafine can be administered orally and accumulates in hair, nails, skin, and fat cells.

Therapeutic Uses

Allylamines can be used to treat infections caused by fungi that affect the fingernails, toenails, or skin.

Adverse Effects

Common mild side effects of terbinafine when taken orally include nausea, diarrhea, headache, cough, and rash. Severe side effects may include liver damage and allergic reactions.

Drug-Drug Interactions

Allylamines have the potential to affect medications metabolized through the CYP450 pathway. Terbinafine can inhibit metabolism of some drugs and in turn is affected by other drugs that affect liver metabolism through the CYP450 pathway.

Summary

Many of the above drugs are used for a variety of systemic fungal infections not discussed above, including Blastomyces, Cryptococcus, Coccidioides, and Histoplasma. Many topical drugs are not included in the above list. For dentists, oral candidiasis is the most common fungal infection encountered.

Antiviral Drugs

Antiviral drugs are classified here by the type of virus that is being targeted. Viruses need to invade mammalian cells to replicate, and viruses possess either RNA or DNA. The viral RNA or DNA can be targeted as well as the mechanisms by which viruses invade cells and set up their replication machinery. Vaccines are available to prevent some viral diseases, although they are not listed here. Vaccines are important prevention strategies. Mechanisms by which many antiviral drugs act are shown in Fig. 13.7.

Drugs to Treat *Herpes Simplex* Virus

Orolabial herpes is a common disorder encountered by dentists. Drugs used for *Herpes simplex* are listed in Table 13.13.

Drugs Used for Three Other Common Viral Infections

See Table 13.14.

Drugs Used to Treat Hepatitis B and Hepatitis C

See Table 13.15.

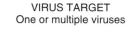
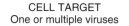
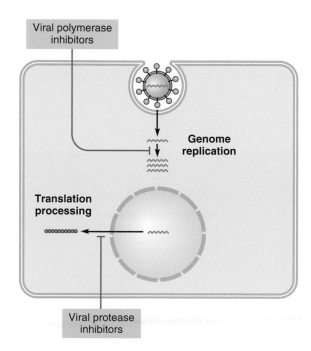
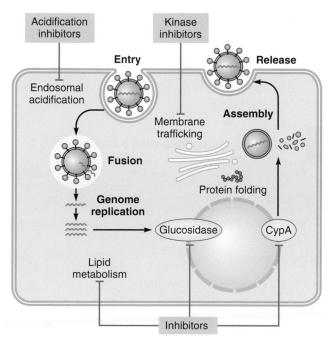

• **Fig. 13.7** The various scientific strategies for development of antiviral drugs. Left panel: direct-acting antivirals that target a specific viral protein and are aimed at a single virus target or a target for multiple viruses. This cartoon shows inhibitors of viral polymerases or proteases, but other viral proteins may also be targeted. Right panel: drugs that target cellular processes that are essential for replication of one or several viruses. The cartoon shows several classes of inhibitors, but there are many other cellular functions that could be targets. *CypA*: cyclophilin A. (From Katze, Michael G., et al. *Viral pathogenesis: From Basics to Systems Biology*. Elsevier; 2016. 3rd ed.)

TABLE 13.13 **Anti-Herpes Simplex Drugs**

Drug	Antiviral Mechanism (See Fig. 13.7)	Adverse Effects
Acyclovir (Oral and topical)	Inhibition of DNA synthesis	(oral use) GI effects, renal toxicity, tremors
Famciclovir (Oral)	Inhibition of DNA synthesis	GI effects
Valacyclovir (Oral)	Inhibition of DNA synthesis	GI effects
Penciclovir (Topical)	Inhibition of DNA synthesis	
Docosanol (Topical)	Fusion inhibitor preventing entrance of virus	

DNA, Deoxyribonucleic acid; *GI*, gastrointestinal.

TABLE 13.14 **Drugs Used for Three Other Common Viral Infections**

Varicella zoster Virus		
Drug	Antiviral Mechanism	Adverse Effects
Acyclovir	See Table 13.13	See Table 13.13
Valacyclovir	See Table 13.13	See Table 13.13
Famciclovir	See Table 13.13	See Table 13.13
Foscarnet	Inhibits DNA polymerase directly	Anemia, renal toxicity, electrolyte disorders
Cytomegalovirus		
Valganciclovir	Inhibits DNA synthesis	Bone marrow suppression, peripheral neuropathy, headache, confusion
Respiratory Syncytial Virus		
Ribavirin	Inhibits replication of RNA	Anemia, nausea, hemolytic anemia, insomnia

DNA, Deoxyribonucleic acid; *RNA*, ribonucleic acid.

TABLE 13.15 **Drug Treatment of Hepatitis B and Hepatitis C**

Hepatitis B		
Drug Class	Examples	Adverse Effects
DNA polymerase inhibitors	Adefovir, entecavir	Adefovir, nephrotoxicity; entecavir, headache, dizziness, nausea
Reverse transcriptase inhibitor	Tenofovir	Nephrotoxicity
Hepatitis C (Used in Combination)		
NS5B polymerase inhibitor	Sofosbuvir,	Fatigue, interacts with several drugs
NS3 Protease inhibitor	Grazoprevir, glecaprevir	GI effects, fatigue
NS5A protein inhibitor	Daclatasvir, velpatasvir	Fatigue, insomnia

(Interferon alpha 2a is used for hepatitis B and hepatitis C.)
DNA, Deoxyribonucleic acid; *GI*, gastrointestinal.

The HIV Life Cycle

HIV medicines in seven drug classes stop (🛑) HIV at different stages in the HIV life cycle.

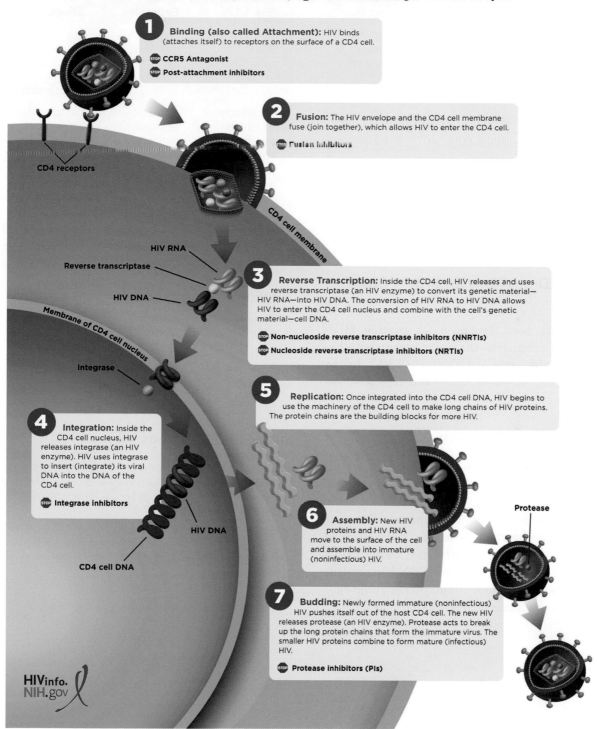

1 Binding (also called Attachment): HIV binds (attaches itself) to receptors on the surface of a CD4 cell.
🛑 CCR5 Antagonist
🛑 Post-attachment inhibitors

2 Fusion: The HIV envelope and the CD4 cell membrane fuse (join together), which allows HIV to enter the CD4 cell.
🛑 Fusion inhibitors

CD4 receptors

CD4 cell membrane

HIV RNA
Reverse transcriptase
HIV DNA

3 Reverse Transcription: Inside the CD4 cell, HIV releases and uses reverse transcriptase (an HIV enzyme) to convert its genetic material—HIV RNA—into HIV DNA. The conversion of HIV RNA to HIV DNA allows HIV to enter the CD4 cell nucleus and combine with the cell's genetic material—cell DNA.
🛑 Non-nucleoside reverse transcriptase inhibitors (NNRTIs)
🛑 Nucleoside reverse transcriptase inhibitors (NRTIs)

Membrane of CD4 cell nucleus

Integrase

5 Replication: Once integrated into the CD4 cell DNA, HIV begins to use the machinery of the CD4 cell to make long chains of HIV proteins. The protein chains are the building blocks for more HIV.

4 Integration: Inside the CD4 cell nucleus, HIV releases integrase (an HIV enzyme). HIV uses integrase to insert (integrate) its viral DNA into the DNA of the CD4 cell.
🛑 Integrase inhibitors

HIV DNA

CD4 cell DNA

Protease

6 Assembly: New HIV proteins and HIV RNA move to the surface of the cell and assemble into immature (noninfectious) HIV.

7 Budding: Newly formed immature (noninfectious) HIV pushes itself out of the host CD4 cell. The new HIV releases protease (an HIV enzyme). Protease acts to break up the long protein chains that form the immature virus. The smaller HIV proteins combine to form mature (infectious) HIV.
🛑 Protease inhibitors (PIs)

HIVinfo.
NIH.gov

• **Fig. 13.8** Human immunodeficiency virus (HIV) is subject to attack by drugs at several stages during the HIV life cycle. Certain agents block the binding of HIV to the CD4 host cells (helper T cells). This can occur by the drug binding to glycoproteins on the virus or by binding to CCR5 chemokine receptors on the host cell or related mechanisms. Some of these drugs block fusion of the virus with the host cell. Collectively these can be classified as entry inhibitors (Steps 1 and 2). The nucleoside/nucleotide and non-nucleoside reverse transcriptase inhibitors prevent the synthesis of new viral DNA from viral RNA (Step 3). Integrase inhibitors prevent the incorporation of viral DNA into host DNA (Step 4). Protease inhibitors prevent the maturation of the HIV virus (Step 7). (From an NIH website: https://hivinfo.nih.gov/understanding-hiv/fact-sheets/hiv-life-cycle)

TABLE 13.16   Drug Treatment for Influenza

Drug Class	Examples	Anti-Influenza Effectiveness
Neuraminidase inhibitors	Oseltamivir, Zanamivir	Many subtypes of influenza A and influenza B
Inhibitors of viral uncoating	Amantadine, Rimantadine	Influenza A
Inhibitors of viral transcription and replication	Baloxavir	Influenza A and B

TABLE 13.17   Anti-HIV Drug Classes with Representative Examples

Mechanism (Fig. 13.8)	Drug Examples	Adverse Effects
Entry inhibitors (Steps 1 and 2 in Fig 13.8)	Enfuvirtide, maraviroc	Enfuvirtide, injection site reactions; maraviroc, hypotension;
Nucleoside/nucleotide reverse transcriptase inhibitors (NRTI)	Abacavir, tenofovir, emtricitabine, lamivudine	Lactic acidosis for the class (NRTI), Abacavir, hypersensitivity; Tenovovir, nephrotoxicity; Others, less toxic
Nonnucleoside reverse transcriptase inhibitors	Efavirenz, rilpivirine; delavirdine, etravirine	CNS toxicity; Rashes
Integrase inhibitors	Raltegravir, elvitegravir	GI effects
Protease inhibitors	Fosamprenavir, ritonavir	GI effects, hyperglycemia, hyperlipdemia

CNS, Central nervous system; *GI*, gastrointestinal.

Drug Treatment for Influenza

See Table 13.16.

Antiretroviral Drugs (Only Anti-HIV-1 Drugs Listed)

Many drugs have been developed for treating HIV-AIDS. Fig. 13.8 summarizes the major antiviral mechanisms within the life cycle of HIV. Table 13.17 list the mechanisms of the anti-HIV drugs and representative examples.

Drugs used to treat COVID -19

Although vaccines are the main agents for dealing with COVID-19, the following are drugs that have some efficacy in treating the disease. !. Nirmatrelvir/Ritonavir (Paxlovid). Nirmatrelvir is a protease inhibitor. Ritonavir is used in this combination to reduce metabolism of nirmatrelvir by inhibiting cytochrome P450 3A4.2. Remdesivir (Veklury). This drug is an RNA-dependent RNA polymerase inhibitor. 3. Molnupiravir (Legevrio). This drug causes mutations of virus RNA.

Suggested Readings

Richman Douglas D., Neal Nathanson. 20 Antiviral therapy. In: Katze, Michael G., ed, et al. *Viral Pathogenesis: From Basics to Systems Biology*. On-Line: Elsevier; 2016: pii: B9780128009642000203/f20-01-9780128009642.

American Dental Association Antibiotic Stewardship. https://www.ada.org/resources/research/science-and-research-institute/oral-health-topics/antibiotic-stewardship; 2019. [Accessed 23 May 2023].

14

Analgesics and Acute Pan Control[a]

Drugs for the treatment of pain are common drugs used in the dental setting. Most dental use of analgesics is short term because of dental pain related to disease (e.g., dental caries) or dental treatment (e.g., dental extraction). Therefore, preoperative and postoperative pain are indications for oral analgesics. Often local anesthetics and, on occasion, general anesthesia are used during dental procedures to control pain.

Nonsteroidal Antiinflammatory Drugs

The most common oral analgesics are nonsteroidal antiinflammatory drugs (NSAIDs), acetaminophen, and opioid drugs.

It is not a coincidence that inflammation and pain are often discussed together because inflammation often accompanies pain and is a major cause of pain. Inflammation is often a feature of dental pain. The NSAIDs inhibit both pain and inflammation.

Introduction

NSAIDs inhibit the enzyme **cyclooxygenase (COX)**, which catalyzes the conversion of arachidonic acid to prostaglandins and thromboxane A_2. These products have important biological effects. COX has more than one isoform, the most important of which are COX-1 and COX-2. Some of the effects of COX-1 and COX-2 enzymes are listed in Fig. 14.1, with varying tissue effects. Most COX inhibitors inhibit both isoforms but differ in the degree to which they inhibit each isoform. By examining Fig. 14.1, one can see, for instance, that a drug that selectively inhibits COX-2 would be useful in inhibiting pain and inflammation but would not prevent the production of thromboxane A_2.

By virtue of their ability to inhibit COX, most NSAIDs have **analgesic, antipyretic, and antiinflammatory** actions.

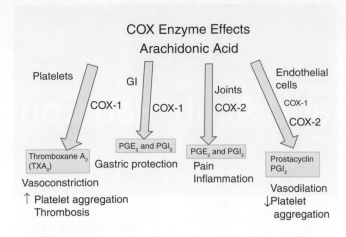

• **Fig. 14.1** Conversion of arachidonic acid to prostaglandins and thromboxane A$_2$. The various biological effects resulting from these conversions are shown. *COX,* Cyclooxygenase; *GI,* gastrointestinal; *PGE$_2$,* prostaglandin E$_2$; *PGI$_2$,* Prostaglandin I$_2$. (Redrawn from Cannon CP, Cannon PJ. COX-2 inhibitors and cardiovascular risk. *Science.* 2012;336:1386–1387.)

Salicylates (Particularly Aspirin)

Mechanism of Action

These drugs are the oldest NSAIDs and, in the form of aspirin, are commonly used. Aspirin has a unique action among the salicylates and indeed other NSAIDs. Aspirin is an irreversible inhibitor of the isoforms of the COX enzymes. The importance of the action of aspirin on COX enzymes is the duration of action on preventing platelet aggregation. More specifically, irreversibly inhibiting the COX-1 enzyme by aspirin prevents platelets from regenerating thromboxane A$_2$. The effects of aspirin on platelet aggregation therefore last much longer than those of other NSAIDs, including other salicylates.

Aspirin should be used with caution during pregnancy. In the third trimester, it may cause premature closure of the *ductus arteriosus*. Aspirin given late in pregnancy may result in prolonged labor and excessive bleeding during delivery.

Metabolism and Elimination

Fig. 14.2 shows the pathways for aspirin metabolism. Aspirin is rapidly metabolized to salicylic acid by plasma esterases and has a short half-life. Salicylic acid is further metabolized to other conjugated products shown. These reactions are saturable at toxic doses of aspirin, accounting for the longer elimination half-life of salicylic acid. Since salicylic acid is an active metabolite of aspirin, toxicity can remain long after aspirin is converted to salicylic acid.

At therapeutic doses, most of the salicylic acid is converted into conjugated products. At higher doses, the percentage of salicylic acid in the urine increases. A strategy to eliminate more salicylic acid in the kidney is to make the urine more basic with IV sodium bicarbonate. This favors a greater formation of the basic (charged) form of salicylic acid in the kidney tubule to reduce reabsorption and increase excretion.

Adverse Effects

A common side effect of salicylates is excessive bleeding. Gastrointestinal (GI) bleeding and dyspepsia are adverse effects commonly associated with aspirin. Anticoagulants and ethanol can increase the toxicity of aspirin.

Chronic toxicity can lead to a condition called **salicylism**. It is characterized by tinnitus, electrolyte disturbances, bleeding, GI irritation, and mental confusion. Higher doses will also lead to hyperthermia and alkalosis, followed by, in severe case, acidosis.

Table 14.1 lists several characteristics of aspirin and another salicylate, diflunisal. Table 14.2 lists drug-drug interactions for aspirin. Table 14.3 presents potential contraindications to the use of aspirin.

Other Nonsteroidal Antiinflammatory Drugs

Ibuprofen and naproxen are the two most commonly used drugs in this group. Ibuprofen is commonly used alone or with an opioid to treat dental pain. As with aspirin, these drugs are nonselective inhibitors of COX. Unlike aspirin, they are reversible inhibitors of COX enzymes.

Adverse effects of the NSAIDs are generally mild, and some are listed in Box 14.1. Table 14.4 lists the half-lives of some NSAIDs.

Celecoxib, a Selective COX-2 Inhibitor

Celecoxib is the only COX-2 selective inhibitor approved in the United States. The advantage to a COX-2 selective

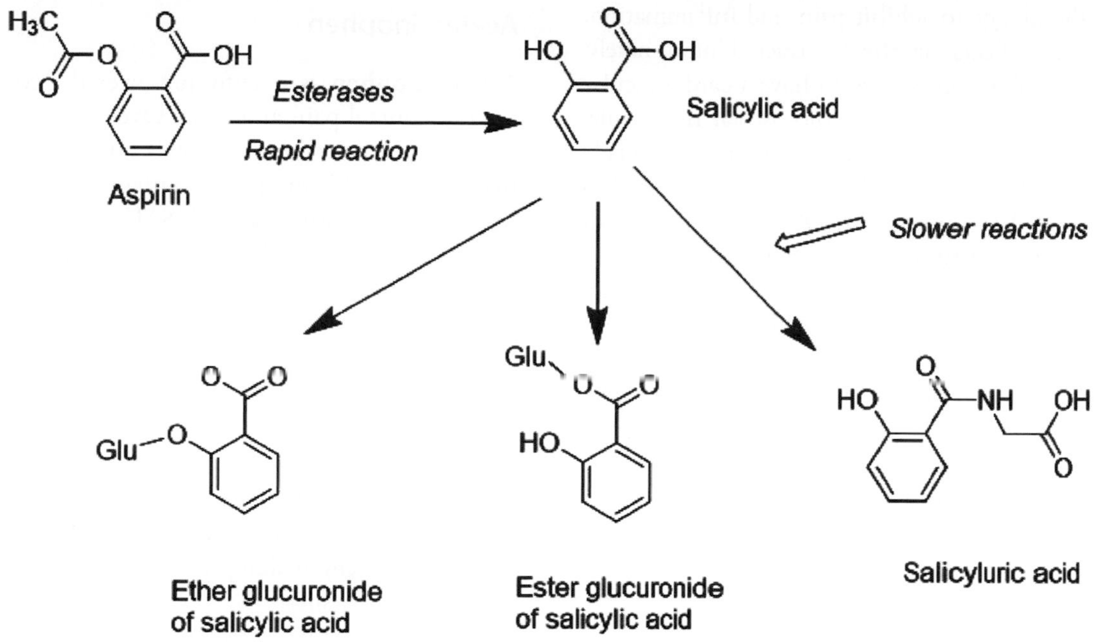

• Fig. 14.2 Aspirin metabolism.

TABLE 14.1	Characteristics of the Aspirin and Another Salicylate, Diflunisal				
Drug	Inhibition of COX	Uses	Duration of Action[a]	Adverse Effects
Aspirin	Irreversible	Pain Inflammation Fever Prophylaxis against platelet aggregation (low dose)	2–3 h including half-life for salicylic acid[b]	Heightened bleeding tendency Gastric bleeding, and ulcers, due to the effect on gastric mucosa Analgesic-associated nephropathy (long-term use) Salicylism with toxicity Hyper-responsive airways in asthmatic patients Reye syndrome in children and teens in the presence of or recent history of a viral infection
Diflunisal	Reversible	Pain Inflammation	8–12 h	Similar to aspirin but less platelet effect

[a]The duration of aspirin's antiplatelet effect lasts about 10 days due to the inability of platelets to form new thromboxane A_2.
[b]The duration can be over 20 hours in cases of acute aspirin poisoning.
COX, Cyclooxygenase.

TABLE 14.2	Some Drug-Drug Interactions Involving Aspirin	
Drug	Possible Interactions With Aspirin
Warfarin, apixaban, and other anticoagulants	Internal bleeding
Insulin	Aspirin may cause a decrease or increase in blood glucose
Phenytoin, valproic acid	Increased free plasma concentration of phenytoin or valproic acid
Methotrexate	Increased free plasma concentration of methotrexate
Ethanol	GI bleeding
Probenecid, sulfinpyrazone	Decreased uricosuric effect of probenecid or sulfinpyrazone
Lithium	Increased lithium toxicity
ACE inhibitors, β-adrenergic receptor blockers, diuretics	Decreased antihypertensive effect of each of these drugs

ACE, Angiotensin-converting enzyme.

inhibitor is the ability to inhibit pain and inflammation, with less adverse effects on the GI tract. Unfortunately, these drugs have also been shown to have a cardiovascular risk, especially in patients with a cardiovascular risk profile. The drug, therefore, must be used with caution especially in these individuals. Further, COX-2 inhibition can lead to renal toxicity. Similar to other NSAIDS, this drug class can also inhibit the effect of some antihypertensive drugs.

Celecoxib has indications for arthritis, but there are no, or very few, dental uses for celecoxib. Although celecoxib is also an analgesic, more effective treatment is usually attained with an NSAID or acetaminophen. The advantage of celecoxib for patients with significant GI risk has to be weighed against the cardiovascular risks. Dosages for celecoxib are more limited than for other analgesics.

TABLE 14.3	Contraindications or Potential Contraindications to the Use of Aspirin
Disease State	**Possible Adverse Effect**
GI ulcer	GI bleeding
Asthma	Asthmatic attack in some asthmatics
Diabetes	Decrease or increase in blood glucose
Gout	Increase in plasma urate at common analgesic doses
Viral infections including influenza[a]	Reye syndrome in children and teens
Hypocoagulation conditions	Excessive bleeding

[a]Particular attention should be paid to avoid Reye's syndrome.
GI, Gastrointestinal.

• BOX 14.1   Typical Adverse Effects of Nonsteroidal Antiinflammatory Drugs

GI symptoms: nausea and vomiting, dyspepsia, ulcers
CNS symptoms: dizziness, headache, tinnitus
Cardiovascular: fluid retention
Hepatic: abnormal liver function tests
Pulmonary: worsening of asthma
Skin: rashes
Kidney: hyperkalemia, renal insufficiency, may antagonize the antihypertensive effects of ACE inhibitors, β-adrenergic receptor blockers, or diuretics

CNS, Central nervous system; *GI*, gastrointestinal.

Acetaminophen

Acetaminophen is a common over-the-counter agent used to control pain and fever. Over 25 billion doses are sold per year. Acetaminophen is an analgesic and antipyretic drug with modest antiinflammatory effects. It is therefore not classified as an NSAID. Because it is a weak inhibitor of COX, it has fewer GI adverse effects compared to aspirin and other NSAIDs.

Mechanism of Action

The mechanism of action of acetaminophen has not been fully established. The following comments address this issue.

1. Acetaminophen inhibits COX enzymes; however, peroxides found in inflammatory tissues inhibit acetaminophen, thereby making it a weak inhibitor of COX at inflammatory sites.
2. Acetaminophen undergoes metabolism in the brain. A key metabolic route is the conversion to p-aminophenol, which in turn can be conjugated to arachidonic acid in the brain. This product, *N*-arachidonoyl phenolamine (compound

TABLE 14.4	Half-Lives of Some Nonsteroidal Antiinflammatory Drugs and Comments	
Drug	**Elimination Half-Life (h)**	**Comments**
Ibuprofen	~ 2	Very commonly used over the counter; Commonly used by prescription with an opioid
Naproxen	~15	Its longer action has advantages.
Fenoprofen	~ 2.5	Less commonly used
Ketoprofen	~2–4	Less commonly used; GI irritation is more likely than with ibuprofen.
Etodolac	~7	Longer acting
Diclofenac	~2	Can be administered in several forms
Ketorolac	5–6	Giving orally after a parenteral dose has been given; commonly used post-surgically for a limit of 5 days because of adverse effects

GI, Gastrointestinal.

AM404), may have analgesic effects by stimulating certain receptors in the brain (Fig. 14.3).

3. Other CNS effects may lead to analgesia.

Metabolism

Fig. 14.3 shows a summary of metabolic routes for acetaminophen. Three general routes are outlined: conjugation to glucuronic acid and sulfate, hydrolysis to p-aminophenol leading to conversion to AM404 in the CNS, and conversion to the metabolite, N-acetyl-p-benzoquinone imine (NAPQI). NAPQI is a chemical that is toxic to the liver.

Adverse Effects

The major serious effect of acetaminophen is liver toxicity. This is a predictable effect of overdose, and it is more likely in patients with preexisting liver disease and in alcoholics. Without intervention, there is a high risk of death. Large doses of acetaminophen can lead to the conversion of acetaminophen to N-acetyl-p-benzoquinone imine (**NAPQI**), a toxic metabolite (see Fig. 14.3). Prompt administration of **acetylcysteine** can neutralize NAPQI, thereby reducing its toxicity. Acetaminophen in overdose is also a risk for acute kidney toxicity.

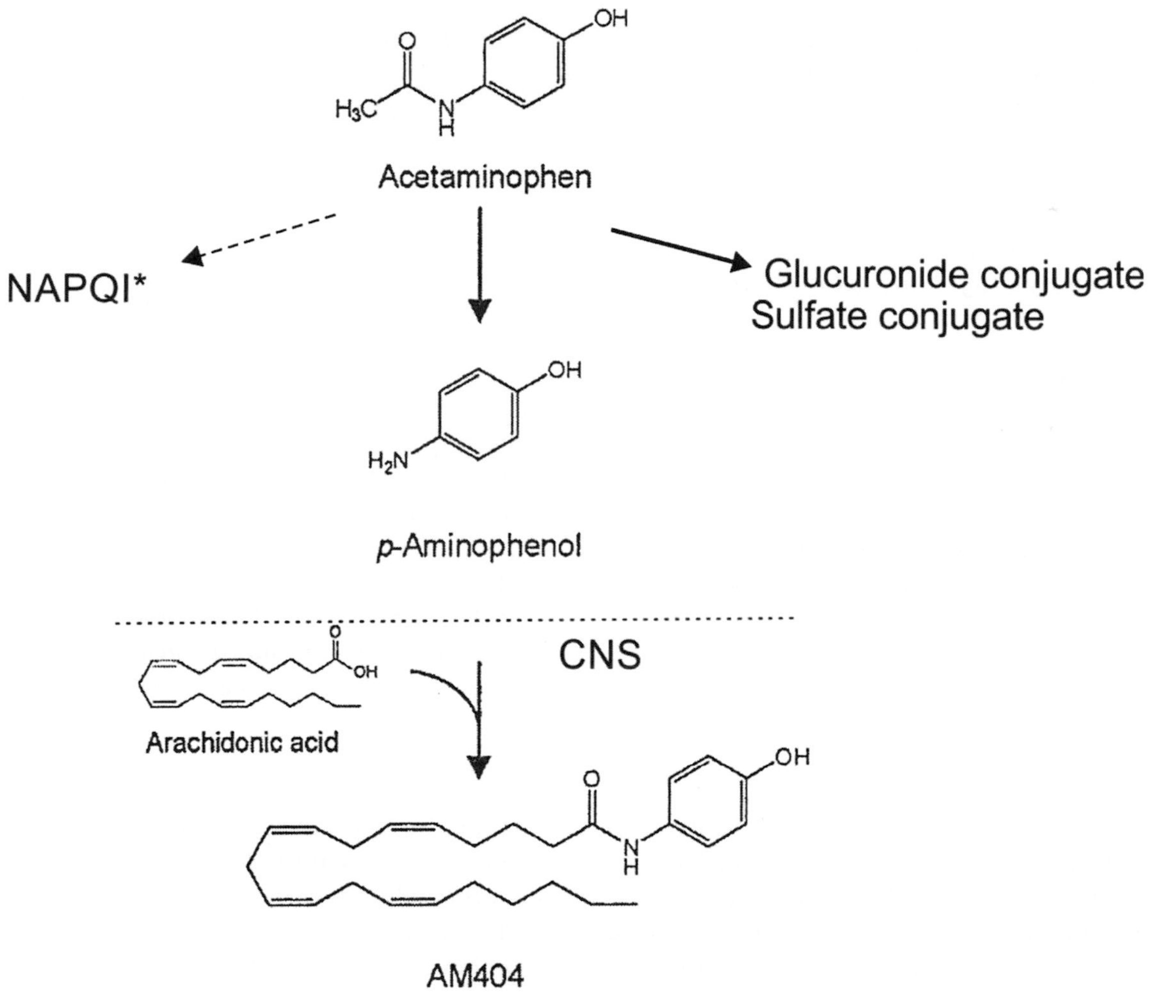

• **Fig. 14.3** Metabolism of acetaminophen. Acetaminophen is mostly metabolized by conjugation to glucuronic acid or sulfate. The conversion to N-acetyl-p-benzoquinone imine (NAPQI) can lead to hepatotoxicity. Conversion of p-aminophenol to arachidonic acid to form N-arachidonoyl phenolamine (compound AM404) occurs in the central nervous system. CNS, Central nervous system. (Figure modified from Högestätt ED, Jönsson BAG, Ermund A, et al. Conversion of acetaminophen to the bioactive N-acylphenolamine AM404 via fatty acid amide hydrolase-dependent arachidonic acid conjugation in the nervous system. J Biol Chem. 2005;280:31406–31412. © 2023 American Society for Biochemistry and Molecular Biology. Published by Elsevier Inc. on behalf of American Society for Biochemistry and Molecular Biology. All rights reserved.)

TABLE 14.5	Comparisons of Three Analgesics		
Condition	Acetaminophen	Aspirin	Ibuprofen
Antiinflammatory	No	Yes	Yes
Analgesic	Yes	Yes	Yes
GI irritation	Least	Most	In between[a]
Reduces platelet aggregation?	Least	Most	In between[a]
Drug-drug interactions	Least	Most	In between[a]
Risk in asthma	Least	Most	In between[a]
Risk for Reye syndrome	Very low	High[c]	Very low
Can be combined with an opioid?	Yes	Yes	Yes
Analgesic half-life	2–3h	2–3 h[b]	~2h
Extensively metabolized?	Yes	Yes	Yes

In young patients with recent or ongoing viral infection.
[a]The risk from ibuprofen is closer to that of aspirin than to that of acetaminophen.
[b]Longer with large doses.
[c]In young patients with recent or ongoing viral infection.

Some Comparisons of Nonsteroidal Antiinflammatory Drugs and Acetaminophen

Table 14.5 compares acetaminophen to aspirin and ibuprofen. Acetaminophen and ibuprofen are commonly used to treat dental pain.

Opioid Analgesics

Morphine and **codeine** are natural opiates and prototypes of opioid analgesics. **Oxycodone** and **hydrocodone** are semisynthetic opioid drugs that are structurally related to morphine and codeine. Other opioids are completely synthetic and include **fentanyl** and **methadone**.

Mechanism of Action

The physiologic effects of opioid agonists occur when opioid receptors are activated. The opioid receptors are located in several sites in the CNS, on peripheral pain fibers, and in the GI tract. Opioid receptors also respond to endogenous agonists that are called **endogenous opioid peptides** (e.g., endorphins, enkephalins, dynorphins, and endomorphins).

There are three types of opioid receptors: **μ (mu), κ (kappa),** and **δ (delta)**. Each receptor is associated with analgesia; however, the μ (mu) receptor is the most important for most opioids. Pharmacologic doses of natural, semisynthetic, or synthetic opioids will affect the different receptors to varying degrees.

Fig. 14.4 shows the result of the stimulation of opioid receptors by morphine and other opioid agonists. At presynaptic sites, morphine inhibits the production of cyclic AMP, thus reducing the influx of calcium and the release of neurotransmitters. At the postsynaptic neuron, morphine acts to increase conduction in potassium channels, thereby causing hyperpolarization of the nerve and inhibiting conduction. Many areas in the central nervous system are affected, including the periaqueductal gray area, the thalamus, and the cerebral cortex.

There is a unique characteristic of pain relief from an opioid. Not only is there inhibition of pain sensation, but opioids also reduce the **motivational-affective** component of pain, reducing the suffering associated with pain.

Metabolism

Opioids undergo extensive metabolism in the liver. Morphine is metabolized to a metabolite, morphine-6-glucuronide, which is a strong analgesic. Morphine-6-glucuronide contributes to the pain-relieving effect of morphine, especially with chronic use (Fig. 14.5). An important aspect of the metabolism of codeine and some other opioids is discussed below.

Adverse and Other Effects

The acute toxicity of opioids is characterized by **stupor, pinpoint pupils, and respiratory depression**. Other adverse effects are indicated in Table 14.6.

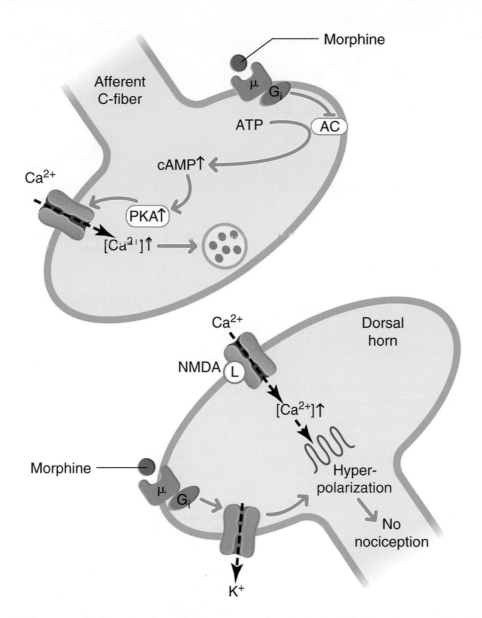

• **Fig. 14.4** Opioids act both presynaptically and postsynaptically on neurons in pain circuits. Activation of presynaptic opioid receptors leads to a reduced intracellular cAMP concentration and decreased Ca^{2+} influx (and thus inhibition of the release of excitatory neurotransmitters such as glutamate and substance P). Opioid receptor binding postsynaptically hyperpolarizes the neuronal membrane, which decreases the probability of the generation of an action potential in response to excitatory input at "L" (such as during pain transmission). *AC*, Adenylyl cyclase; *AMP*, adenosine monophosphate; *ATP*, adenosine triphosphate; *cAMP*, Cyclic AMP; *NMDA*, N-methyl-D-aspartate; *PKA*, protein kinase A.

Characteristics of Individual Opioids

As with other opioids, codeine undergoes metabolism involving a number of reactions. These are shown in Fig. 14.6. Conversion to morphine accounts for a large part of its analgesic effect. Since cytochrome P450 2D6 (see Fig. 14.6) is genetically determined, the degree to which codeine is converted to morphine varies between patients. Thus, the analgesic effect of codeine varies among individuals. Moreover, cytochrome P450 2D6 can be inhibited or induced by some drugs, further reducing the predictability of codeine's effect. The genetic metabolizer scale shows the

range of activity of P450 2D6 throughout the population (Fig. 14.7). What further complicates the clinical response is that the percentage of people in each range of activity varies among races.

Other opioids such as oxycodone, hydrocodone, and tramadol (Table 14.7) are subject to P450 2D6, but the clinical implications are less than with codeine. Some deaths have occurred with codeine administered to children. Codeine, and other opioids, should be avoided in children and also in adolescents with underlying health risk factors.

Morphine

Morphine-6-glucuronide

• **Fig. 14.5** Structures of morphine and morphine-6-glucuronide.

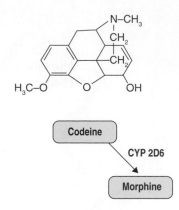

Codeine

CYP 2D6

Morphine

• **Fig. 14.6** Metabolism of codeine to morphine. Other routes of metabolism of codeine are not shown.

TABLE 14.6	Effects of Morphine and Other Opioid Receptor Agonists
Effect	**Comments**
Analgesia	See above
Respiratory depression	Dose-related, often the cause of lethality
Histamine release	May cause hypotension, rash, and breathing problems
Constriction of pupils	Due to central mechanism of opioids
Nausea and vomiting	Due to stimulation of the chemoreceptor trigger zone. This effect wanes after initial doses.
Constipation	Direct effect on GI tract opioid receptors
Cough suppression	Due to inhibition of cough center in the brainstem
Tolerance	Reduced effect of the drug with continued therapy, due to adaptive changes in CNS
Physical dependence	Characterized by withdrawal symptoms if the drug is abruptly removed
Abuse	Associated with inappropriate non-medical use. Habitual abuse is characterized by cravings and physical dependence.
Dysphoria	Associated especially with κ (kappa) receptor stimulation.

CNS, Central nervous system; *GI*, gastrointestinal.

CYP2D6 Metabolizer Scale

Slow ——————————————— Fast

PM   IM   EM   UM

PM=Poor Metabolizers
IM=Intermediate Metabolizers
EM= Extensive Metabolizers ("normal")
UM=Ultra Rapid Metabolizers

• **Fig. 14.7** Cytochrome P450 2D6 metabolizer scale. (Data from Lötsch J, Geisslinger G. A critical appraisal of human genotyping for pain therapy. Trends Pharmacol Sci. 2010;31:312–317.)

useful in cases of overdose from an opioid receptor agonist. Quick action is important, making the immediate availability of an antagonist essential. Naloxone is often the one most prescribed. One caution with the use of naloxone is that its half-life may be shorter than the opioid causing the toxicity (see Tables 14.7 and 14.8). Therefore, the patient must be observed for the return of signs of toxicity.

Opioid Addiction

Addiction is the irresistible cravings for a drug with compulsive and continued use despite harmful consequences and accompanied by physical dependence. The addictive nature of opiates can affect anyone, and certain physiologic and psychologic factors can increase the risk of addiction. Opioids can become addictive because they activate powerful reward centers in the brain. Continued use of opioids often causes drug tolerance, creating an ever-increasing demand of drug for the same sense of physical and psychological well-being.

If for recreational use or as a result of addiction, approximately 50,000 US citizens died from opioid overdose in 2019. The misuse of opioids is a serious national crisis that affects the social and economic welfare of the country. In

Some Other Drugs That Have Mixed Actions or Other Actions

Opioid Receptor Antagonists

Naloxone and naltrexone are pure opioid receptor antagonists. Their ability to reverse respiratory depression and other effects of opioid receptor agonists makes them very

TABLE 14.7 Comparisons of Opioid Receptor Agonists

Opioid	Half-Life	Used Orally	Comments
Morphine	~ 2 h	Not often	Used for severe pain
Codeine	~ 3 h (see below)	Yes	Used for moderate pain, often in combination[a]
Hydrocodone	~5 h	Yes	Used for moderate pain, often in combination
Oxycodone	~2.5 h	Yes	Used for moderate pain, often in combination
Fentanyl	~4 h	No[b]	80–100 times as potent as morphine
Methadone	Variable ~30 h	Yes	Analgesia, also used for maintenance therapy in the treatment for addiction

[a]See metabolic routes and comments above.
[b]Fentanyl is used IV and by epidural administration. Transdermal and trans-buccal administration can be used for breakthrough pain in opioid-tolerant patients.

TABLE 14.8 Comparison of Five Additional Drugs

Drug	Comments
Buprenorphine	A mixed-action drug, an agonist at μ receptors and an antagonist at κ (kappa) receptors, used in chronic addiction control.
Tramadol	Weak μ agonist, also inhibits reuptake of norepinephrine and serotonin. All these actions are analgesic. It is available alone or in combination with acetaminophen.
Tapentadol	Moderate μ agonist, inhibits reuptake of norepinephrine.
Naloxone	A pure antagonist at opioid receptors, used as an antidote in cases of opioid overdose. It has a half-life of about 1 h.
Naltrexone	A pure antagonist at opioid receptors, used as an antidote for opioid overdose, with a longer half-life (~10 h) than naloxone.

addition to the devastating effects of these drugs on individuals, the Centers for Disease Control and Prevention estimates misuse of opioids accounts for almost $79 billion a year in healthcare, opioid treatment, lost productivity, and criminal justice involvement.

Dental Analgesia

To reduce acute pain for patients, dentists must be acutely aware of opioid risks. **NSAIDs and/or acetaminophen** should be the first line of treatment for the management of acute dental pain since these drugs have been shown to be more effective than opioids in reducing most dental acute pain. If opioids are prescribed to enhanced the effect of NSAIDS or acetaminophen, the dentist must carefully consider if increasing an opioid dose or renewing a prescription for opioids offers any advantage.

Safe and effective management of acute pain is an important goal for dentists. The best available evidence suggests that combining NSAIDs with acetaminophen balances the benefits of pain relief while minimizing harmful effects. Due to the different pharmacologic mechanisms of NSAIDs and acetaminophen, the additive effects of these drugs optimize efficacy. Opioids should be reserved for acute pain not relieved by NSAIDs alone, and only for a limited time, that is, 2 to 3 days. Suggested doses and treatment regimens for pain medications are available in Essentials Chapter 19.

Suggested Reading

Hersh EV, Moore PA, Grosser T, et al. Nonsteroidal anti-inflammatory drugs and opiods in postsurgical dental pain. *J Dent Res.* 2020;99(7):777–786. https://doi.org/10.1177/0022034520914254.

[a]Note: The following topics are reserved for the larger edition of "Pharmacology and Therapeutics for Dentistry":
- Drugs used for the treatment of chronic pain and neuropathic pain
- Drugs used for autoimmune inflammatory conditions such as rheumatoid arthritis
- Antigout drugs

15

Bone-Sparing Drugs: Bisphosphonates and RANKL Inhibitors

KEY POINTS

- Selection of an appropriate antiresorptive bone therapy for a specific patient must consider relevant factors such as efficacy, adverse effects, dosing regimen, cost, and the patient preferences.
- Bisphosphonates and RANKL inhibitors are first-line drug therapies for patients susceptible to bone fracture due to disease.
- The bisphosphonate molecule attaches to bone and disrupts osteoclast function.
- RANKL inhibitors are proteins that prevent osteoclast maturation.
- A rare oral condition of bisphosphonates and RANKL inhibitors is medication-related osteonecrosis of the jaw (MRONJ).

DEFINITIONS

- Osteoblasts are cells that secrete matrix for bone formation.
- Osteoclasts are large multinucleated bone cells that resorb bone tissue.
- Osteoporosis is a bone disease that results in fracture when bone strength weakens and bones become brittle.
- RANK is the receptor activator of nuclear factor kappa B. RANK is expressed on osteoclast precursors and is a key regulator for osteoclastogenesis.
- RANKL is the ligand for receptor activator of nuclear factor kappa B. The secretion of RANKL from osteoblasts causes osteoclasts to proliferate and break down bones.

Introduction

Drugs that preserve bone from resorption, antiresorptive or bone-sparing drugs, are used to reduce the risk of bone fracture by increasing bone strength in individuals with osteoporosis or cancer metastases to bone. The five principal classes of agents used to spare bone and reduce fracture risk include bisphosphonates, estrogens, selective estrogen receptor modulators (SERMs), calcitonin, and monoclonal antibodies, such as RANKL inhibitors.

In postmenopausal women, a low-dose regimen of estrogen treatment can be considered for women with postmenopausal symptoms, including osteoporosis. Due to the potential adverse effects of estrogens (e.g., uterine cancer, thromboembolism, etc.) in postmenopausal women, only short-term management has been advocated. Another antiresorptive drug class is the selective estrogen receptor modulators or SERMs. SERMs are used sparingly due to their modest efficacy and are currently not considered as first-line therapy. Similar to SERMs, there is limited antifracture efficacy of the hormone calcitonin, and it is only recommended when the patient is unable to take other antiresorptive agents. Considering the limitations of antiresorptive drugs, only bisphosphonates or RANKL inhibitors should be recommended as first-line therapy for patients susceptible to bone fracture due to disease.

Bisphosphonates

In the mid-1960s, inorganic pyrophosphates were found to prevent calcification in body fluid by binding to hydroxyapatite crystals. This discovery led investigators to find stable analogs of inorganic pyrophosphates, which are now called bisphosphonates. As a family of pyrophosphate analogs, bisphosphonates contain a common chemical configuration: two phosphate groups attached to a central carbon atom that forms a three-dimensional structure.

Over time, bisphosphonate structure has been modified to increase efficacy (Table 15.1). First-generation bisphosphonates (e.g., etidronate) had minimally modified side chains of the pyrophosphate molecule or contained a chlorophenyl group. With the addition of a nitrogen group in the side chain, second-generation bisphosphonate (e.g., alendronate) potency increased by 10- to 100-fold. Third-generation bisphosphonate (e.g., risedronate) potency increased by 10,000 times when a heterocyclic ring containing nitrogen was inserted into the drug molecule.

TABLE 15.1	Antiresorptive Potency of Bisphosphonates Currently on U.S. Market				
Generic Name	Trade Name	Manufacturer	Side Chain	Relative Potency	Administered
Etidronate	Didronel	Procter & Gamble	Short alkyl or halide	1	Orally/intravenously
Tiludronate	Skelid	Sanofi-Aventis	Cyclic chloro	10	Orally
Pamidronate	Aredia	Novartis	Aminoterminal	100	Intravenously
Alendronate	Fosamax	Merck	Aminoterminal	100–1000	Orally
Risedronate	Actonel	Procter & Gamble	Cyclic nitrogen	1000–10,000	Orally
Ibandronate	Boniva	Roche	Cyclic nitrogen	1000–10,000	Orally
Zoledronic acid	Zometa	Novartis	Cyclic nitrogen	>10,000	Intravenously

The value of bisphosphonates resides in their ability to inhibit bone resorption. These drugs are employed for the treatment of osteoclast-mediated bone diseases, which include osteoporosis, steroid-induced osteoporosis, Paget disease, tumor-associated osteolysis, multiple myeloma, and malignancies associated with hypercalcemia. With regard to the prevention of bone metastases, bisphosphonates are important adjunctions commonly used in patients with many types of neoplasms, especially breast and prostate cancer. In dentistry, they have been shown to prevent dental calculus formation and may be beneficial in modulating host responses in the management of periodontal diseases.

Mechanism of Action

The molecular construct of bisphosphonate enables the molecule to attach to bone and disrupt osteoclast function. More specifically, bisphosphonates are released into the acidic environment of the resorption lacunae where they impede osteoclast action by either inhibiting cholesterol biosynthetic pathways, accelerating apoptosis, or disrupting the cell cycle (Fig. 15.1). In addition to the effects on bone, they also have antiinvasive, antiangiogenic, and antiproliferative properties.

Pharmacokinetics

Bisphosphonates are highly polar compounds and as a result are poorly absorbed after oral ingestion (e.g., ibandronate [Boniva], alendronate [Fosamax], or risedronate [Actonel]). More specifically, the bioavailability of the drug is less than 5% after oral administration. Because food can reduce absorption, timing of meals is important to enhance the bioavailability of the drug. To increase the

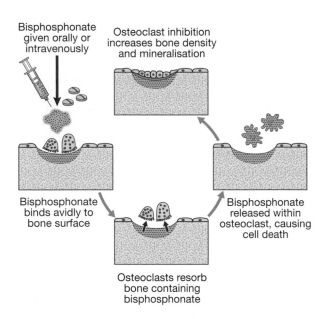

• Fig. 15.1 Mechanism of action of bisphosphonates.

amount of bisphosphonates introduced to bone, drug delivery can be accomplished via intravenous administration (e.g., pamidronate [Aredia], zoledronic acid [Zometa], or ibandronate [Boniva]). Once in the bloodstream, almost the entire dose is either absorbed by the bone or eliminated in urine. As a result of their negative charge and chemical structure, bisphosphonates can be retained by the bone for as long as 10 years.

Adverse Effects

Bisphosphonates can have toxic properties and some of the adverse effects include osteomalacia, esophagitis, mild fever, aches, renal toxicity, fracture of the subtrochanteric or diaphyseal femur, and medication-related osteonecrosis of the jaw (MRONJ).

Drug to Drug Interactions

Food and many drugs will inhibit the absorption of bisphosphonates.

RANKL Inhibitors

Biologic drugs, such as monoclonal antibodies, are synthesized in the laboratory to recognize a specific virus, bacterium, human cell, or biologic process. The first monoclonal antibody, anti-CD3 muromonab, was approved for use in 1986 for the management of acute transplant rejection. Since that time, the synthetic manufacture of monoclonal antibodies has rendered important biologic compounds to combat disease. In 2010, **denosumab** was approved for use as a RANKL inhibitor for treatment of osteoclast-related bone diseases.

Mechanism of Action

Similar to bisphosphonates, a RANKL inhibitor affects the bone-remodeling process but by an entirely different mechanism. For osteoclastogenesis, the secretion of RANKL (receptor activator of nuclear factor kappa ligand) from osteoblasts is essential. RANKL is a member of the tumor necrosis factor (TNF) family and binds to cell surface receptors, known as RANK (receptor activator of nuclear factor kappa) on the preosteoclast. Once bound to RANK, RANKL stimulates the production of numerous proteins that are necessary for osteoclast formation, function, and survival. A RANKL inhibitor is a protein that binds to RANKL, preventing the binding of RANKL to RANK. This prevents stimulation of RANK on the osteoclast and prevents osteoclast maturation (Fig. 15.2). The value of a RANKL inhibitor resides in the ability to inhibit bone resorption. This drug is employed for the treatment of osteoclast-mediated bone diseases, which include osteoporosis, and prevention of skeletal-related events in cancer patients.

Pharmacokinetics

Currently the only approved RANKL inhibitor for treatment and prevention of osteoporosis is denosumab, a human monoclonal antibody that binds to RANKL and prevents its action on RANK (Fig. 15.2). For treatment of osteoporosis, denosumab is known as Prolia, and for cancer bone metastasis it is called Xgeva, the difference being the dose used for osteoporosis versus cancer. Denosumab is administered by subcutaneous injection. The half-life of denosumab is approximately 32 days, and clearance is by the reticuloendothelial system followed by excretion by the kidneys.

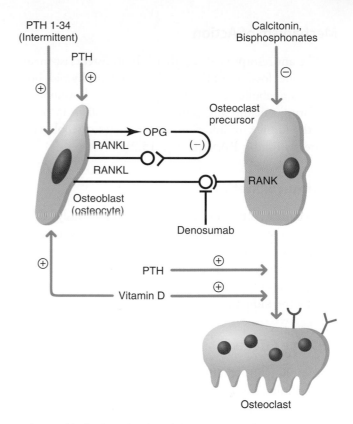

• **Fig. 15.2** Mechanism of action of denosumab and bisphosphonates. Denosumab binds to RANKL and prevents its action on RANK, resulting in a lower production of osteoclasts and their activity. Bisphosphonates get incorporated into osteoclasts and inhibit osteoclast activity. *OPG*, Osteoprotegerin; *PTH*, parathyroid hormone; *RANK*, receptor activator of nuclear factor kappa-B; *RANKL*, ligand for receptor activator of nuclear factor kappa-B. (Osteoprotegerin, after being released by osteocytes, inhibits RANKL). (Modified from Dowd F: Mosby's review for the NBDE, Part 2, ed 2, St. Louis, 2015, Mosby.)

Adverse Effects

Adverse effects reported for denosumab include back, arm, muscle and leg pain, allergic reactions, hypocalcemia, bladder infection, fractures of the femoral shaft, and osteonecrosis of the jaw.

Recombinant Human Parathyroid Hormone

Teriparatide (Forteo) is a recombinant portion (amino acids 1 to 34) of human parathyroid hormone that stimulates bone formation and has anabolic properties (Fig. 15.2). It was approved for use in the United States in 2002. Teriparatide is an expensive drug that must be injected daily to treat bone fractures related to osteoporosis. Although gains in bone density have been reported using recombinant human parathyroid hormone, these gains are lost once drug administration is stopped, unless other means of osteoporosis prevention are used.

Mechanism of Action

Unlike antiresorptive drugs that inhibit osteoclast-mediated bone loss, recombinant human parathyroid hormone is anabolic and mimics parathyroid hormone by regulating calcium and phosphate metabolism in bones and the kidney. In addition, it stimulates osteoblasts to indirectly inhibit RANKL (Fig. 15.2).

Pharmacokinetics

Teriparatide must be injected subcutaneously daily. It reaches a peak serum concentration approximately 30 minutes after administration, and decreases within 3 hours. Peripheral metabolism is believed to occur by nonspecific enzymatic mechanisms in the liver and excretion by the kidneys.

Adverse Effects

Common reported untoward effects include hypotension, palpitations, nausea, vomiting, dyspepsia, pain in limbs, sciatica, dizziness, dyspnea, rash, and anemia. In rat safety studies, this drug has shown to cause osteosarcoma.

Dental Management of a Patient Using a Bone-Sparing Drug

A side effect of oral and intravenously administered bisphosphonates and RANKL inhibitors in the jaws of patients is known as **medication-related osteonecrosis of the jaw (MRONJ)** (Fig. 15.3). There is no evidence that routine use of oral bisphosphonates for treatment or prevention of osteoporosis increases risk of MRONJ; however, oncologic (i.e., high) doses increase the risk of developing an MRONJ spontaneously or following invasive dental treatment (e.g., extractions). Appropriate bisphosphonate or RANKL inhibitor administration should be encouraged for appropriate disease control; however, it seems reasonable to do necessary oral surgery before beginning high-dose bisphosphonate therapy, to encourage good oral hygiene at home and to schedule regular care with a dentist while patients are taking bisphosphonates.

All patients who are going to begin treatment with bone-sparing drugs should receive a dental examination

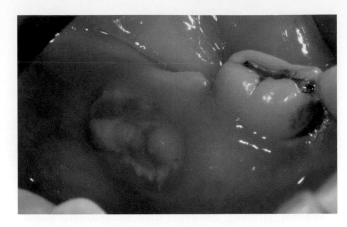

• **Fig. 15.3** Osteonecrosis of the jaw distolingual to tooth #18.

and be informed about the potential adverse oral effects of these drugs. Patient management should be directed at reducing future needs of dentoalveolar surgery. This means eliminating active sites of infection by periodontal, prosthodontic, and/or endodontic treatment or with appropriate dental extractions, if possible, before beginning therapy with these drugs. It is also very important to establish meticulous preventive dental regimens for patients. Each preventive dental regimen should be customized to patient needs. In general, these regiments should include patient education, oral hygiene home care routines to reduce dental caries and periodontal disease, elimination of habits that can increase dental disease (e.g., smoking, alcohol, etc.), and a schedule for routine visits to a dentist. Delaying initiation of bisphosphonate therapy until dental treatment is completed is probably not necessary, since there appears to be a 3-month window prior to when the first oral pathological outcomes of high-dose bisphosphonates were observed.

There is limited use of recombinant parathyroid hormone (PTH 1-34) due to cost, method of administration, transient effect, and putative carcinogenic effects.

Suggested Reading

American Dental Association Website Osteoporosis and medication-related osteoporosis of the jaw. https://www.ada.org/resources/research/science-and-research-institute/oral-health-topics/osteoporosis-medications, 2023. [Accessed 28 May 2023].

16

Drugs Affecting the Cardiovascular System

KEY POINTS

- Diuretics stimulate excretion of water by the kidney and are classified according to site of action in the kidney tubule and their action on those membranes.
- Reduction in peripheral vascular resistance is an important strategy in treating hypertension, heart failure, and angina pectoris.
- Antihypertensive drugs include angiotensin converting enzyme (ACE) inhibitors, angiotensin II receptor blockers (ARBS), renin inhibitors, adrenergic receptor blockers, calcium channel blockers, vasodilators, diuretics, and centrally acting antihypertensive agents.
- Antiarrhythmic drugs act by blocking specific ion channels in the heart or by actions on autonomic receptors.
- Drugs for treating heart failure include angiotensin converting enzyme (ACE) inhibitors, angiotensin II receptor blockers, aldosterone antagonists, diuretics, digoxin, as well as other medications.
- Anticoagulant drugs inhibit important clotting factors, especially IIa (thrombin) and Xa.
- Antiplatelet drugs reduce blood clotting by preventing platelet aggregation and adhesion.

DEFINITIONS

- Cotransporter is a membrane protein able to move more than one ion or other substance at the same time.
- Hypokalemia is a lower-than-normal potassium level in the plasma.
- ACE is an acronym for angiotensin-converting enzyme.
- Angiotensinogen is converted to angiotensin I by the enzyme, renin.
- Angiotensins are proteins that increase blood pressure and promote aldosterone secretion from the adrenal cortex.
- Angioedema is an adverse vascular reaction resulting in edema, swelling, and giant wheals.
- Afterload is the load on the heart due to arterial resistance.
- Preload is the load on the heart from stretching of heart muscle due to return of venous blood to the heart.
- International normalized ratio (INR) is the standardized method of normalizing results of prothrombin time tests (PT) from various labs.

Diuretics

Introduction

The kidneys play a crucial role in regulation of fluids and electrolyte balance and excretion. Fluid is filtered through the glomerulus, and during the passage of fluid in the kidney tubule, about 99% of the fluid and solute is reabsorbed from the lumen of the tubules back into the systemic circulation. It is these processes of reabsorption that are the target of the diuretic drugs discussed below. More specifically, these diuretics block reabsorption of Na^+ and H_2O. Other ions are also affected by the diuretics, but the ability of a diuretic to increase the excretion of H_2O is dependent on the ability of these drugs to inhibit reuptake of Na^+ from the renal tubule.

Although diuretics are used to treat edema and other conditions, they are also useful medications for the treatment of hypertension and heart failure.

Classification of diuretics is based on their site of action in specific sections of the kidney tubule. Their action on reabsorption mechanisms accounts for their ability to increase urine flow.

Fig. 16.1 shows the target location of four diuretic drug classes, which include the loop diuretics, thiazide drugs, and potassium-sparing diuretics.

Loop Diuretics

The loop diuretics are the group of drugs that affect reabsorption in the long U-shaped portion of the kidney tubule (i.e., loop of Henle). Four common loop diuretics are **furosemide**, torsemide, bumetanide, and ethacrynic acid.

Mechanism of Action

Loop diuretics, also referred to as high ceiling diuretics, act at the thick ascending limb of the loop of Henle.

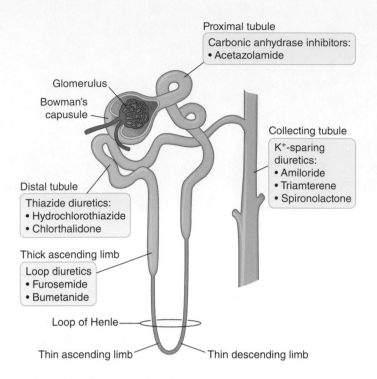

• **Fig. 16.1** Diuretics and Their Sites of Action Along the Nephron. (From Walsh EC, Seifter JL, Sloane DE. *Integrated Physiology and Pathophysiology.* Philadelphia: Elsevier; 2022. 1st ed.)

They block the **Na⁺, K⁺, 2Cl⁻ cotransporter** (NKCC2) (Fig. 16.2) by binding to the chloride binding site on this cotransporter. The net effect is to excrete more Na⁺, K⁺, and Cl⁻ in the urine. This mechanism leads to a large increase in urine volume. As Na⁺ increases in the downstream tubule fluid from the action of loop diuretics, K⁺ is prevented from being reabsorbed through the Na⁺/K⁺ exchange. This can lead to hypokalemia, necessitating correction using potassium supplementation or by coadministration of a potassium-sparing diuretic (see below).

Pharmacokinetics

The loop diuretics are metabolized in the liver but also depend on renal elimination. Each member of this class can be administered orally or parenterally. The loop diuretics have short half-lives in the range of 1 to 4 hours.

Adverse Effects

Due to their diuretic effects, the loop diuretics can cause hyponatremia, hypokalemia, and extracellular volume depletion. Hypomagnesemia can also occur. Other potential untoward effects can also occur in the central nervous system, including vertigo, tinnitus, and hearing loss.

Drug Interactions

The loop diuretics can cause ototoxicity and can enhance the ototoxicity of other drugs such as the aminoglycosides. Because the loop diuretics can cause hypokalemia, they can enhance the toxicity of digoxin. Corticosteroids may enhance the hypokalemia caused by loop diuretics. Nonsteroidal anti-inflammatory drugs may reduce the effects of loop diuretics.

Thiazide Diuretics

The thiazide class of diuretics reduce blood volume by acting on the kidney tubule (i.e., distal convoluted tubule). Five common thiazide diuretics include hydrochlorothiazide, chlorothiazide, chlorthalidone, bendroflumethiazide, and metolazone.

Mechanism of Action

The thiazide diuretics inhibit the Na⁺-Cl⁻ cotransporter in the distal convoluted tubule (see Fig. 16.2). This leads to an increased delivery of Na⁺ to distal segments and greater excretion of Na⁺ with diuresis. The increased delivery of Na⁺ to the downstream Na⁺/K⁺ exchange mechanism causes this to be a K⁺-losing diuretic.

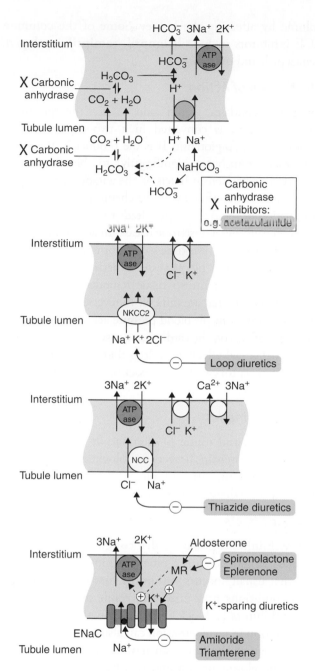

• **Fig. 16.2** Sites of Action of Diuretics. Osmotic diuretics increase osmotic pressure through the tubule, reducing electrolyte reabsorption across the luminal membrane. Other drugs gain access to their sites of action after secretion into the tubule by the organic anion transporters (OATs) in the proximal tubule. Acetazolamide inhibits carbonic anhydrase and is a weak, self-limiting diuretic, now largely used for other conditions such as glaucoma. Loop diuretics such as furosemide block the luminal $Na^+/K^+/2Cl^-$ co-transporter (NKCC2) and inhibit up to 20% to 25% of filtered Na^+ reabsorption. The thiazide diuretics inhibit the luminal Na^+/Cl^- co-transporter (NCC) and reduce reabsorption of 3% to 5% of filtered Na^+. The aldosterone antagonists spironolactone and eplerenone compete with aldosterone for the mineralocorticoid receptor (MR), blocking the induction by aldosterone of the expression and activity of the epithelial Na^+ channel (ENaC) and the basolateral Na^+/K^+-ATPase pump. Amiloride and triamterene act directly on ENaC to block Na^+ reabsorption. Potassium-sparing diuretics inhibit the reuptake of less than 2% of filtered Na^+. (Adapted from: Hitchings A, Sampson A, Waller DG. *Medical Pharmacology and Therapeutics*. London: Elsevier; 2022. 6th ed.)

TABLE 16.1 Thiazide Diuretics

Thiazide	Half-Life (h)	Site of Elimination
Chlorothiazide	1–2	Renal
Chlorthalidone[a]	35–50	Mostly renal
Bendroflumethiazide	8–9	Mostly hepatic
Hydrochlorothiazide	6–15	Renal
Metolazone[a]	14	Mostly renal

[a]Thiazide-like diuretics.

Pharmacokinetics

Table 16.1 lists five thiazide diuretics, their half-lives, and site of elimination.

Adverse Effects

Adverse effects of the thiazides include hypokalemia, hyperuricemia, hyponatremia, and volume depletion.

Drug-Drug Interactions

Hypokalemia caused by these diuretics increases the risk of toxicity from digoxin. Corticosteroids may enhance the hypokalemia caused by thiazides. Thiazides reduce the renal clearance of lithium which may result in lithium toxicity. Nonsteroidal anti-inflammatory drugs tend to reduce the effects of thiazide diuretics.

Potassium-Sparing Diuretics

Mechanism of Action

The potassium-sparing class of diuretics functions by altering the way kidney nephrons produce urine. Some of the more common potassium-sparing diuretics include spironolactone, amiloride, eplerenone, and triamterene.

The aldosterone antagonists, spironolactone and eplerenone, compete with aldosterone for the mineralocorticoid receptor (MR), blocking the induction by aldosterone of the expression and activity of the epithelial Na^+ channel (ENaC) and the basolateral Na^+/K^+-ATPase pump. Amiloride and triamterene act directly on ENaC to block Na^+ reabsorption. By blocking the entry of Na^+, the potassium-sparing diuretics prevent the release of K^+ into the lumen (see Fig. 16.2). Potassium-sparing diuretics inhibit the reuptake of less than 2% of filtered Na^+.

Pharmacokinetics

Amiloride is not metabolized and is solely dependent on the kidney for elimination. The other potassium-sparing diuretics undergo metabolism in the liver.

Adverse Effects

Spironolactone is also an antagonist at androgen receptors and can cause gynecomastia and decreased libido in males and menstrual irregularities in females. The other potassium-sparing diuretics do not have this adverse effect.

Drug-Drug Interactions

When used in the presence of an angiotensin-converting enzyme (ACE) inhibitor or an angiotensin II receptor blocker, hyperkalemia is a risk with any of the potassium-sparing diuretics.

Antihypertensive Drugs

Regulation of Blood Pressure

Pressure in a hydraulic system is the product of flow through the system and the resistance to such flow. The relationships between mean arterial blood pressure (MAP), cardiac output (CO), and total peripheral resistance (TPR) can be described in the following equation:

$$MAP = CO \times TPR$$

CO is determined by the load presented to the heart (venous return or preload) and the inotropic and chronotropic state of the myocardium. TPR depends on the diameter and compliance (stiffness) of the arterioles. These factors are regulated by the resting vascular smooth muscle tone, intrinsic reactivity of the vasculature, vasoactive substances in the blood, and sympathetic nervous system activity. Another important factor in the governance of blood pressure is the blood volume, which is regulated by the kidneys. Blood volume is reduced by **diuretics**.

Overview of Antihypertensive Drugs

There are various sites at which blood pressure can be potentially affected by targeted drug therapy (Fig. 16.3). The drugs more commonly used to treat hypertension are ACE inhibitors, angiotensin II receptor blockers, renin inhibitors, adrenergic receptor blockers, calcium channel blockers, vasodilators, and, to a lesser degree, centrally acting antihypertensive agents.

Angiotensin Converting Enzyme Inhibitors and Angiotensin II Receptor Blockers

ACE inhibitors are a class of antihypertensive drugs that cause relaxation of blood vessels and reduce blood volume by affecting the kidney. Some of the common ACE inhibitors include **lisinopril, ramipril, enalapril,** benazepril, and quinapril.

Mechanism of Action

By two peptidases, renin and ACE, the precursor, angiotensinogen, is converted in a two-step process to angiotensin II. Angiotensin II is the product in this pathway that contributes significantly to blood pressure (Fig. 16.4). Angiotensin II acts on the angiotensin$_1$ receptor (AT$_1$) (not to be confused with the chemical, angiotensin I). Stimulation of the AT$_1$ receptor leads to a rapid increase in blood pressure and aldosterone release. In addition, stimulation of this receptor over time has important chronic effects such as cardiac and blood vessel hypertrophy. These and other effects contribute to tissue remodeling that results in adverse effects that are difficult to reverse. The use of an ACE inhibitor controls blood pressure acutely, but also the long-term effects on the cardiovascular system.

The beneficial effects of a drug that blocks the angiotensin II receptors (AT$_1$) are essentially the same as an ACE inhibitor.

Pharmacokinetics

The half-lives and routes of elimination of ACE inhibitors and angiotensin II receptor blockers (ARBS) vary depending on the drug (Table 16.2). (ACE inhibitors end in "pril," whereas ARBS end in "sartan.")

Adverse Effects

The ACE inhibitors cause a **dry cough** in up to 20% of patients. Angioedema is a rarer but more serious condition that usually occurs within the first days of therapy. Both conditions may arise as a result of the ability of ACE inhibitors to block the breakdown of bradykinin. An alteration in taste sensation can also occur. Given during pregnancy, the fetus can have significant defects in kidney development and may die. For this reason, ACE inhibitors are **contraindicated in pregnancy**.

ARBS are not associated with cough and angioedema because they do not affect the bradykinin pathway. ARBS should not be given during pregnancy.

Drug-Drug Interactions

ACE inhibitors and ARBS should be used with caution with other drugs that may cause an increase in potassium plasma concentrations. These include potassium-sparing diuretics. Hyperkalemia may result.

Inhibitors of Renin

Aliskiren is an inhibitor of renin and therefore interrupts the renin-angiotensin pathway (Fig. 16.3). It is similar to

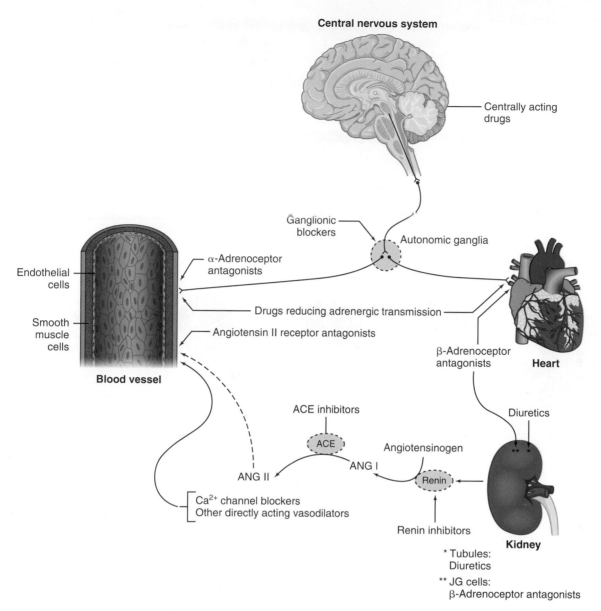

• **Fig. 16.3** Sites of Action of Antihypertensive Drugs. The diagram indicates by drug class the targets for antihypertensive action. *ACE,* Angiotensin-converting enzyme; *ANG,* Angiotensin; *JG,* juxtaglomerular.

TABLE 16.2	Elimination Characteristics of Some Angiotensin-Converting Enzyme Inhibitors and Angiotensin II Receptor Blockers	
Drug	**Elimination Half-Time (h)**	**Elimination Route**
Captopril	2	Metabolism and renal
Enalapril	11	Mostly renal
Lisinopril	12	Only renal
Trandolapril	20	Biliary excretion and renal
Losartan	4	Metabolism, renal, biliary
Valsartan	6	Mostly biliary excretion
Eprosartan	6	Biliary and renal
Telmisartan	24	Biliary excretion

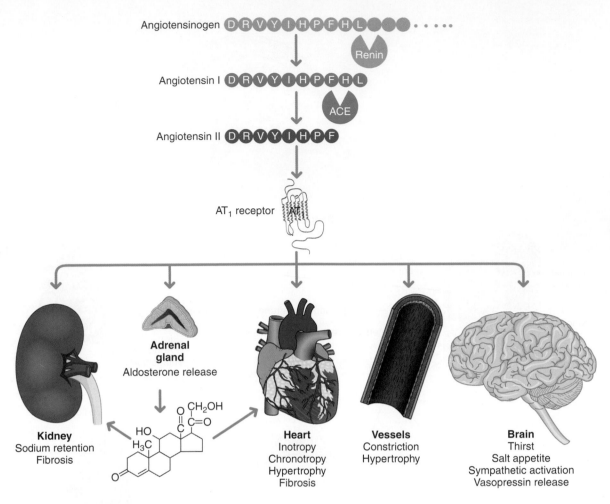

• **Fig. 16.4** Classical Renin-Angiotensin-Aldosterone System. Angiotensin expressed in the liver is cleaved by renin from the kidney to release angiotensin I in plasma. Angiotensin converting enzyme *(ACE)* on endothelial cells catalyzes the conversion of angiotensin I to angiotensin II. Angiotensin II binds to angiotensin II receptors *(AT₁)* in the organs and tissue shown, leading to the effects listed.

ACE inhibitors and ARBS in its antihypertensive effects. Its adverse effects are similar to those of ARBS.

β-Adrenergic Receptor Blockers

The β-blockers are discussed in Chapter 8. **Metoprolol and atenolol** are two β-blockers that are commonly used. Regarding hypertensin, they are valuable drugs and work by more than one mechanism to lower blood pressure. By blocking β-adrenergic receptors, they inhibit the release of renin from the kidney (Fig. 16.3). They also reduce cardiac output. Central sympathetic output can also be reduced. Other mechanisms may occur as well.

α₁-Adrenergic Receptor Blockers

The α₁-adrenergic receptor blockers block the sympathetic effect on blood vessels (Fig. 16.3). **Prazosin, terazosin,** and **doxazosin** are commonly used. Blood pressure is lowered by a decrease in peripheral resistance.

Although adverse effects of α-blockers are discussed in Chapter 8, one should be emphasized here. The **first dose effect** refers to the sensitive drop in blood pressure at the start of therapy. This hypotensive effect wanes as therapy continues and it can be avoided by starting therapy with lower than maintenance doses.

Other Adrenergic Receptor Blockers

The mechanisms of action of adrenergic receptor blockers with multiple actions and used to treat hypertension are listed in Table 16.3.

Calcium Channel Blockers

Calcium channel blockers are a class of drugs that lower blood pressure by preventing calcium from entering cells of the heart and arteries. Some common calcium channel blockers include **nifedipine**, amlodipine, diltiazem, felodipine, and verapamil.

TABLE 16.3   **Characteristics of Three Receptor Blocking Drugs With Unique Mechanisms**

Drug	Blocks α_1-Adrenergic Receptors	Blocks β- Adrenergic Receptors	Other Action
Labetalol	Yes	Yes	
Carvedilol	Yes	Yes	
Nebivolol	No	Yes	Releases nitric oxide in blood vessels

Mechanism of Action

The antihypertensive effect of calcium channel blockers is due to their ability to block influx of calcium through L-type calcium channels in blood vessels. Calcium channel blockers can be divided into two groups: those that have near equal effect on blood vessel calcium channels, and cardiac calcium channels (for example, verapamil and diltiazem). The second group have greater effect on vascular smooth muscle calcium channels compared to heart calcium channels. These are represented by nifedipine, a dihydropyridine. Nifedipine-like drugs are the calcium channel blockers that are used to treat hypertension

The first group of calcium channel blockers (above) is used for their cardiac effect, making them useful for treating angina pectoris.

The nifedipine-like drugs lower blood pressure by causing vasodilation without as much effect on the heart (Fig. 16.5).

Pharmacokinetics

Calcium channel blockers are extensively metabolized and elimination half-times for these drugs vary dramatically (Table 16.4).

For chronic therapy, extended-release preparations of short half-life drugs are used. This is to avoid large fluctuations in plasma levels of these drugs. Therefore, calcium channel blockers with long half-lives or extended-release preparations are used for chronic treatment of hypertension.

Adverse Effects

Therapy with calcium channel blockers in which there are large fluctuations in plasma levels is associated with an increased risk of myocardial infarction, necessitating a more constant blood level of the drug. Calcium channel blockers can cause coronary steal in patients with angina. This is due to shifting of blood away from ischemic vessels in the heart due to vasodilation. The nifedipine-drugs can cause reflex tachycardia, unlike verapamil and diltiazem which are not associated with this effect. Flushing, dizziness, and nausea may occur with any of the calcium blockers. In the mouth, the calcium channel blockers have also been implicated in causing enlargement of gingival tissues.

Drug-Drug Interactions

Inducers of **cytochrome P450 enzymes** may decrease plasma levels of nifedipine-like drugs. Inhibitors of cytochrome P450 enzymes may increase plasma levels of nifedipine-like drugs.

Other Vasodilators

There are numerous drugs that act on blood vessels (see Fig. 16.5). Table 16.5 gives a brief summary of the other drugs that have special indications for vasodilation.

Centrally Acting Antihypertensive Drugs

These drugs stimulate α_2-adrenergic receptors in the central nervous system resulting in a reduction in sympathetic outflow from the central nervous system and decreased vascular resistance. **Clonidine**, methyl dopa, guanabenz, and guanfacine are members of this class. They are seldom used. Clonidine can cause dry mouth. These drugs may cause rebound hypertension if withdrawn too rapidly.

Antiarrhythmic Drugs

Introduction

A properly functioning heart requires a coordinated process of heart contraction. This is dependent on the cells in each section of the heart depolarizing and repolarizing at precise intervals. These electrical properties are dependent on the action of ion channels, including channels for Na^+, K^+, and Ca^{2+}. Autonomic input is another related factor. The action on ion channels and autonomic receptors is a basis for the action of antiarrhythmic drugs. Drug therapy is often required to correct or control abnormal

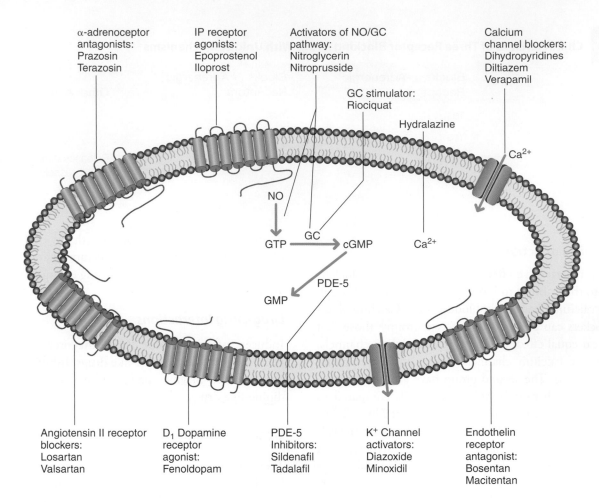

α-adrenoceptor
antagonists:
Prazosin
Terazosin

IP receptor
agonists:
Epoprostenol
Iloprost

Activators of NO/GC
pathway:
Nitroglycerin
Nitroprusside

Calcium
channel blockers:
Dihydropyridines
Diltiazem
Verapamil

GC stimulator:
Riociquat

Hydralazine

Ca²⁺

NO

GC

GTP → cGMP   Ca²⁺

PDE-5

GMP

Angiotensin II receptor
blockers:
Losartan
Valsartan

D₁ Dopamine
receptor
agonist:
Fenoldopam

PDE-5
Inhibitors:
Sildenafil
Tadalafil

K⁺ Channel
activators:
Diazoxide
Minoxidil

Endothelin
receptor
antagonist:
Bosentan
Macitentan

• **Fig. 16.5** Sites of Action of Drugs That Relax Vascular Smooth Muscle. Various drug types that act on the vascular smooth muscle cell are depicted. Individual drug examples are given with each drug class. Drugs shown in red are drugs that are typically used in chronic therapy. The others are used in hypertensive emergencies, refractory cases, or in pulmonary hypertension. Hydralazine inhibits the release of intracellular calcium. *cGMP,* Cyclic guanosine monophosphate; *GC,* guanylyl cyclase; *GMP,* guanosine monophosphate; *GTP,* guanosine triphosphate; *IP,* prostacyclin; *NO,* nitric oxide; *PDE-5,* phosphodiesterase-5.

TABLE 16.4	Five Calcium Channel Blockers and Their Elimination Half-Times	
Drug	**Elimination Half-Time (h)**	
Nifedipine	2	
Nimodipine	1.5	
Felodipine	13	
Nisoldipine	10	
Amlodipine	40	

electrical properties in various disorders. Classification of antiarrhythmic drugs has been based on these actions.

Fig. 16.6 is an image of the electrocardiogram. Segment intervals and configuration of ECG tracings are helpful in determining abnormalities as well as effects of drugs. It is important to remember that the ECG is not a tracing of the electrical activity of a single heart cell but rather the summation of the electrical activities of the whole heart. These two electrical perspectives are compared in Fig. 16.7. Membrane action potentials are positioned to correspond to the ECG tracing.

Individual cell action potentials are composed of phases as shown in Fig. 16.8. Fig. 16.8A, the SA node action potential corresponds to the "P" wave on the ECG tracing in Fig. 16.8C. The ventricular action potential in Fig. 16.8C corresponds to the "QRS" complex on the ECG, followed by the "T" wave on the ECG in Fig. 16.8C. The Purkinje fiber action potential also contributes in a manner similar to the ventricular action potential on the ECG. The five phases, 0, 1, 2, 3, and 4, are shown in Fig. 16.9 representing individual cells in the sinoatrial (SA) node, Purkinje fibers, and ventricular myocardium. The ion currents responsible for each phase are identified. The effects of antiarrhythmic drugs on action potentials are shown in Fig. 16.9.

TABLE 16.5	Summary of Pharmacology of Drugs Shown in Fig. 16.5	
Drug	**Vasodilator Mechanism**	**Comment**
Hydralazine	May inhibit calcium release or increase nitric oxide (NO)	Acts selectively on arteries, may cause palpitations, flushing, lupus erythematosus
Nitroglycerin	Generates NO	Leads to increase in cGMP, short-term use
Nitroprusside	Generates NO	For hypertensive emergencies
Diazoxide	Activates potassium channels	For hypertensive emergencies
Sildenafil	Inhibits PDE-5	Useful in pulmonary hypertension
Fenoldopam	Stimulate D_1 dopamine receptors	For hypertensive emergencies, has short action
Epoprostenol	Stimulates IP receptor	Useful in pulmonary hypertension

cGMP, Cyclic guanosine monophosphate; *IP*, prostacyclin; *PDE*, phosphodiesterase.

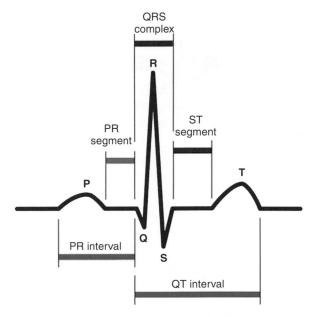

• **Fig. 16.6** Normal Electrocardiogram. The P wave corresponds with atrial depolarization; the QRS complex corresponds with ventricular depolarization; the T wave corresponds with ventricular repolarization. The atrial repolarization is "lost" in the QRS complex. The PR segment is the pause at the atrioventricular node to allow ventricular filling with blood. The ST segment corresponds to phase 1 and 2 (refractory period) of the ventricular myocardium. (From Workman ML, LaCharity LA. Understanding Pharmacology: Essentials for Medication Safety. St. Louis: Saunders; 2016. 2nd ed.)

The phases of each action potential account for certain characteristics of each cardiac cell.

Phase 0: The slope of this phase indicates the degree of conduction velocity in that cell.

Distance between Phase 0 and Phase 3 of the ventricle: This is directly proportional to the refractory period in those cells.

Phase 4: A slope in phase 4 indicates the degree of automaticity of the cell.

Mechanism of Action

The action of antiarrhythmics involves the **blockade** of one or more **ion channel** or **receptor**. Table 16.6 indicates the major ion channel or receptor blocked for each drug class.

The effects of antiarrhythmic drugs on each segment of the heart are displayed in Fig. 16.9 resulting from the mechanisms in Table 16.6.

In Fig. 16.9A, slowing of the heart rate due to reduced automaticity of the SA node is shown. Fig. 16.9B shows major drugs that slow atrioventricular (AV node) conduction. In Fig. 16.9C, abnormal automaticity in Purkinje can be inhibited by lidocaine and the β-blockers. Fig. 16.9D shows the effect of IA drugs and lidocaine (IB) on the ventricular action potential. Fig. 16.9E shows the effect of class IC and class III drugs on the ventricular action potential.

Since these drugs are used to treat tachyarrhythmias (rapid rhythms), the benefit of the drugs is to **reduce automaticity, slow conduction rate, or increase the refractory period** by increasing the action potential duration.

Atrial fibrillation and ventricular tachycardia are two examples of disorders treated with antiarrhythmic drugs.

Adverse Effects

The adverse actions of antiarrhythmic drugs depend on the agent and the length of time it is used (Table 16.7).

Drug-Drug Interactions

Amiodarone, by inhibiting cytochrome CYP2D6, may decrease the therapeutic effect of codeine, hydrocodone, and tramadol. Amiodarone may inhibit the metabolism of warfarin and thereby increase the effect of warfarin.

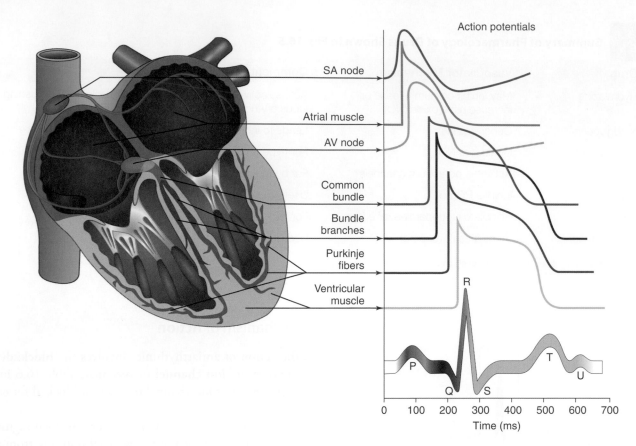

• **Fig. 16.7** Characteristic membrane action potentials from a sinoatrial *(SA)* nodal cell *(top)* down to ventricular myocardium *(bottom)*. The differences between leaky phase 4 s and rapid versus slower phase 0 s can easily be seen. Note that the atrioventricular node resembles the SA node because it can assume the pacemaking functions of the heart should the SA node become damaged. All of the action potentials are related to the various phases of the ECG in the lower part of the figure.

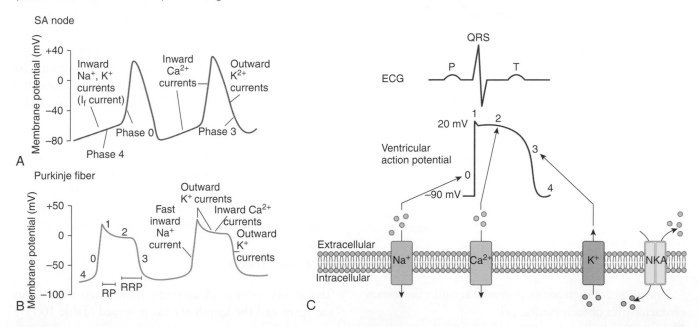

• **Fig. 16.8** A Comparison of the "Leaky" Sinoatrial (SA) Node (A) and the Action Potential of a Ventricular Myocyte. In the SA node, phase 4 is leaky and allows slow depolarization until the firing threshold is reached. There is then a more rapid depolarization (phase 0) and a nebulous phase 1 and 2. Phase 3 is repolarization. In comparison, these phases are much more defined in the Purkinje fiber (B) and ventricular myocardium (C) and demonstrate a clear refractory period (phases 1 and 2 and part of 3). Conduction velocity is directly related to the slope of phase 0, and the refractory period is directly related to the duration of the action potential. Note that in the SA (and atrioventricular [AV]) node, phase 0 is slower than in the Purkinje fibers and ventricular myocardium because phase 0 in the SA and AV nodes primarily depends on Ca^{2+} influx. In C, the temporal relationship between the electrocardiogram tracing and the ventricular action potential is shown, as well as important ion conductances for the ventricular action potential. NKA, Na^+, K^+-ATPase pump. (A and B, Modified from Waller DG, Sampson, AP, Hitchings A. *Medical Pharmacology and Therapeutics*. 4th ed. St. Louis: Saunders; 2014; C, From Goldman L, Schafer AI. *Goldman-Cecil Medicine*. 25th ed. Philadelphia: Elsevier; 2016.)

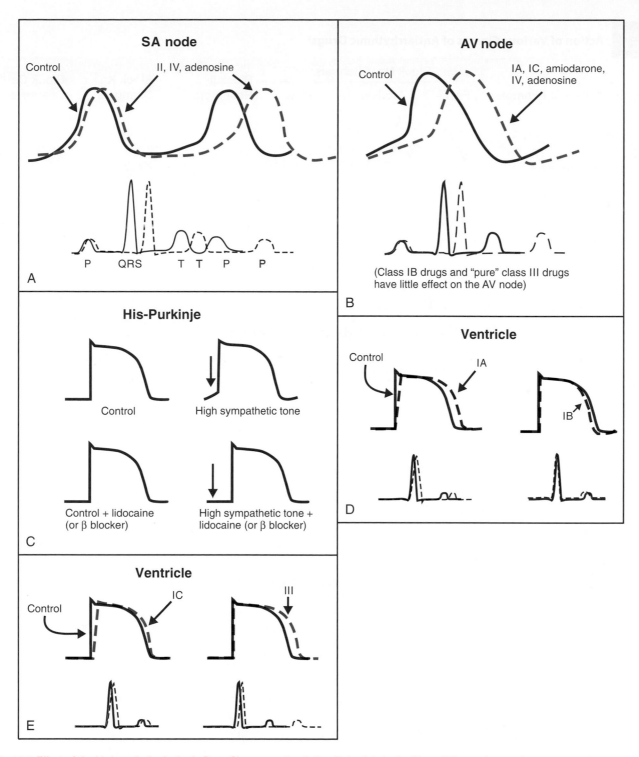

• **Fig. 16.9** Effect of the Various Antiarrhythmic Drug Classes on the Action Potentials in the Heart. Where relevant, the corresponding electrocardiogram (ECG) pattern is also shown. Omitted drug classes have less effect on the action potentials depicted. The changes shown do not imply the same magnitude of change for each drug class. Amiodarone is specifically identified because, although it is classified as a class III drug, it has additional actions. (A) Sinoatrial node. Note the delay in appearance of the QRS complex, T wave, and subsequent P wave caused by the identified drugs. (B) Atrioventricular node. Various drugs delay conduction through the node with certain drugs. (C) His-Purkinje system. Active drugs reduce phase 4 depolarization *(arrows)*. (D) and (E), Ventricular muscle. In D, class IB drugs minimally alter the ECG pattern in normal cardiac rhythms. *AV,* Atrioventricular; *SA,* sinoatrial.

Drugs Used to Treat Heart Failure

Heart failure is characterized by a decreased ability of the heart to pump blood in adequate amounts. It may be due to an underlying heart disorder and/or excessive load placed on the heart. Diseases contributing to heart failure include hypertension, valvular abnormalities, and myocardial infarction. Initial therapy for heart failure involves

TABLE 16.6   Action of Various Classes of Antiarrhythmic Drugs[a]

Drug Class and Examples	Block Na⁺ Channels			Block β-Receptors	Block K⁺ Channels	Block Ca⁺⁺ Channels
	Fast	Medium	Slow			
IA Procainamide		√				
IB Lidocaine, mexiletine	√					
IC flecainide			√			
II Metoprolol				√		
III Amiodarone, Dofetilide					√	
IV Verapamil, Diltiazem						√
Adenosine[b]	Adenosine stimulates adenosine A₁ in the heart.					

[a]The distinguishing characteristics for the main classes of antiarrhythmic drugs are the following: class I drugs block Na⁺ channels. The subclassification is based on the characteristics of the block. The terms *slow, medium*, and *fast* refer to the rates of onset of, and recovery from, Na⁺ channel blockade. Class II drugs block β-adrenergic receptors. Class III drugs block K⁺ channels. Class IV drugs block Ca²⁺ channels. This table only shows the major action of the drugs. Most drugs have more than one action.
[b]Adenosine has a very short duration of action.

TABLE 16.7   Notable Adverse Effects of Antiarrhythmic Drugs

Drug	Adverse Effects
Procainamide	Mental changes, *Torsades de pointes*[a] Lupus erythematosus[b]
Lidocaine	Convulsions
Flecainide	Cardiac risk with recent myocardial infarction
Metoprolol	See β-blockers
Amiodarone	Pulmonary fibrosis, thyroid abnormalities, skin discolorations, corneal deposits, peripheral neuropathy
Verapamil, diltiazem	Flushing, gingival hyperplasia, AV node conduction defects, reduced contractility of the heart
Adenosine[b]	Flushing, asthma, dyspnea, SA nodal arrest, AV nodal block

[a]A tachyarrhythmia preceded by a long QT interval.
[b]The ultrashort duration of adenosine reduces the severity of the adverse effects.
AV, Atrioventricular; *SA*, sinoatrial.

control of underlying causes such as hypertension and coronary artery disease, eliminating smoking, restricting sodium intake, improving diet, and appropriate exercise.

Drug therapy is aimed at **reducing the load on the heart and/or improving cardiac contractility**. Drug therapy is aimed at improving the pumping efficiency of the heart and to reduce remodeling of the heart. Over time remodeling involves fibrosis and cardiac hypertrophy which worsen heart failure.

Overview of Drugs

The drugs used to treat chronic heart failure have wide ranges in their mechanisms of action (Table 16.8). The only two that target the heart itself are digoxin and ivabradine.

Angiotensin-Converting Enzyme Inhibitors and Angiotensin II Receptor Blockers

The pharmacology of these drugs is discussed with the antihypertensive drugs above.

β-Blockers

With careful dosing, β-blockers can have beneficial effects (see Table 16.8) without depressing the heart (negative inotropy).

Aldosterone Antagonists

The potassium-sparing diuretic effect of spironolactone and eplerenone account for only part of the beneficial effects of these drugs (see Table 16.8).

TABLE 16.8	Drug Treatment of Chronic Heart Failure
Drug or Drug Class	**Mechanism**
Angiotensin converting enzyme inhibitors	Reduce effect of angiotensin II, reduce load on the heart, reduce remodeling
Angiotensin II receptor blockers	Reduce effect of angiotensin II, reduce load on the heart, reduce remodeling
β-blockers	Reduce sympathetic effect on heart, prevent arrhythmias, reduce remodeling
Aldosterone antagonists (spironolactone, eplerenone)	Inhibit Na$^+$ and water retention, reduce K$^+$ loss, reduce sympathetic activation, reduce baroreceptor reflex, reduce ischemia, reduce cardiac fibrosis
Loop and thiazide diuretics	Reduce fluid volume, reduce load on the heart
Hydralazine/ isosorbide dinitrate	Reduce afterload and preload
Digoxin	Direct cardiotonic effect
Ivabradine	Inhibits cardiac pacemaker current reducing heart rate and heart rate variability
Sacubitril (combined with valsartan)	Sacubitril inhibits the enzyme, neprilysin, leading to an increase in natriuretic peptides. (result = vasodilation, increased renal blood flow and natriuresis)

Hydralazine/Isosorbide Dinitrate

Hydralazine is presented in the section on hypertension. It may block Ca^{2+} release and/or generate nitric oxide (NO) inside blood vessels, leading to vasodilation. It acts selectively on arterioles. Hydralazine therefore reduces afterload and reduces vascular resistance on the arteriole side. Isosorbide nitrate reduces preload which is the stretch of the heart due to venous return. It also reduces afterload at higher doses. Nitrates are discussed in the section on antianginal drugs.

Digoxin

Digoxin is a steroid glycoside and a potent compound found in the foxglove plant. In small doses it is used as a cardiac stimulant.

Mechanism of Action

Digoxin is the main example of a cardiac glycoside. It increases the force of contraction of the heart (positive inotropy). It is a specific inhibitor of the sodium/potassium pump (Na^+, K^+- ATPase). Inhibition of this enzyme leads to an increase in intracellular sodium. This in turn reduces Na^+-Ca^{2+} exchange at the cell membrane resulting in more calcium at the contractile apparatus of heart muscle and greater force of contraction.

Pharmacokinetics

Digoxin is usually given orally. It is excreted in the kidney largely without metabolism. The half-life of digoxin is about 36 hours.

Adverse Effects

Digoxin has a very low therapeutic index. (The toxic dose is close to the therapeutic dose.) Toxicity is therefore is more likely to occur with this drug.

Anorexia, nausea, and vomiting may occur, as well as dizziness, mental changes, and visual disturbances. Cardiac toxicity is of special concern. Heart block may occur because of slowing of the AV nodal conduction rate. Ventricular tachyarrhythmias may occur due to increased automaticity of Purkinje fibers and a decrease in the refractory period of the myocardium. Ventricular fibrillation may occur.

Drug-Drug Interactions

Any drug that can cause hypokalemia, such as several diuretics, can enhance the toxicity of digoxin. Certain antibiotics may increase the amount of digoxin that is absorbed orally. Sympathetic drugs may enhance the toxic effects of digoxin, whereas antimuscarinic drugs may inhibit certain cardiac effects of digoxin.

Ivabradine

Mechanism of Action

Ivabradine is a hyperpolarization-activated, cyclic nucleotide-gated (HCN) channel blocker with a negative effect on heart rate. Ivabradine has the ability to slow the heart rate by inhibiting pacemaker current (see Table 16.8). This slows the rate of phase 4 depolarization.

Pharmacokinetics

Ivabradine is absorbed orally and is metabolized in the liver. The combined half-life of ivabradine and its metabolites is about 6 hours.

Adverse Effects

Bradycardia (slowing of the heart), fetal toxicity, and phosphenes (i.e., bright visual flashes) are some of the side effects.

Drug-Drug Interactions

Drugs that cause bradycardia will enhance the effects of ivabradine.

Sacubitril

Mechanism of Action

Sacubitril inhibits the enzyme, neprilysin. The inhibition of neprilysin leads to an increase in atrial natriuretic peptide and other peptides that cause natriuresis and vasodilation. Since sacubitril is **combined with valsartan**, the combination has a dual effect in reducing the load on the heart.

Pharmacokinetics

Sacubitril is absorbed orally and metabolized by esterases in the plasma. The half-life of the combined sacubitril and its metabolite is about 11 hours. This is similar to the half-life of valsartan.

Adverse Effects

Hypotension can occur.

Drug-Drug Interactions

Most drug-drug interactions occur as a result of the valsartan component in the combined medication, (sacubitril/valsartan) (Entresto).

Antianginal Drugs

Anginal pectoris pain occurs when coronary arteries cannot supply sufficient oxygen to the myocardium to meet the workload of the heart. Vasodilation of coronary blood vessels adapts to increased demands. However, when coronary artery sclerosis occurs, these vessels are unable to adapt to the increase in energy needs. This description is typical of classic (chronic stable, exertional) angina.

The three major drug groups used to treat angina are organic nitrites and nitrates, calcium blockers, and β-adrenergic receptor blockers (Fig. 16.10).

Organic Nitrites and Nitrates

Nitroglycerin is commonly used for acute attacks and sustained release forms are available to counter the very short duration of action of the drug. Other organic nitrates used to treat angina are **isosorbide dinitrate** and isosorbide mononitrate. Amyl nitrate is available as an inhalant.

Mechanism of Action

These drugs generate nitric oxide, which then leads to the production of cyclic guanosine monophosphate (cGMP). Relaxation of vascular smooth muscle occurs. Relaxation occurs in coronary vessels as well as peripheral vessels. The latter effect reduces both preload and afterload.

Pharmacokinetics

Sublingual nitroglycerin is highly effective for the treatment of acute anginal episodes. A transdermal patch is available. It releases nitroglycerin over 24 hours. Nitroglycerin used as an ointment is applied every 3 to 4 hours. Metabolism takes place in the liver. The metabolites are excreted by the kidney.

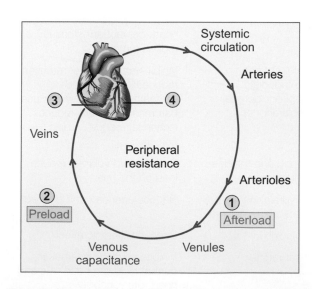

• **Fig. 16.10** Sites of Action of Antianginal Drugs. Site 1: reduce afterload—calcium channel blockers (CCB), beta blockers, nitrates. Site 2: reduce preload—nitrates. Site 3: negative inotropic action—beta blockers, CCB (verapamil and diltiazem). Site 4: coronary dilators—nitrates and CCB. (From Satoskar RS, Tripathi RK, Rege NN, et al. *Pharmacology and Pharmacotherapeutics*. New Delhi: Elsevier; 2021. 26th ed.)

Adverse Effects

The nitrates and nitrites cause hypotension and a reflex tachycardia that can be pronounced. β- Blockers are often given concurrently with these vasodilators to reduce this response. Flushing and syncope can also occur.

Nitrites and nitrates can cause methemoglobinemia.

Drug-Drug Interactions

Other vasodilators can augment the hypotension and reflex tachycardia resulting from the nitrites and nitrates.

Calcium channel blockers and β-blockers are discussed in the section on antihypertensive drugs. β-Blockers are also discussed in Chapter 8. Atenolol and metoprolol are commonly used β-blockers for treating angina. Verapamil, diltiazem, and nifedipine-like drugs are calcium channel blockers that can be used in angina.

Anticoagulant, Antiplatelet Drugs, Fibrinolytic Drugs, and Antifibrinolytic Drugs

Blood Coagulation Pathways

Drugs that reduce blood coagulation are used for a number of reasons. These include prevention of an occlusive stroke and to reduce the risk of coronary artery clotting. This section will concentrate on drugs that inhibit clotting at sites along the coagulation pathway, as well as drugs that reduce the aggregation and adhesion of platelets. Table 16.9 lists the factors, by number, in the coagulation pathway and the alternative names for each factor.

Fig. 16.11 shows the flow chart for blood coagulation.

Heparin

Mechanism of Action

Heparin is a mixture of linear sulfated mucopolysaccharides. It binds to antithrombin III (ATIII). ATIII is an anticoagulant whose effect is enhanced 1000-fold in the presence of heparin. This accounts for its ability to inhibit factors IIa and Xa (Fig. 16.11). The "a" refers to an activated factor. For instance, factor II refers to prothrombin, whereas factor IIa refers to thrombin. Inhibition of the coagulation cascade at a point along the pathway will eventually reduce fibrin formation and reduce clotting. Heparin -ATIII also inhibits some other clotting factors.

In addition to the original unfractionated heparin, newer fractionated heparins have become available. These are smaller molecules and these do not have the broad

TABLE 16.9	Blood Clotting Factors
Factor	**Alternative Names**
I	Fibrinogen
II	Prothrombin
III	Tissue factor, thromboplastin
IV	Calcium
V	Proaccelerin
VII	Proconvertin
VIII	Antihemophilic factor A (AHF A)
IX	Antihemophilic factor B (AHF B), Christmas factor
X	Stuart-Prower factor
XI	Plasma thromboplastin antecedent
XII	Hageman factor
XIII	Fibrin stabilizing factor

Thrombin is factor IIa. Factor VI has been abandoned.

capability that the unfractionated heparin do, but are effective anticoagulants in many clinical settings. They are more selective for factor Xa. The unfractionated heparins include: **tinzaparin, enoxaparin,** and **dalteparin**.

Pharmacokinetics

The heparins have to be injected to avoid destruction in the GI tract. Unfractionated heparin is given by IV or subcutaneous administration. The fractionated heparins (low molecular weight heparins) are used subcutaneously and excreted in the kidney. Unfractionated heparin is removed through the liver. Half-lives range from about 1 to 5 hours for fractionated and unfractionated drugs. These drugs are usually given over a short time period.

Adverse Effects

Bleeding is an obvious adverse effect. Allergic reactions can occur. An immune response can occur to the heparin-ATIII complex which can lead to thrombocytopenia. Osteoporosis and hair loss have been reported. These adverse effects are not as likely to occur with the low molecular weight heparins. Toxicity due to heparins is treated with protamine, which is a chemical antagonist, reacting directly with heparins.

Drug-Drug Interactions

Bleeding is more likely when used with other anticoagulants.

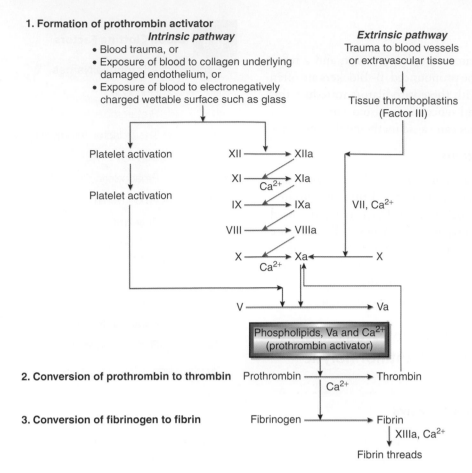

1. Formation of prothrombin activator

Intrinsic pathway
- Blood trauma, or
- Exposure of blood to collagen underlying damaged endothelium, or
- Exposure of blood to electronegatively charged wettable surface such as glass

Extrinsic pathway
Trauma to blood vessels or extravascular tissue

Tissue thromboplastins (Factor III)

Platelet activation   XII ⟶ XIIa

Platelet activation   XI ⟶ XIa   Ca²⁺

IX ⟶ IXa   VII, Ca²⁺

VIII ⟶ VIIIa

X ⟶ Xa ⟵ X   Ca²⁺

V ⟶ Va

Phospholipids, Va and Ca²⁺ (prothrombin activator)

2. Conversion of prothrombin to thrombin   Prothrombin ⟶ Thrombin   Ca²⁺

3. Conversion of fibrinogen to fibrin   Fibrinogen ⟶ Fibrin   XIIIa, Ca²⁺

Fibrin threads

• **Fig. 16.11** The blood coagulation cascade. Factors IIa (thrombin) and Xa are important sites of drug action. (Modified from Kowlgi NG, Khurana A, Khurana I. *Textbook of Medical Physiology*. 2020. 3rd ed.)

Fondaparinux

Fondaparinux is a synthetic inhibitor of factor Xa. More specifically, fondaparinux binds to and activates ATIII and this complex inhibits factor Xa (see Fig. 16.11). The drug is given subcutaneously and is excreted unchanged in the kidney. Its half-life is about 20 hours.

Oral Direct Factor Xa Inhibitors ("Xaban" Drugs)

Xabans are direct factor Xa inhibitors. Common examples of this class of anticoagulants include apixaban and rivaroxaban.

Mechanism of Action

This group of drugs, represented by **apixaban** and **rivaroxaban**, directly inhibits factor Xa, thereby preventing the conversion of prothrombin to thrombin (see Fig. 16.11). The oral effectiveness makes them very useful for chronic therapy and treatment does not require monitoring as is the case with warfarin (see below).

Pharmacokinetics

The drugs are all effective orally. The half-life of apixaban is approximately 12 hours and that of rivaroxaban is approximately 5 to 9 hours. Both drugs undergo metabolism in the liver by cytochrome P450 3A4. Most of the drug gets metabolized with some unmetabolized drug removed through the kidney.

Adverse Effects

Bleeding is the most likely adverse effect. Less common adverse effects include thrombocytopenia and hypotension. Inappropriate sudden withdrawal of a "xaban" drug can lead to thrombosis.

Although not commonly used, andexanet alfa, a factor Xa decoy, can be used as an antidote in life-threatening bleeding.

Drug-Drug Interactions

Other anticoagulants will enhance the adverse bleeding effects of the "xabans." Drugs that increase or decrease the activity of CYP450 3A4 enzymes will likely decrease or increase, respectively, the effect of the "xabans."

Dabigatran

Dabigatran is an oral drug that directly inhibits thrombin. The prodrug, a dabigatran etexilate ester, is converted to active dabigatran after GI absorption. After metabolism to metabolites, which have near equal anticoagulant activity, dabigatran and its metabolites are excreted in the urine.

Warfarin

Mechanism of Action

Warfarin is an anticoagulant that acts differently from the drugs discussed above, in that warfarin inhibits the **synthesis** of 4 clotting factors shown in Fig. 16.11. The synthesis of factors II (prothrombin), VII, IX, and X is inhibited in their final steps (Fig. 16.12). Measurement of the effect of warfarin is monitored using the **prothrombin time (PT)** test. The results of the PT tests are normalized between labs by converting them to the **International normalized ratio (INR)**.

Pharmacokinetics

Warfarin is an oral drug that has about a 36-hour half-life. Withdrawal of the drug results in a long delay in the return to normal clotting for two reasons. First the drug has a long half-life and second, levels of clotting factors are dependent on resynthesis of these factors. The indirect action of warfarin, and its dependence on inhibiting clotting factor synthesis, pose a disadvantage compared to other oral drugs, such as the "xabans." Warfarin is almost completely metabolized.

Adverse Effects

Bleeding is the major risk and it is complicated by the slow reversal of warfarin's effects. Since warfarin is a competitive inhibitor of vitamin K, vitamin K can be used to prevent episodes of bleeding, however this does not represent a rapid reversal. Clotting factor infusions are a more rapid means of reversal of excessive bleeding; however these are not usually needed. Warfarin monitoring on a continual basis is needed because of the difficulty in controlling warfarin plasma levels.

Drug-Drug Interactions

Drugs that increase or decrease the liver cytochrome metabolism of warfarin likely will lead to the decrease

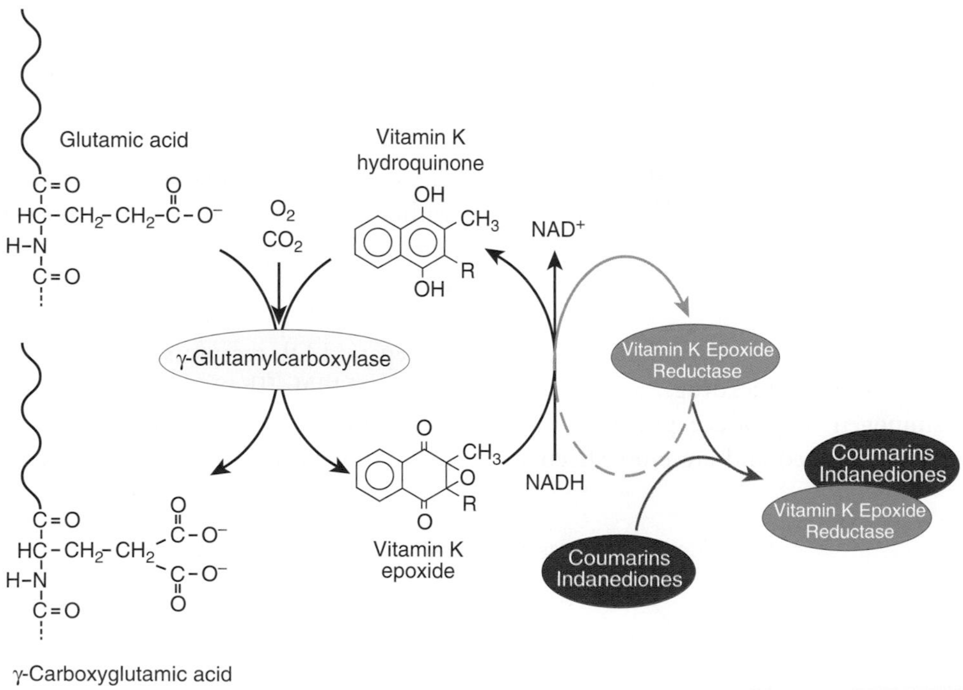

• **Fig. 16.12** Inhibition of synthesis of vitamin K–dependent clotting factors by warfarin and similar anticoagulants (brown oval). In the final post-translational modification of factors II (prothrombin), factor VII, factor IX, and factor X, vitamin K is oxidized to the epoxide in the process of carboxylating glutamic acid residues on the amino end of each protein. The resultant γ-carboxyglutamic acid groups serve to chelate Ca^{2+} ions and conformationally change to expose a hydrophobic domain that settles into phospholipid membranes, anchoring the factors for normal hemostasis. Warfarin, a coumarin, prevents the restoration of vitamin K by competitively inhibiting vitamin K epoxide reductase, the enzyme responsible for reducing vitamin K epoxide by nicotinamide adenine dinucleotide *(NADH)*. *R*, Hydrocarbon side chain of vitamin K.

or increase of warfarin levels, respectively. Bacteria in the intestine synthesize vitamin K. Antibiotic therapy can depress these bacteria and thus reduce absorption of vitamin K leading to an enhanced effect of warfarin. This can be problematic for patients who have a diet low in vitamin K. Likewise, the level of vitamin K in the diet can have a significant effect on the effect of warfarin.

Antiplatelet Drugs

There are three receptors on platelets that are targets for drugs designed to reduce platelet aggregation (binding of one platelet to another) and reduce adhesion (binding of a platelet to the vessel wall). These drugs are used to reduce clotting that is largely platelet in composition. For example, these drugs can prevent coronary artery occlusion.

Drug Class	Example(s)	Mechanism
Cyclooxygenase inhibitors	**Aspirin**	Prevents synthesis of thromboxane A$_2$, which causes aggregation and adhesion
Adenosine diphosphate (ADP) receptor inhibitors	**Clopidogrel, prasugrel**	Are irreversible antagonists at P2Y12 receptors, preventing the effect of ADP
Glycoprotein IIb/IIIa (GP IIb/IIIa) receptor inhibitors	Abciximab, tirofiban	Inhibit GP IIb/IIIa receptors preventing the near final step in platelet aggregation

Fibrinolytic Drugs

Fibrinolytic drugs, or thrombolytic drugs, are capable of stimulating plasminogen to produce plasmin. (Fig. 16.13). Fibrinolytics are injected and are most effective

soon after the clot has formed. Antifibrinolytics are used to aid in clot formation such as after surgery. They act by binding to plasminogen and plasmin to prevent breakdown of fibrin (see Fig. 16.13).

Drugs Used for Blood Lipid Disorders

Hypercholesterolemia is a major risk factor for cardiovascular disease. Elevated low-density lipoprotein (LDL) cholesterol is used as an indicator of risk, whereas elevated high-density lipoprotein (HDL) is interpreted as offering cardiovascular protection.

Another common blood lipid disorder is hypertriglyceridemia. Elevated levels of very low density lipoproteins (VLDL) are used as a measure of triglyceride levels.

The choice of drug(s) used to treat a particular patient's hyperlipidemia depends on the type of hyperlipidemia, risk factors, severity of the disorder, and other considerations. Drugs may be effective against more than one type of lipid disorder. Fig. 16.14 shows the pathways for the exogenous and the endogenous pathways for lipids.

3-Hydroxy-3-Methylglutaryl-Coenzyme A Reductase Inhibitors

3-hydroxy-3-methylglutaryl-coenzyme A (HMG-CoA) reductase inhibitors are a group of drugs that act to reduce blood levels of lipids, including cholesterol and triglycerides. Some common HMG-CoA inhibitors include **atorvastatin**, lovastatin, simvastatin, and rosuvastatin.

Mechanism of Action

HMG-CoA reductase inhibitors (also called "statins") act within the liver and they inhibit the synthesis of cholesterol by blocking the rate limiting enzyme, HMG-CoA reductase, in the synthesis of cholesterol (Fig. 16.15). The reduced synthesis also results in greater synthesis of hepatic LDL receptors, resulting in increased hepatic uptake of LDL. The net result of these changes is a reduction in LDL plasma concentration, and a related decrease in lipoprotein cholesterol and triglyceride concentrations.

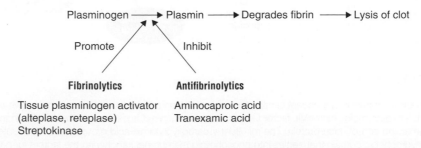

• **Fig. 16.13** Sites of Action of Fibrinolytic and Antifibrinolytic Drugs. (Modified from Shanbhag TV, Shenoy S. *Pharmacology for Medical Graduates.* New Delhi: Elsevier. 4th ed.)

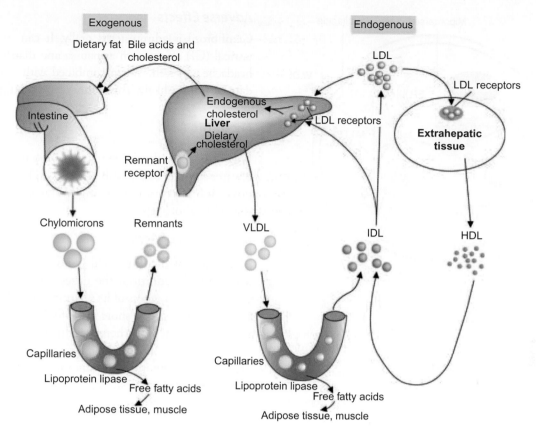

• **Fig. 16.14** Exogenous and Endogenous Pathways for Lipids, Including Cholesterol. Fat is ingested and processed into chylomicrons in the intestine; the chylomicrons are absorbed into the circulation where lipoprotein lipase releases some fatty acids from the chylomicrons and the free fatty acids form a complex with albumin and are carried to adipose and muscle tissues. The partially degraded chylomicrons (chylomicron remnants) are taken up into the liver by a membrane remnant receptor and the cholesterol is packaged into VLDLs. These enter the circulation where lipoprotein lipase releases more fatty acids that are carried to peripheral tissues as before and the IDLs (partially degraded VLDLs) are carried to the liver through the LDL receptor on the hepatocyte. Some IDLs are partially degraded by the phosphoprotein lipase to form LDLs and these are carried to peripheral tissues and enter cells by way of the LDL receptor. HDLs from the peripheral tissues bind cholesterol in the circulation forming IDLs, and return to the liver by way of LDL receptors. Some of the cholesterol in the liver is converted to bile acids and discharged, along with some cholesterol into the intestine. A small amount of the bile acids are excreted in the feces but most are recirculated to the liver (enterohepatic circulation). *HDL,* High-density lipoprotein; *IDL,* intermediary density lipoprotein; *LDL,* low-density lipoprotein; *VLDL,* very-low-density lipoprotein. (Reproduced form Figs. 9.5 to 9.17 of Litwack, G. Human Biochemistry and Disease. Academic Press/Elsevier;2008: 204.)

Pharmacokinetics

All the statins are given orally. The half-life of lovastatin ranges from 1 to 4 hours. The half-life of simvastatin is approximately 12 hours, while the half-lives of atorvastatin and rosuvastatin are about 20 hours. Most statins are metabolized and excreted by the liver.

Adverse Effects

Myopathy is the most common and potentially serious adverse effect. The risk is higher if the patient is concomitantly taking a drug that has skeletal muscle toxicity or a drug that inhibits the metabolism of the statin. Hepatotoxicity is a serious but rare toxicity and more likely when combined with another drug with the same adverse effect profile. Statins are contraindicated in pregnancy.

Drug-Drug Interactions

Drugs that increase the risk of myopathy with the statins include gemfibrozil. amiodarone, itraconazole, and erythromycin.

Bile Acids-Binding Resins

These drugs are cholestyramine, colestipol, and colesevelam.

Mechanism of Action

These drugs are non-absorbable resins that bind bile acids in the gut. Preventing bile acids from being reabsorbed results in the liver synthesizing more bile acids from cholesterol. This results in lowering of the circulating cholesterol.

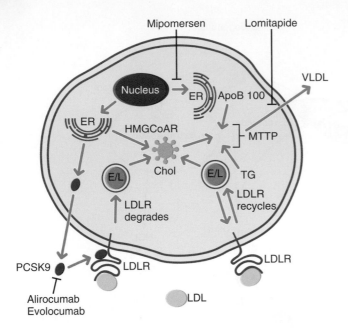

• **Fig. 16.15** Sites of action of lipid-lowering drugs acting on the hepatocyte. 3-hydroxyl-3-methylglutaryl coenzyme A reductase inhibitors inhibit the synthesis of cholesterol from the ER. The synthetic pathway for proprotein convertase subtilisin/kexin type 9 *(PCSK9)* is shown. Alirocumab and evolocumab are monoclonal antibodies directed against PCSK9, inhibiting its action on the low-density lipoprotein *(LDL)* receptor. PCSK9 causes the LDL receptor to be degraded once it is internalized. (The LDL receptor is recycled to the cell surface in the absence of PCSK9.) Other inhibitors, mipomersen and lomitapide, are shown as they prevent cholesterol release from the liver. *Chol,* Cholesterol; *E/L,* endosome/lysosome; *ER,* endoplasmic reticulum; *MTTP,* microsomal triglyceride transfer protein; *TG,* triglyceride; *VLDL,* very low-density lipoprotein. (Modified from Page MM, Stefanutti C, Sniderman A, et al. Recent advances in the understanding and care of familial hypercholesterolemia: significance of the biology and therapeutic regulation of proprotein convertase subtilisin/kexin type 9. Clin Sci. 2015;129:63–79.)

Adverse Effects

Adverse effects are generally limited to the GI tract. Nausea, bloating, and constipation are likely. These resins may prevent absorption of some drugs from the GI tract. Hyperchloremic acidosis may result as the chloride ion from the resin is released as bile acids are bound.

Fibric Acid Derivatives

Fibric acid derivatives, or fibrates, are a drug class that exert a variety of effects on lipoprotein metabolism. Gemfibrozil is an example of a fibrate.

Mechanism of Action

Gemfibrozil modifies synthesis of certain enzymes at the transcription level. These enzymes are important in controlling the level of fatty acids. The drug is effective in reducing blood triglycerides (VLDL) and cholesterol.

Adverse Effects

Gemfibrozil is administered orally. It can cause gastrointestinal (GI) effects such as nausea and diarrhea, as well as headache and rash. When combined with a statin, muscle damage is more likely. This combination should not be used.

Nicotinic Acid

Nicotinic acid, also known as niacin and vitamin B3, is a water soluble, essential B vitamin. When given in high doses, it is effective in lowering LDL cholesterol and raising HDL cholesterol.

Mechanism of Action

The action of nicotinic acid is not related to its role as a vitamin. In addition, the doses used for its anti-lipid effects are far in excess of its vitamin doses. Nicotinic acid is an oral drug with a short half-life. It reduces delivery of fatty acids to the liver thereby reducing production of triglycerides for VLDL particles. It may also increase clearance of VLDL by increasing lipoprotein lipase. Nicotinic acid raises HDL cholesterol.

Adverse Effects

Flushing, itching, and GI effects are common. Liver toxicity is a risk. Given during pregnancy, birth defects can occur. The drug may cause insulin resistance in diabetic patients.

Ezetimibe

Ezetimibe is an azetidinone derivative that inhibits the uptake of cholesteryl esters by inhibiting their uptake transporter in the GI tract. It is well tolerated.

Proprotein Convertase Subtilisin/Kexin Type 9 Blockers

Monoclonal antibody drugs are composed of a specific type of antibody to attach to a specific receptor or destroy a particular tissue target. Two monoclonal antibodies are available clinically, alirocumab and evolocumab to inhibit the proprotein convertase subtilisin/kexin type 9 (PCSK9) plasma protein. By blocking PCSK9, these drugs prevent the breakdown of the LDL receptors on the surface of the liver cell. This action provides more receptors to remove LDL from the blood (see Fig. 16.15).

Drugs That Inhibit Liver Very-Low-Density Lipoproteins Release

Lomitapide and mipomersen are two drugs used to treat hypertriglyceridemia (see Fig. 16.15). Lomitapide inhibits an enzyme on the endoplasmic reticulum of hepatocytes, called microsomal triglyceride transfer protein, necessary for very low-density lipoprotein assembly and secretion. Mipomersen, an antisense oligonucleotide, inhibits apo B-100 synthesis, which is an essential component of very-low-density and low-density lipoproteins.

Suggested Readings

Hypertension, https://www.ada.org/resources/research/science-and-research-institute/oral-health-topics/hypertension. [Accessed 24 May 2023].

Oral Anticoagulant and Antiplatelet Medications and Dental Procedures. https://www.ada.org/resources/research/science-and-research-institute/oral-health-topics/oral-anticoagulant-and-anti-platelet-medications-and-dental-procedures. [Accessed 24 May 2023].

17
Endocrine Drugs

KEY POINTS

- Insulin and Hypoglycemic Agents
  - Insulin's actions involve increasing glucose uptake into cells, increasing glucose use, and decreasing glucose production.
  - Insulin acts on cell surface receptors that have tyrosine kinase activity.
  - Insulin is used to treat both type 1 and type 2 diabetes.
  - Oral hypoglycemic drugs (sulfonylureas, meglitides, metformin, thiazolidinediones, incretin-related drugs, sodium-glucose co-transporter 2 [SGLT2] inhibitors, amylin analogues, etc.) act by a variety of different mechanisms.
  - The major sign of toxicity from insulin or oral hypoglycemic agents is hypoglycemia.
- Glucocorticoids and Synthetic Analogues
  - Synthetic glucocorticoids are administered for various reasons. They are used for replacement (e.g., treatment of insufficient production of corticosteroids). Another indication is for a palliative approach to systemic illnesses or conditions (e.g., to suppress inflammation and immune reactions).
  - The long-term use of synthetic glucocorticoids may affect circulatory cortisol levels as well as the function of the adrenal glands, among other organs.
  - Synthetic glucocorticoids are available in various forms for local, oral, and parenteral administration.
  - Synthetic compounds are classified based on the differences in duration of action compared to natural hydrocortisone (short-, intermediate-, and long-acting).
  - Glucocorticoid drugs are used in dentistry mainly to treat oral ulcerations, temporomandibular joint disorders, postoperative edema, as well as allergic reactions.
- Contraceptive Agents
  - Sex steroid hormones, or their precursors, are secreted from the ovary, testis, and inner layer of the adrenal medulla cortex.
  - Estrogens and progesterone produce numerous physiologic actions. The most common pharmacologic uses of these hormones or their antagonists are for contraception, menopausal therapy, infertility, and hormone-responsive breast cancer.
  - Numerous synthetic estrogens and progestins are used for contraception.
  - Estrogen and progesterone agonists and/or selective estrogen receptor modulators (SERMs) are used in the management of menopause and osteoporosis in women.
  - Although the dentist will not prescribe sex steroid hormones or the antagonists, the pervasive presence of these drugs requires the dentist to be aware of:
  - biologic responses in the oral cavity.
  - drug interactions (especially concerning antibiotics).
  - direct effects on the oral cavity

DEFINITIONS

- Hormones are stimulatory molecules produced by specific tissues that are transported in tissue fluids and affect specific cells distant from the secreting tissue.
- The pancreas is a glandular organ that contains enzymes for digestion and several important hormones, including insulin and glucagon.
- Hyperglycemia (or high blood sugar) is when plasma glucose rises above 180 mg/dL (postprandial) and 125 mg/dl (fasting). Depending on severity, it causes frequent urination, increased thirst, blurred vision, fatigue, confusion, and may result in a coma.
- Hypoglycemia (or low blood sugar) is when blood glucose drops below 70 mg/dL (fasting). It causes an irregular/rapid heartbeat, pale skin, confusion, and unconsciousness.
- Insulin is a hormone produced by the β-cells in the pancreatic islets of Langerhans. It regulates the amount of glucose in the blood and generally lowers blood glucose levels.
- Glucagon is a hormone produced by the α-cells in the islets of Langerhans in the pancreas. Glucagon regulates the amount of glucose in the blood by raising blood glucose levels.
- Oral hypoglycemic agents can be taken by mouth and lower blood glucose.
- The adrenal cortex is the outer part of the adrenal gland that produces steroid hormones such as cortisol, aldosterone, and other anabolic steroid hormones.
- Corticosteroids consist of two types of steroid hormones (glucocorticoids and mineralocorticoids) that are produced by the adrenal cortex.

- Estrogens are a family of steroid hormones that include estrone, estradiol, and estriol. Estrogens are secreted primarily from the ovary, and estradiol is the most potent naturally occurring estrogen.
- Progesterone is released from the ovary, placenta, and its precursor, and from the adrenal cortex. Synthetic progesterone-like compounds are called progestins.
- SERMs is an abbreviation for selective estradiol receptor modulators because they are selective for certain estrogen receptors and have tissue-selective actions.
- Follicle stimulating hormone (FSH) is released from the pituitary gland and regulates the growth of eggs in the ovary.
- Luteinizing hormone (LH) is released from the pituitary gland and stimulates ovulation and the development of the corpus luteum.
- Nidation is the implantation of the fertilized egg into the uterus.

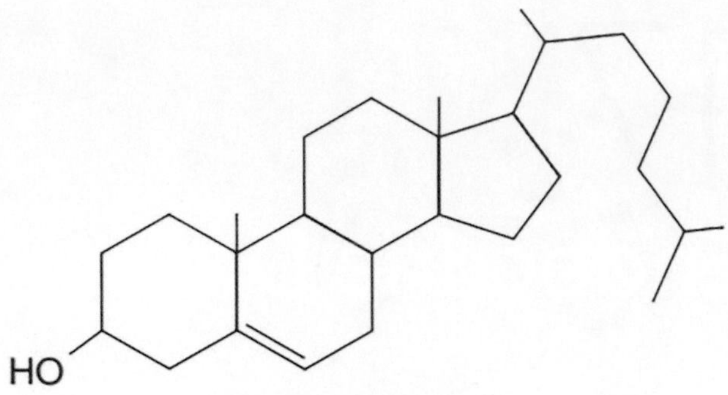

• **Fig. 17.1** Molecular structure of cholesterol.

General Principles of Endocrinology

The central focus of endocrinology revolves around specific regulatory molecules (i.e., hormones) that govern reproduction, growth and development, maintenance of the internal environment, as well as energy production, utilization, and storage. As a result of these global demands within the organism, it is not surprising that the actions of hormones are complex and diverse in nature. Despite the complex and diverse nature of hormones, it is possible to categorize these compounds into two classes depending on their chemical structure: the peptide/amino acid derivative hormones and the steroid hormones. Steroid hormones are derivatives of **cholesterol** (Fig. 17.1) and consist of a complex hydrogenated cyclopentanoperhydrophenanthrene ring system. Steroid hormones can be further divided into **three principal sets**: corticosteroid hormones (glucocorticoids and mineralocorticoids), calcium-regulating steroid hormones (vitamin D and its metabolites), and gonadal or sex steroid hormones (estrogens, androgens, and progesterone).

Most proteins and peptide hormones are the result of the transcription of a gene. Often more than one pro-hormone, due to post-transcriptional modifications, may result from a single gene with post-translational processing of pro-hormones having different biologically active peptide units. Usually proteins and peptide hormones are stored in, as well as secreted from, secretory granules. The amine hormones are formed by side-chain modifications of amino acids. Steroid hormones result from synthesis in the mitochondria and rough endoplasmic reticulum, and due to the presence of specific enzymes, cholesterol is converted into the appropriate steroid.

Steroid hormones and thyroid hormones are primarily bound to specific plasma globulins or albumin. For all hormones to act, it is the unbound or free hormone that is biologically active. The metabolism rates for hormones will vary depending on the hormone. For example, catecholamines have half-lives in seconds, proteins in minutes, and steroids/thyroid in hours.

Hormones induce changes in cell function by activating receptors either on the cell surface or via intracellular receptors. Since water-soluble proteins and peptide hormones do not diffuse across the cell membrane, these hormones activate cell surface receptors, resulting in a cascade of intracellular signal transduction. For example, insulin binding to cell surface insulin receptors stimulates tyrosine kinase activity of the receptor. Steroid hormones diffuse across the cell membrane and either bind to receptors in the nucleus or to cytoplasmic receptors which translocate to the nucleus. Once the hormone is in the nucleus, the steroid hormone-receptor complex recognizes hormone responsive elements on the deoxyribonucleic acid (DNA) to activate transcription (Fig. 17.2).

The endocrine drugs reviewed in this chapter deal with medications that dentists prescribe, or medications commonly prescribed to dental patients by their physicians. As such, this chapter will focus on corticosteroids (related to the adrenal gland), insulin, oral hypoglycemic drugs, glucagon (related to the pancreas), and oral contraceptives (related to the gonads). A more thorough explanation of these drugs and other endocrine drugs can be found in the *Pharmacology and Therapeutics for Dentistry, eighth edition.*

The Pancreas: Insulin, Glucagon, and Hypoglycemic Agents

The pancreas has exocrine and endocrine functions (Fig. 17.3). The exocrine system comprises the acinar cells, which secrete digestive enzymes. The endocrine system comprises the islets of Langerhans, which contain four types of cells. Each of these cell types synthesizes

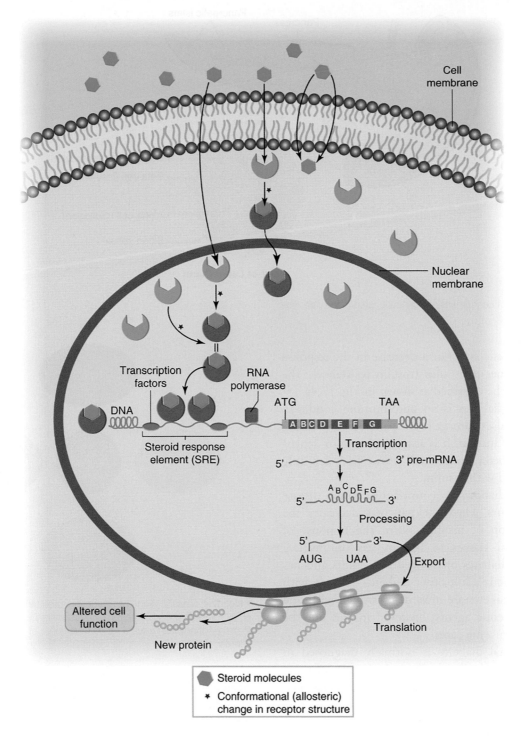

• **Fig. 17.2** The current hypothesis of sex steroid hormone action. Deoxyribonucleic acid (DNA) domains are shown (ABCDEFG). ATG and U are the nitrogen bases that stand for *A*, adenine, *G,* guanine, T, thymine and U, uracil. *RNA*, ribonucleic acid. Groups of combinations of three bases pictured represent codons.

and secretes different polypeptide hormones. Insulin is produced by the β cells, which constitute most (60% to 80%) of the islet and form its central core. Glucagon is produced by the α cells of the islets of Langerhans.

Diabetes Mellitus

Diabetes mellitus (DM) is a group of syndromes characterized by hyperglycemia. Virtually all forms of DM are due to either a decrease in the circulating concentration of

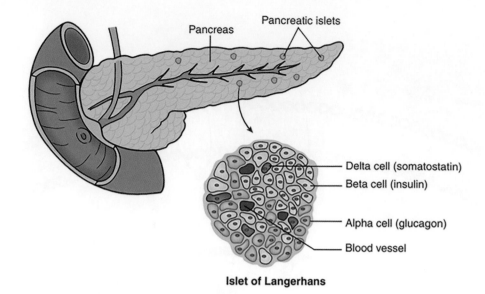

• **Fig. 17.3** The islets of Langerhans, which are located in the pancreas.

insulin (insulin deficiency) or a decrease in the response of peripheral tissues to insulin (insulin resistance). The disease forms can be classified as shown in Fig. 17.4.

(A) Type 1 diabetes is an autoimmune condition which causes damage to the pancreas, preventing release of insulin. It is also called insulin-dependent diabetes. Individuals with type 1 can only be treated with insulin.

(B) Type 2 diabetes is a non-autoimmune disease that occurs when the pancreas decreases the production of insulin and/or the response of peripheral tissues to insulin has diminished. Type 2 diabetes often occurs in adults and has been called "adult-onset diabetes." People with type 2 diabetes are most often treated with oral hypoglycemic agents; however, insulin may be needed in some cases.

(C) Gestational diabetes is normally diagnosed in the mother during the second trimester of pregnancy. Treatment involves lifestyle changes (i.e., diet and appropriate exercise). Insulin or oral hypoglycemics may be needed.

(D) Other specific types of diabetes include drug-induced diabetes, diseases of the exocrine pancreas, and many others.

Drugs for the Treatment of Diabetes Mellitus

Insulins

Insulin is the mainstay for the treatment of virtually all type 1 and many type 2 diabetic patients. Type 1 diabetes must be treated with insulin. Type 2 diabetes may be

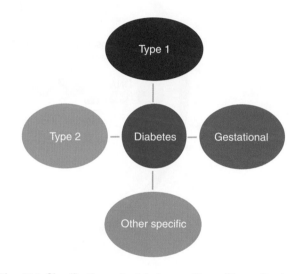

• **Fig. 17.4** Classification of diabetes mellitus. (From Dureja, H. et al. *Drug Delivery Systems for Metabolic Disorders*. Chapter 29 Phytonanoparticles toward the treatment of diabetes. London: Elsevier; 2022.)

treated with diet and exercise as well as oral anti-hyperglycemic agents, parenteral anti-hyperglycemic agents, or insulin.

Available preparations include human insulin and insulin analogues. Human insulins, so called because they have the same structure as normal human insulin, are made by genetic engineering (recombinant DNA). In ultra-short-acting insulin analogues (insulin aspart, glulisine, and lispro), amino acids are substituted or reversed. Long-acting insulin analogues (e.g., insulin detemir and glargine) have groups added. Insulin analogues have been developed to alter the pharmacokinetics of insulin. Other preparations are also available.

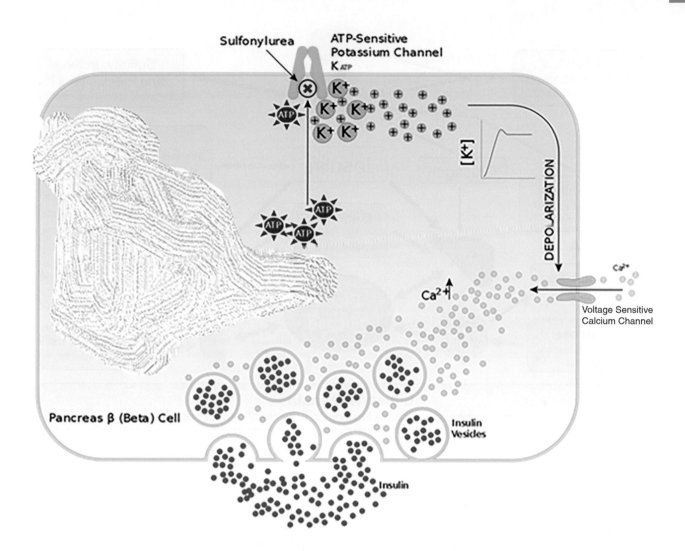

• **Fig. 17.5** Mechanism of action of sulfonylureas and meglitinides. *ATP*, Adenosine 5′-triphosphate.

Insulin preparations are classified according to **their duration of action** into rapid-acting (ultra-short-acting and short-acting), intermediate-acting, and long-acting preparations.

All insulin agents should be used in combination with appropriate diet and exercise to lower blood glucose.

Oral Hypoglycemic Agents

The therapeutic uses of hypoglycemic agents are primarily to reduce plasma glucose levels. Depending on the drug, some can be administered as monotherapy while others are used in combination with other oral hypoglycemic drugs. Further, the various treatment modalities affect not only the pancreas but also other tissues in the body.

All oral hypoglycemic agents should be used in combination with appropriate diet and exercise to lower blood glucose.

Sulfonylureas

Sulfonylureas are sulfonamide derivatives. They are traditionally divided into two groups or generations of agents. Second-generation sulfonylureas, glipizide and glimepiride, are considerably more potent than the earlier drugs and are the most commonly used sulfonylureas.

Mechanism of Action

Sulfonylureas are effective only in patients with functioning pancreatic β cells. These drugs stimulate the release of insulin by blocking the adenosine 5′-triphosphate (ATP)–dependent K+ current in pancreatic β cells. The effects of sulfonylureas are initiated by their binding to and **blocking an ATP-sensitive K+ channel** (Figs. 17.5 and 17.6). This leads to depolarization of β cells and calcium entry into the cells, followed by enhanced insulin release.

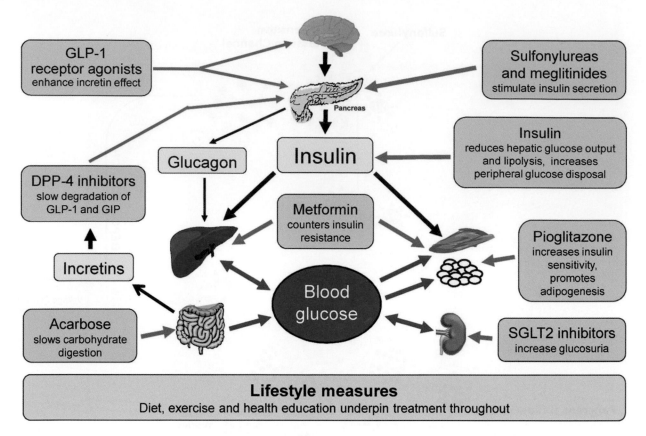

• **Fig. 17.6** Glucose lowering therapies. *DDP4*, Dipeptidyl peptidase IV; *GIP*, glucose-dependent insulinotropic peptide; *SGLT2*, sodium-glucose co-transporter 2 inhibitors.

Pharmacokinetics

Sulfonylureas are well absorbed after oral administration. All sulfonylureas are highly bound to plasma proteins (90% to 99%). Sulfonylureas are metabolized in the liver and excreted in the urine. The half-lives and extent of metabolism vary considerably among first-generation sulfonylureas.

Adverse Effects

The most important adverse effect is hypoglycemia, which, if severe, can lead to coma. Hypoglycemia is a particular problem in elderly patients with impaired hepatic or renal function who are taking longer-acting sulfonylureas.

Drug Interactions

Numerous drugs interact with sulfonylureas by enhancing or decreasing their effect on blood glucose concentration (Table 17.1).

Meglitinides

The meglitinides that are approved for use in the United States are repaglinide and nateglinide. These drugs are effective only in patients with functioning pancreatic β cells.

TABLE 17.1	Drugs That Interact With Sulfonylurea Hypoglycemic Drugs
Sulfonylurea Drug Interactions	
Increase Effect of Sulfonylureas	**Decrease Effect of Sulfonylureas**
Antihistamines	Calcium salts
Azole antifungals	Corticosteroids
Clofibrate	Diazoxide
Magnesium salts	Estrogens
Methyldopa	Phenothiazines
Monoamine oxidase inhibitors	Sympathomimetics
Oral anticoagulants	Thiazide diuretics
Salicylates	Thyroid hormones
Sulfonamide antibiotics	
Tricyclic antidepressants	
β-adrenergic receptor blockers	

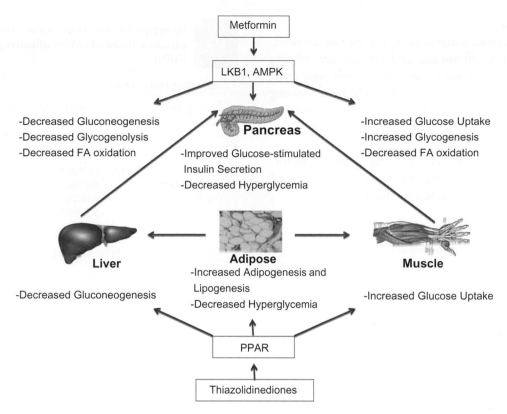

• **Fig. 17.7** Mechanism of action of metformin and thiazolidinediones. *AMPK*, AMP-dependent protein kinase; *FA*, fatty acid; *LKB1*, liver kinase B1; *PPAR*, peroxisome proliferator-activated receptor.

Mechanism of Action

Similar to sulfonylureas, they stimulate the release of insulin by blocking ATP-dependent K^+ channels in pancreatic β cells (Figs. 17.5 and 17.6).

Pharmacokinetics

Repaglinide and nateglinide are rapidly absorbed after oral administration. They are metabolized primarily by the liver. Repaglinide peak plasma levels occur within 1 hour, and the plasma half-life is 1 hour. It is recommended that this drug be taken just before each meal. Nateglinide is most effective if taken 1 to 10 minutes before a meal. These drugs offer the advantage of rapid and short-term control over blood glucose.

Adverse Effects

Hypoglycemia is the major adverse effect of repaglinide and is most likely to occur if a meal is delayed or skipped or in patients with hepatic insufficiency. Nateglinide is less likely to cause hypoglycemia.

Drug Interactions

Certain cytochrome p450 enzyme inhibitors may decrease biotransformation and potentiate the effect of the meglitinides. Nonsteroidal anti-inflammatory drugs, salicylates, sulfonamides, and other highly protein-bound drugs may potentiate the hypoglycemic effects of the meglitinides.

Biguanides

Biguanide refers to a class of antihyperglycemic drugs, of which metformin is currently the only biguanide approved for use in the United States.

Mechanism of Action

Biguanides stimulate AMP-dependent protein kinase (AMPK), thereby decreasing blood glucose concentrations by reducing hepatic gluconeogenesis, improving tissue sensitivity to insulin, increasing peripheral glucose uptake and use, and decreasing intestinal absorption of glucose (Fig. 17.7).

Pharmacokinetics

Approximately half of an oral dose of metformin is absorbed after oral administration. Protein binding is minimal, and metformin is excreted unchanged in the urine by tubular secretion with a plasma half-life of approximately 6 hours. Biguanides do not cause hypoglycemia. The action of biguanides does not depend on functioning pancreatic β cells.

Adverse Effects

Gastrointestinal tract symptoms, such as nausea, anorexia, vomiting, diarrhea, flatulence, and cramps, are adverse effects associated with metformin. Metformin may cause a decrease in vitamin B_{12} levels, possibly by decreasing absorption from the vitamin B_{12} intrinsic factor complex.

Drug Interactions

Because of overlapping toxicities, drugs that are significantly toxic to the gastrointestinal tract, should be used with caution in patients taking metformin.

Thiazolidinediones

Thiazolidinediones (TZD), also known as glitazones, are a class of heterocyclic compounds. This family of drugs was introduced in the late 1990s for the management of diabetes mellitus.

Mechanism of Action

Thiazolidinediones (rosiglitazone and pioglitazone) act by increasing insulin sensitivity in tissues. They are agonists at the nuclear peroxisome proliferator-activated receptor γ (PPARγ). PPAR-γ stimulates the transcription of many of the genes responsive to insulin. The thiazolidinediones depend on the presence of insulin for their activity. They decrease hepatic gluconeogenesis and increase insulin-dependent glucose uptake in muscle and fat (see Fig. 17.6).

Pharmacokinetics

Thiazolidinediones are taken orally, once a day. The maximal effect is not seen for 6 to 12 weeks. They are metabolized by the cytochrome P450 oxidative enzyme system.

Adverse Effects

Thiazolidinediones carry a warning of contributing to congestive heart failure and myocardial ischemia. The risk is greater with rosiglitazone. There is also weight gain and a risk of edema, osteoporosis, fractures, and hepatotoxicity.

Drug Interactions

Rifampin induces CYP 450 enzymes and can enhanced the effects of thiazolidinediones.

Incretin-Related Drugs

Incretin-related drugs are a class of agents related to molecules from the enteric nervous system,   e.g., glucagon-like peptide-1 (GLP-1). These drugs act by stimulating GLP-1 receptors, resulting in insulin release, inhibition of glucagon release, and delayed gastric emptying (Table 17.2). This drug class includes dulaglutide, semaglutide, and liraglutide. Another similar group of drugs is the class

TABLE 17.2	Function of Incretion Hormones (GLP-1 and glucose-dependent insulinotropic peptide [GIP])
Incretion Hormones	
Glucagon-like peptide-1 (GLP-1)	Released from gastrointestinal track in reaction to food. Promotes insulin secretion in a glucose-dependent manner.
Glucose-dependent insulinotropic peptide (GIP)	Released when glucose contacts cells in the small intestine. Promotes insulin secretion as well as β cell expansion and survival.
Metabolism of Incretin Hormones	
Dipeptidyl peptidase-4 (DPP4)	Expressed on surface of most cell types. Responsible for degradation of incretin hormones.

of inhibitors of dipeptidyl peptidase-IV, including sitagliptin, saxagliptin, alogliptin, and linagliptin. Inhibiting this enzyme leads to an increase in GLP-1 (Table 17.2).

Mechanism of Action

Incretin-related drugs work by mimicking the incretin hormones from the gastrointestinal tract to stimulate the release of insulin in response to a meal. Others in this group, the gliptins, block the metabolism of the incretins by inhibiting dipeptidyl peptidase IV (DPP-4) (see Fig. 17.6).

Pharmacokinetics

Incretin-related drugs may be administered orally or by subcutaneous injection, depending on the specific drug. As an injectable, incretin-related drugs should only be used when other oral hypoglycemic drugs (e.g., metformin, sulfonylureas, etc.) have failed to be effective in controlling blood glucose levels.

Adverse Effects

In general, incretin-related drugs may cause minor side effects, such as constipation, diarrhea, abdominal pain, dizziness, etc. However, the various incretin-related drugs have more serious adverse effects that are dependent on the specific drug. Some of the more severe reported adverse reports are rare cases of hemorrhagic or necrotizing pancreatitis.

Drug Interactions

Many herbal drugs affect the metabolism of incretin mimetics. Furthermore, incretin-related drugs can cause

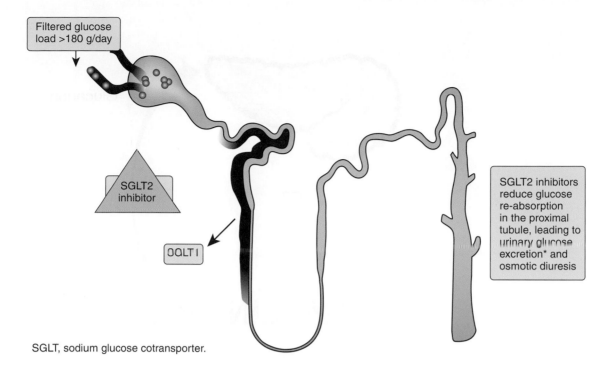

SGLT, sodium glucose cotransporter.

• **Fig. 17.8** Mechanism of action of SGLT2 inhibitor.

hypoglycemia if used with other oral hypoglycemic agents.

Sodium-Glucose Co-Transporter 2 Inhibitors

Sodium-glucose co-transporter 2 (SGLT2) inhibitors were first isolated from the root bark of the apple tree. Unlike many other oral hypoglycemic drugs, SGLT2 does not primarily affect the pancreas or insulin receptors but rather reduces plasma glucose by increasing the excretion of glucose by the kidneys. This class of drugs includes canagliflozin, dapagliflozin, empagliflozin, and ertugliflozin.

Mechanism of Action

The SGLT2 inhibitors block the sodium-glucose co-transporter 2, which facilitates glucose reabsorption in the kidney. As a result, reabsorption of glucose from the kidney is decreased, renal excretion of glucose is increased, and blood glucose levels are lowered (Figs. 17.6 and 17.8).

Pharmacokinetics

SGLT2 inhibitors are administered orally and are tightly bound to plasma proteins. The drug half-life (ranging between 11 and 13 hours) makes these drugs appropriate for once-daily dosing. SGLT2 inhibitors are eliminated by fecal and renal routes.

Adverse Effects

As the drugs cause more glucose to be excreted in the urine, there is a higher chance of getting genital and urinary tract infections. These side effects are more common in women than in men. They may increase the incidence of bladder cancer. They may cause hyperkalemia.

Drug Interactions

No significant interactions with other drugs have been reported; however, taking SGLT2 inhibitors with insulin, sulfonylureas, or meglitinides may increase the risk of hypoglycemia.

Analogues of Amylin

Analogues of amylin are synthetic compounds that have a similar function to amylin, a polypeptide hormone that is secreted with insulin from β cells. Amylin analogues can be used to treat type I or type II diabetes mellitus. Pramlintide is the soluble form of amylin. Pramlintide is primarily an adjunct treatment for diabetes.

Mechanism of Action

Pramlintide is an amylinomimetic. Pramlintide functions to lower blood sugar in three ways: (1) it decreases glucagon secretion, which lowers blood glucose released from the liver, (2) it slows gastric emptying by a vagal-mediated mechanism; and (3) it decreases appetite centrally.

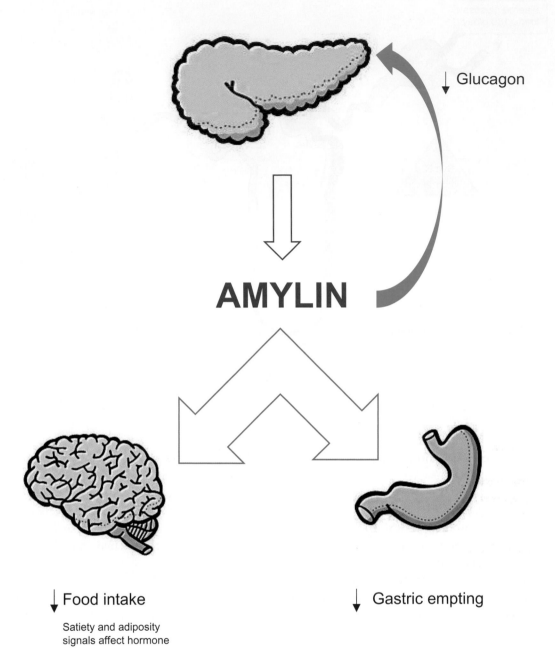

↓ Glucagon

AMYLIN

↓ Food intake

Satiety and adiposity
signals affect hormone

↓ Gastric empting

• **Fig. 17.9** Effects of amylin.

Three receptor activity-modifying proteins are involved in the mechanism of action (Fig. 17.9).

Pharmacokinetics

Pramlintide is given as a subcutaneous injection with a half-life of 48 minutes. Pramlintide is primarily an adjunct treatment for diabetes. Metabolism and excretion are primarily by the kidney.

Adverse Effects

The most important adverse effect is hypoglycemia, which, if severe, can lead to coma. Hypoglycemia is a

particular problem in elderly patients with impaired hepatic or renal function who are taking longer-acting sulfonylureas.

Drug Interactions

Amylin analogues can cause hypoglycemia when administered with insulin.

Glucagon

Glucagon is a 29-amino acid peptide that binds to specific G protein–linked receptors in the liver, causing

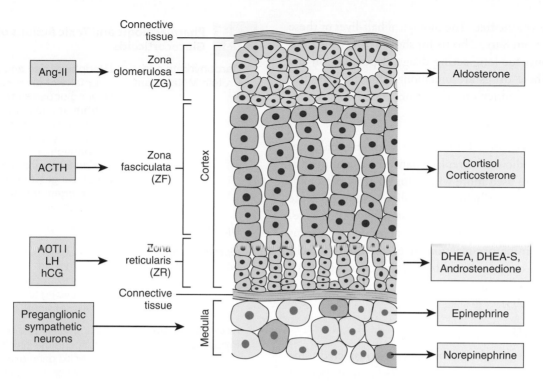

• **Fig. 17.10** The adrenal gland with zones and sources of adrenal hormones. *ACTH*, Adrenocorticotropic hormone; *Ang II*, angiotensin II; *DHEA*, dehydroepiandrosterone; *DHEA-S*, DHEA sulfate; *hCG*, human chorionic gonadotropin; *LH*, luteinizing hormone.

an increase in adenylyl cyclase activity and the production of cyclic adenosine 3′,5′-monophosphate (cAMP). This ultimately results in an increase in glycogen phosphorylase activity and a decrease in glycogen synthase. Glucagon increases blood glucose concentration by decreasing glycogen synthesis, stimulating breakdown of stored glycogen, and increasing gluconeogenesis in the liver. It does not affect skeletal muscle glycogen, although it can cause skeletal muscle wasting.

Glucagon is rapidly degraded in the plasma, liver, and kidney. Its half-life is 3 to 6 minutes. Glucagon may be used in the emergency treatment of severe hypoglycemic reactions (sufficient to cause unconsciousness). It is given parenterally. Adverse effects include nausea (usually transient) and vomiting. Glucagon may cause transient tachycardia and hypertension.

Adrenal Gland: Glucocorticoid Hormones

The adrenal glands are located in the retroperitoneum superior to the kidneys. Despite their small size, the secretions from these glands play an integral role in the function, development, and growth of the body and the ability to deal with stress. Production of all corticosteroids is highly compartmentalized in the adrenal cortex (Fig. 17.10). The glucocorticoids are produced by the middle layer (zona fasciculata) of the adrenal cortex. The glucocorticoids are not stored to any extent in the adrenal

gland but are continuously synthesized and secreted. The total daily production of the major glucocorticoid, cortisol, is normally 9.5 to 10 mg with a strong diurnal variation.

Glucocorticoids and Synthetic Analogues

Synthetic glucocorticoids have related structural properties to the endogenous hormones. Synthetic glucocorticoids are widely used in medicine and dentistry. The mechanism of action, pharmacokinetics, therapeutic effects, adverse effects, and drug interactions for glucocorticoids and synthetic analogues are listed below for this drug class.

Mechanism of Action

Glucocorticoids diffuse through cell membranes and bind to intracellular receptors found in the cytoplasm. The hormone-receptor complex then enters the nucleus. The steroid-receptor complex binds to regulatory elements of the DNA to allow gene activation and protein synthesis.

Pharmacokinetics

Glucocorticoids may be administered orally, topically, or by intramuscular injections. Similar to other lipid-soluble drugs, glucocorticoid analogues are transported in the blood principally bound to carrier proteins, leaving only

2% of the hormone free. The biological half-lives of these drugs range from 8 to 12 hours for short-acting drugs and 36 to 72 hours for long-acting drugs, depending on the analogue. These drugs are metabolized in the liver and excreted by the kidney into the urine.

Therapeutic Effects

Exogenous glucocorticoids and their synthetic analogues are used in medicine for replacement in adrenal insufficiency. They are used more widely for an array of nonadrenal diseases, primarily for their ability to suppress acute or chronic inflammation. In dentistry, glucocorticosteroids are used mainly to reduce the signs and symptoms of excess inflammatory reactions (e.g., for the treatment of oral ulcers, temporomandibular joint disorders, postoperative symptoms, anaphylaxis, and other allergic reactions) (Table 17.3).

Adverse Effects

Glucocorticoids and their analogues are considered to be safe when given at recommended doses for short periods of time. Even large doses given over a short course of less than 1 week have few harmful effects. Similarly, topical oral application of glucocorticoids has a limited number of adverse effects. (Long-term use of glucocorticoids is associated with several adverse effects.)

Drug Interactions

Since glucocorticoids affect numerous tissues in the body, taking these drugs can provoke many drug interactions. In particular, administration of glucocorticoids is not recommended if you are receiving a bacterial or viral vaccine or being treated for an active bacterial, fungal, or viral infection.

Topical Glucocorticoid Drugs

Successful therapeutic outcomes for topically applied glucocorticoid drugs are dependent on an accurate diagnosis and choosing the correct potency and frequency of drug in an appropriate vehicle. The potency of topical glucocorticoids can be categorized into classes ranging from Class I (the most potent) to Class VII (the least potent). Table 17.4 lists some of the glucocorticoids' synthetic analogues for each class.

The Ovary: Estrogens and Progestins

Steroidal and nonsteroidal compounds with the properties of sex steroid hormones are extensively used in the prophylaxis or treatment of disease and for birth control. Although dentists do not typically prescribe these agents, their ubiquitous presence in the population requires a

TABLE 17.3	Pharmacologic and Toxic Actions of Glucocorticoids
Carbohydrate and Protein Metabolism	↓Peripheral use and cellular uptake of glucose ↑Liver glucose synthesis from amino acids (gluconeogenesis) ↓Protein synthesis in muscle, connective tissues, and skin (antianabolic effect) ↑In blood glucose, liver glycogen, urinary nitrogen excretion
Lipid Metabolism	↓Fatty acid synthesis
Electrolyte and Water Balance	↑Reabsorption of Na^+ from the tubular fluid ↑Urinary excretion of K^+ and H^+ (leading to edema and hypertension)
Anti-inflammatory Properties	↓Inflammatory response (through the inhibition of specific gene expression) ↓Production of cytokines
Immune Responses	↓T-lymphocyte activation and proliferation ↓Production of plasma cells ↓Phagocytosis of antigen by macrophages ↓Antibody production

TABLE 17.4	Classification of Glucocorticoid Synthetic Analogues	
Class	Potency	Drug
I	Highest	Clobetasol propionate 0.05% in any vehicle
II	High	Fluocinonide 0.05% cream, gel, or ointment
III	High to medium	Betamethasone dipropionate 0.05% cream
IV	Medium	Fluocinolone acetonide 0.025% cream or ointment
V	Medium to low	Triamcinolone acetonide 0.025% cream, lotion, or ointment
VI	Low	Fluocinolone 0.01% cream
VII	Least	Hydrocortisone 1% cream, lotion, or ointment

careful understanding of the actions and interactions of sex steroids with other pharmacologic agents and how they affect structures in the oral cavity. Reports of the effects of sex steroid hormones in the oral cavity have been noted for more than a century.

Estrogens

Estrogens are a biologically important hormone class. Estradiol is the most potent estrogen and is secreted by the ovary, testes, placenta, and peripheral tissues.

Mechanism of Action

Estrogens diffuse through cell membranes and bind to intracellular receptors found in the nucleus. The steroid-receptor complex binds to regulatory elements on the DNA to allow gene activation and protein synthesis.

Pharmacokinetics

Estrogens may be administered orally, topically, or through intramuscular injections. Although estradiol is available for enteral administration, it is generally not used in this manner since concentrations in the bloodstream remain low because of extensive hepatic metabolism. The half-life of estrogenic compounds can be increased by synthetic substitutions on the estrogen molecule. For example, the half-life of estradiol is a few minutes, whereas the half-life of ethinyl estradiol (ethinyl substitution at the C17 position) may be more than 13 hours. Nonsteroidal compounds may also have estrogenic activity; examples of such compounds include diethylstilbestrol, flavones, isoflavones, certain pesticides (e.g., p,p′-DDT) and plasticizers (e.g., bisphenol A). Similar to other lipid-soluble hormones, estrogens are transported in the blood principally bound to carrier proteins, leaving only 2% of the hormone free.

Adverse Effects

The side effects for estrogen drugs can vary depending on the reason(s) for use, biologic sex, and age of the patient. Some of the more significant adverse events in women include an increased risk of endometrial cancer. Hormone replacement therapy during menopause has also been associated with stroke and breast cancer.

Drug Interactions

Estrogens may increase the effect of corticosteroids. Rifampin, barbiturates, carbamazepine, phenytoin, and topiramate all tend to decrease the effects of estrogens because these drugs induce the liver metabolism of estrogens. Rifampin is a well-known inducer that inhibits the effect of birth control medications.

Progestins

Progestins are a biologically important hormone class. Progesterone is the most potent naturally occurring progestin and is secreted by the ovary, placenta, and adrenal cortex.

Mechanism of Action

Progestins diffuse through cell membranes and bind to intracellular receptors found in the nucleus. The steroid-receptor complex binds to regulatory elements on the DNA to allow gene activation and protein synthesis.

Pharmacokinetics

Progestins may be administered orally, topically, or by intramuscular injections. Similar to other lipid-soluble hormones, progestins are transported in the blood principally bound to carrier proteins, leaving only 2% of the hormone free.

Drug Interactions

Hepatic enzyme–inducing medications decrease the effect of progestins.

Hormone Antagonists and Partial Agonists

Hormone antagonists and partial agonists modulate estrogen or progesterone activity by selective receptor activation (e.g., SERMs), antagonism of receptors, or inhibition of steroid hormone synthesis. Selective estrogen receptor modulators (SERMs) provide agonist activity in tissues where estrogen action is desired and antagonize or elicit no activity in tissues where estrogen activity may be harmful. The selective modulation of estrogenic activity in tissues is possible because of the presence of two distinct estrogen receptors (α and β forms) with variable tissue distribution and variable drug affinity for these estrogen receptor forms. Drugs in this class can be used to treat cancer, infertility, and osteoporosis.

Pharmacologic Contraceptives

Various methods of pharmacologic contraception have been used to allow couples to plan the timing of pregnancy. Modern pharmacologic methods include oral contraceptives, implants, injectable drugs, contraceptive sponges, spermicides, and hormonal pills (Table 17.5).

Long-Acting Reversible Contraception

Hormonal Intrauterine Device

A hormonal intrauterine device (IUD) is a small device inserted into the uterus that releases levonorgestrel (a progestin hormone). The progestin prevents pregnancy by thickening cervical mucous and preventing sperm motility and fertilization, thinning the uterine lining, and potentially preventing ovulation. The failure rate for a hormonal IUD is less than 1%.

TABLE 17.5 Drug Classes of Pharmacologic Contraception

Drug Class	Types	Administered	Agent or Agent Class
Long-acting reversible contraception	Hormonal intrauterine device	Uterine implant	Progestin
	Hormonal implants	Subcutaneous implant	Progestin
Short-acting reversible contraception	Injectable progestins	Subcutaneous injection	Progestin
	Progestin-only pills	Orally	Progestin
	Combined oral contraceptives	Orally	Estrogen and progestin
	Contraceptive patch	Transdermal patch on skin	Estrogen and progestin
	Vaginal ring	Placed in vagina	Estrogen and progestin
Barrier contraception	Contraceptive sponges	Placed in vagina	Nonoxynol 9
	Spermicides	Placed in vagina	Nonoxynol 9
	Vaginal pH modulators	Placed in vagina	Lactic acid/citric acid/potassium bitartrate
Emergency contraception	Tablets	Orally	Selective progesterone modulator or progestin

Hormonal Implants

This form of contraception involves the surgical placement of a flexible rod containing etonogestrel (a progestin hormone) under the skin of a woman's upper arm. The rod releases the hormone for 5 years and has a failure rate of less than 1%.

Short-Acting Reversible Contraceptive Progestins

Injectable Progestins

The subcutaneous injection of medroxyprogesterone acetate (a progestin hormone) in the arm or buttocks every 3 months regulates or stops ovulation. Injectable progestins can cause a temporary loss of skeletal bone that is regained after discontinuation of the drug.

Progestin-Only Pills

This pill is taken daily and interferes with ovulation and sperm function. Progestin-only pills are not associated with an increased risk of thromboembolic disorders but may result in breakthrough bleeding.

Combined Oral Contraceptives

Combined oral contraceptives have also been called birth control pills. The formulary in this class of contraceptives contains both an estrogen and a progestin to prevent conception (Table 17.6).

TABLE 17.6 Oral Contraceptives (Daily Dosing)

Preparation	Description
Monophasic	A fixed dose of estrogen and progesterone is used over a 21-day period.
Biphasic	A fixed dose of estrogen is used but the progestin dose is increased once over a 21-day period.
Triphasic	Preparations change the dose of progestin every 7 days for 21 days.
Quadriphasic	Preparations change the dose of progestin four times in the cycle of use.
Extended-cycle	Preparations involve 84 days of drug treatment with a combination of ethinyl estradiol and a progestin (usually levonorgestrel), followed by a placebo for 7 days or 7 pill-free days.
Continuous	Oral contraceptives involve no drug-free period.

Mechanism of Action

Estrogen and progesterone prevent pregnancy by several mechanisms. The principal mechanism is that these sex steroid hormones prevent follicular development in the

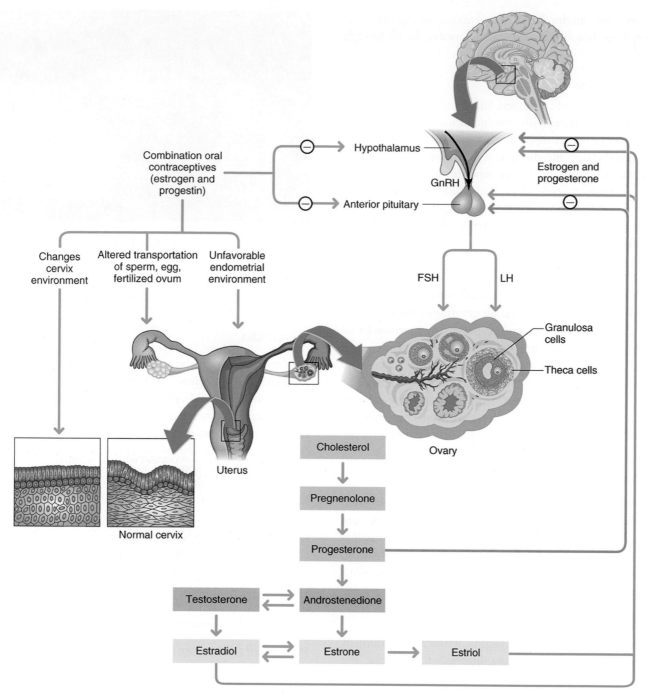

• **Fig. 17.11** Combination oral contraceptives principally affect conception by inhibiting the release of follicle-stimulating hormone *(FSH)* and suppressing the surge of luteinizing hormone *(LH)* from the anterior pituitary, which consequently suppresses ovulation. *GnRH,* Gonadotropin-releasing hormone.

ovary and they inhibit ovulation. This occurs because this hormone combination inhibits the secretion of follicle-stimulating hormone (FSH) and luteinizing hormone (LH). Further, progesterone can change the composition of cervical mucous to make sperm movement difficult. These hormones can also affect the endometrium, thus preventing nidation (Fig. 17.11).

Administration

Prescription of combination oral contraceptives can include either monophasic, biphasic, triphasic, or quadriphasic preparations. Biphasic and triphasic oral contraceptives were designed to approximate more closely the ratios of estrogen and progesterone during the menstrual cycle. In addition, quadriphasic pills can also be used for women with menorrhagia. Continuous dosing oral contraceptives (see Table 17.6) may involve breakthrough bleeding.

Adverse Effects

Most side effects of combined oral contraceptives are mild and often disappear with continued use. The most common adverse effect of combined oral contraceptive pills is break-through bleeding, as well as nausea, headaches, abdominal cramping, breast tenderness, an increase in vaginal discharge, and decreased libido. Risk of venous thromboembolism is increased among oral contraceptive users and the risk is even greater in those over 35 who smoke.

Drug Interactions

Oral contraceptives may increase the effects of glucocorticoids. Numerous anecdotal observations have suggested that antibiotics (e.g., rifampin, penicillins, tetracyclines, metronidazole, etc.) may reduce oral contraceptive efficacy. There is clear evidence that rifampin will reduce the efficacy of oral contraceptives. Rifampin is an inducer of liver microsomal enzymes. However, administration of any antibiotic to a patient using an oral contraceptive should involve informed consent and discussion of the possible interaction between the drugs.

Contraceptive Patch

The contraceptive patch is a thin, transdermal patch attached to the skin of the abdomen, buttocks, or arm that releases ethinyl estradiol (an estrogen) and norelgestromin (a progestin) for 3 weeks to prevent ovulation. Risks and efficacy of this form of contraception are similar to combined oral contraceptives.

Vaginal Ring

The ring is inserted into the vagina, where it continuously releases ethinyl estradiol and a progestin for 3 weeks. The risks and efficacy of this form of contraception are similar to combined oral contraceptives.

Barrier Methods

Contraceptive Sponges

These are soft, disposable, spermicide-filled foam sponges that are inserted into the vagina prior to intercourse. The sponge contains 1000 mg of a surfactant called non-oxynol-9, a non-hormonal drug that immobilizes or kills sperm on contact. The sponge should be in place for at least six hours following intercourse. Chemical spermicides are the least reliable method for birth control (85% effective).

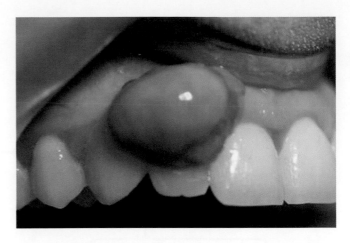

• **Fig. 17.12** The effects of sex steroid hormones in pregnancy can cause proliferation in the periodontium, in this case a pyogenic granuloma. (The Ohio State University, College of Dentistry, Advanced Education in Periodontology Postdoctoral Program Archives.)

Spermicides

Spermicides contain nonoxynol 9 in the form of foam, jelly, cream, suppository, or film and should be used in combination with a diaphragm or cervical cap. A spermicide is vaginally inserted close to the uterus 30 minutes prior to intercourse and left in place 6 hours after intercourse. The use of chemical spermicides alone method for birth control is about 85% effective.

Vaginal pH Modulator

Unlike other spermicides, a lactic acid/citric acid/potassium bitartrate gel reduces the pH in the vagina and takes advantage of sperm vulnerability to acidic environments. The gel is placed vaginally prior to intercourse. The most common adverse reactions include vulvovaginal burning sensations and vaginal infections. This method of contraception has been reported to be 86% effective.

Postcoital Contraception

Prevention of postcoital pregnancy using a selective progesterone modulator (ulipristal acetate) or a progestin (levonorgestrel) pill is given as soon as possible after intercourse. These drugs function by preventing or delaying ovulation and preventing nidation.

Influence of Estrogens on the Oral Cavity

The homeostasis of tissues in the mouth is a complex, multifactorial relationship that involves, at least in part, the endocrine system. The assertion that hormone-sensitive periodontal tissues exist relies on several salient observations, including the retention and metabolic conversion of sex steroid hormones in the periodontium and the presence of **steroid hormone receptors in periodontal tissues** (Fig. 17.12). These biologic findings correlated with clinical observations confirm an increased prevalence of gingival inflammation with fluctuating sex steroid hormone levels that would be consistent with the protective nature of sex steroid hormones in the periodontium.

Suggested Readings

Diabetes.   https://www.ada.org/resources/research/science-and-research-institute/oral-health-topics/diabetes.   [Accessed 26 May 2023].

Women's hormones and dental health. https://www.mouth-healthy.org/all-topics-a-z/womens-hormones-and-dental-health. [Accessed 26 May 2023].

18

Drugs Acting on the Respiratory System

KEY POINTS

- β-Adrenergic receptor agonists, adrenal corticosteroids (more specifically glucocorticoids), and antimuscarinic drugs comprise the principal drugs used to treat asthma and chronic obstructive pulmonary disease (COPD).
- Most drugs used for asthma and COPD are given by inhalation.
- β-Adrenergic receptor agonists are of two types: short-acting and long-acting.
- Tissue remodeling of the respiratory airways is an adverse effect of chronic asthma and COPD.
- Bronchoconstriction and inflammation are two targets of drugs used to treat asthma and COPD.
- Targeted therapys using monoclonal antibodies for immunoglobulin E and interleukin-5 are recently developed therapies for the treatment of asthma.

DEFINITIONS

- COPD includes diseases, such as emphysema and chronic bronchitis, that constrict airways, causing difficulty or discomfort in breathing.
- Phosphodiesterase is an enzyme that breaks down cyclic nucleotides (e.g., cyclic adenosine monophosphate).
- Monoclonal antibodies are antibodies formed from a single cloned line of cells. These antibodies attack a single specific protein or cell type.
- Cytokines are small proteins secreted by cells of the immune system that stimulate cytokine receptors on other cells.
- Tachyphylaxis is the rapidly diminishing responsiveness to successive doses of a drug.

Two significant respiratory diseases are chronic obstructive pulmonary disease (COPD) and asthma. It has been estimated that approximately 334 million people worldwide have asthma, and the prevalence is estimated to increase by 100 million by 2025.

Asthma is characterized by inflammation, bronchoconstriction and, over time, remodeling of the airways. This limits the amount of air in and out of the lungs. The acute phase of bronchoconstriction and inflammation is responsive to drug therapy. Preventing the remodeling of the airway is not easily managed since drug therapy is slow and only modestly effective, if at all. Control of airway remodeling is difficult because it involves multiple processes, including fibrosis, thickening of the airway wall due to smooth muscle thickening, thickening of the bronchial wall, hyperplasia of secretory cells, inflammation, and mucus accumulation. Collapsed alveoli also occur. The effectiveness of drugs for asthma depends on several factors, since the disease may vary in intensity, number of episodes, and underlying causes or triggers.

Fig. 18.1 compares the normal with the asthmatic bronchial tubes.

COPD is a chronic inflammatory disease that often occurs as a result of exposure to environmental irritants and toxins. Cigarette smoke is a common cause, but other inhaled chemicals can also be involved. COPD is progressive over time and is less responsive than asthma to inhaled corticosteroid therapy. COPD is associated with early mortality, high death rates, and significant costs to the health care system. COPD has been projected to be the third leading cause of death worldwide. Further, this disease is associated with considerable comorbidities.

Several drugs can be used to treat asthma or COPD. The drug classes involved include β-adrenergic receptor agonists, corticosteroids, and antimuscarinic drugs, as well as other selective agents.

β-Adrenergic Receptor Agonists

Mechanism of Action

For the treatment of asthma and COPD with β-adrenergic receptor agonists (β-receptor agonists or simply, β-agonists) (Chapters 7 in *Essentials*), selective β_2-agonists are preferred, because they are effective bronchodilators, but with less stimulation of the β-receptors (β_1-receptors), which are the predominant β-receptors in the heart (Fig. 18.2). Depending on the clinical situation, **both short-acting β_2-receptor agonists (SABA) and long-acting β_2-receptor agonists (LABA) are used**.

SABA drugs are used to **treat** bronchospasms and achieve immediate relief in patients with acute episodes of asthma and COPD. SABA should be used only

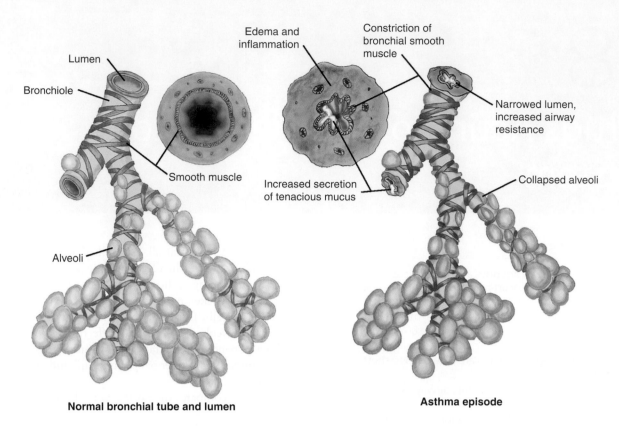

• **Fig. 18.1** Asthma is a chronic inflammatory disorder of the airways. There is an airway hyperresponsiveness with symptoms of wheezing, breathlessness, chest tightness, and coughing. (From Christensen BL, Kockrow EO. *Foundations of Nursing*. 6th ed. St Louis: Mosby; 2011.)

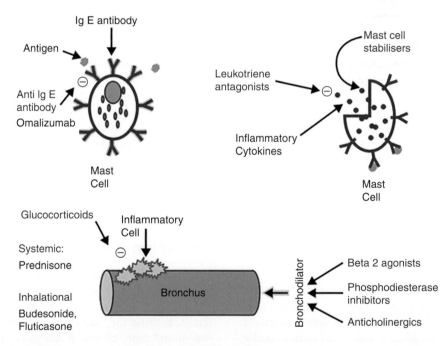

• **Fig. 18.2** Target sites for anti-asthmatic drugs. The action of the anti IgE antibody, leukotriene antagonists, and glucocorticoids are shown in small circles. (Modified from Tripathi RK, Satoskar RS, Bhandarkar SD, et al. *Pharmacology and Pharmacotherapeutics*. 25th ed. Chapter 27— Pharmacotherapy of bronchial asthma, COPD and rhinitis, 2015, Elsevier.)

for treating acute episodes because constant use leads to desensitization and downregulation of β-receptors (Chapter 1 of *Essentials*). This would significantly reduce the effectiveness of the β-agonists, because of tachyphylaxis. LABA drugs are useful in **preventing** acute attacks and are not associated with major desensitization and downregulation.

β-Receptor agonists increase the production of intracellular cyclic AMP, leading to dilation of bronchial smooth muscle (Chapter 7 of Essentials).

Pharmacokinetics

For asthma and COPD, the β-receptor agonists are given by inhalation, which reduces the potential for toxicities.

Adverse Effects

The adverse effects of β-receptor agonists are minimized by being administered by inhalation (Table 18.1).

Drug-Drug Interactions

Other drugs, such as corticosteroids and antimuscarinic drugs work together to improve symptoms. **Corticosteroids increase the sensitivity of the β-receptors** to stimulation by β-receptor agonists. Adverse drug-drug interactions include the effects of other sympathetic drugs adding to the effect of inhaled β-receptor agonists. Non-selective β-receptor blockers antagonize the effects of the β_2-receptor agonists.

Corticosteroids

Mechanism of Action

Refer to Chapter 17 for a discussion of the corticosteroids.

In addition to increasing the effect of β-receptor agonists at the receptor level, corticosteroids reduce **inflammation** (see Fig. 18.2). They inhibit the proliferation of eosinophils, mast cells, and lymphocytes, which contribute in a major way to asthma. Furthermore, cytokine production is inhibited. Hyperresponsiveness of the airways and acute episodes of asthma are reduced by the corticosteroids. COPD is not as responsive to corticosteroids, but these drugs are indicated in severe cases of COPD.

Pharmacokinetics

In normal circumstances, steroids are inhaled when treating asthma and COPD. Inhalation provides access to the respiratory tract with minimal systemic effects. Most corticosteroids administered by inhalation are given in the active form. Drugs absorbed from the lung undergo rapid metabolism in the liver.

There are several inhaled corticosteroids (ICUs) used for the management of asthma and COPD (Table 18.2).

Adverse Effects

Oropharyngeal candidiasis is one of the most common adverse effects of inhaled corticosteroids. Hoarseness is also typical. Long-term use presents a risk of cataracts and osteoporosis. There is a minor risk of weight gain, thinning of the skin, decreased growth in children, and adrenal suppression. Oral administration of corticosteroids, given in severe cases, is associated with the classic systemic effects of corticosteroids (Chapter 17).

Drug–Drug Interactions

Inhibitors of cytochrome P-450 3A4 (e.g., ritonavir, itraconazole, and clarithromycin) may increase blood levels in some inhaled corticosteroids.

Antimuscarinic Drugs (Anticholinergics)

Mechanism of Action

These drugs block muscarinic cholinergic receptors innervated by the vagus nerve in the respiratory tract. In the lung and bronchi, this leads to a decrease in the tone of smooth muscle, resulting in **bronchodilation** (see Fig. 18.2). The mechanism of action of muscarinic receptor antagonists is more fully discussed in Chapter 5.

Table 18.3 compares the half-lives of different inhaled antimuscarinic drugs.

Pharmacokinetics

Similar to other drugs for asthma or COPD, antimuscarinic drugs are given by inhalation. Since the drugs are quaternary amine derivatives, the charge on the drugs prevents systemic absorption. The approximate durations range from 2 to 24 hours (see Table 18.3).

TABLE 18.1 β-Receptor Agonists Used in Asthma and Chronic Obstructive Pulmonary Disease		
β-Receptor Agonists	**Examples**	**Adverse Effects**
Short-acting	Albuterol, terbutaline	Tachycardia, cardiac arrhythmias, hypokalemia, decreased β-receptor effect with continual use
Long-acting	Salmeterol, formoterol	Tachycardia, cardiac arrhythmias, hypokalemia

TABLE 18.2 Representative Inhaled Corticosteroids	
Drug	**Characteristics**
Fluticasone propionate	Flovent is one brand name.
Beclomethasone	More systemic effects than other ICU's
Ciclesonide	Fewest systemic adverse effects among ICUs
Budesonide	Available in a jet nebulizer useful for young children
Fluticasone furoate	Suitable for once-a-day dosing

TABLE 18.3 Four Inhaled Antimuscarinic Drugs and Their Durations	
Drug	**Approximate Duration (h)**
Ipratropium	2
Aclidinium	6
Umeclidinium	11
Tiotropium	24

TABLE 18.4 Other Drugs Used for Asthma and Chronic Obstructive Pulmonary Disease

Drug Class	Examples	Mechanism of Action
PDE-4 inhibitors	Roflumilast	Reduces release of inflammatory mediators such as cytokines, due to an increase in cyclic AMP from the PDE-4 inhibitor
Leukotriene modifiers	Zileuton	Inhibits 5-lipoxygenase thus blocking the synthesis of cysteinyl leukotrienes
	Zafirlukast, montelukast	Block the cysteinyl leukotriene receptor
Mast cell release inhibitors	Cromolyn, nedocromil	Inhibit the release of inflammatory mediators from mast cells and other cells
IgE targeting drugs	Omalizumab	Binds to IgE and prevents its binding to IgE receptors
Interleukin-5 (IL-5) targeting drugs	Mepolizumab	Binds to the cytokine, IL-5, preventing its binding to the IL-5 receptor on eosinophils, thus inhibiting the recruitment and activation of eosinophils
	Benralizumab	Binds to and blocks the IL-5 receptor

IgE, Immunoglobulin E; *PDE*, phosphodiesterase; drugs ending in "mab" are monoclonal antibodies.

Adverse Effects

Antimuscarinic drugs given by inhalation may cause dry mouth, blurring of vision, mydriasis, and an increase in intraocular pressure. Patients with narrow angle glaucoma are most susceptible. Allergic reactions may occur, and angioedema has been reported.

Other Drugs

Additional drugs, such as phosphodiesterase-4 (PDE-4) inhibitors, leukotriene modifiers, mast cell release inhibitors, IgE targeting drugs, and interleukin-5 targeting drugs, have all been used for the treatment of COPD and asthma (Tables 18.4 and 18.5). Due to the different approaches to managing these diseases, the mechanism of action and adverse effects will vary with each drug class (see Tables 18.4 and 18.5).

The action of leukotriene modifiers is shown in Fig. 18.3.

Note: Further discussion of the respiratory drugs with clinical applications is given in Chapter 27 of *Pharmacology and Therapeutics for Dentistry*, 8th edition.

TABLE 18.5 Characteristics of Five Additional Drug Classes Targeting Asthma

Drug Class	Pharmacokinetics	Adverse Effects
PDE-4 inhibitor (used for COPD)	Roflumilast—given orally, metabolized in the liver, half-life ~30 h	Insomnia, behavior problems, anxiety, dyspepsia, rash, rhinitis
Leukotriene modifiers (used prophylactically in asthma)	Zileuton—given orally, metabolized in the liver, half-life ~2.5 h	Potential for liver disease, rash
	Montelukast—given orally, metabolized in the liver, half-life ~5 h	Headache, fever, otitis media, rhinorrhea
Mast cell release inhibitors _(used in asthma as a prophylactic only)	Cromolyn, Nedocromil, given by inhalation, low systemic absorption	Dry throat, cough, wheezing
IgE targeting drugs (used in asthma)	Omalizumab—given sc, metabolized by proteolysis, half-life ~24 days	Rash, fever, hypersensitivity reactions, anaphylaxis (rare)
Interleukin-5 (IL-5) targeting drugs (used in asthma, targeting eosinophilia)	Mepollizumab is given sc, metabolized by proteolysis, half-life—16–22 days	Rash, myalgia, headache, dyspnea, angioedema
	Benralizumab—see mepollizumab	Headache, fever, erythema

IgE, Immunoglobulin E; *PDE*, phosphodiesterase; *sc*, subcutaneously; drugs ending in "mab" are monoclonal antibodies.

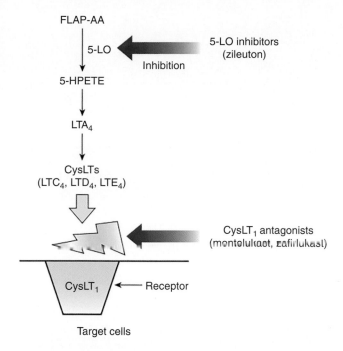

• **Fig. 18.3** Illustration of the mechanism and site of action of the antileukotriene agents zileuton, zafirlukast, and montelukast. Zileuton inhibits the 5-lipoxygenase *(5-LO)* enzyme to prevent leukotriene production, and zafirlukast and montelukast antagonize the action of the cysteinyl leukotrienes *(CysLTs)* at the leukotriene receptor, CysLT1. *FLAP-AA*, 5-Lipoxygenase-activating protein complexed with arachidonic acid; *5-HPETE*, 5-hydroperoxyeicosatetraenoic acid; *LTA4*, LTC4, LTD4, LTE4, leukotrienes A4, C4, D4, E4. (Modified from Gardenhire DS. *Rau's respiratory Care Pharmacology*, 10th ed. Chapter 12, Nonsteroidal antiasthma agents, 2020, Elsevier.)

Suggested Reading

McIntyre A, Busse WW Asthma exacerbations: the Achilles heel of asthma care. Trends Mol Med. 2022;28(12):1112–1127. In this issue.

19
Dental Therapeutics

Depending on the needs of the patient, there are a variety of drugs dentists can prescribe. The nine principal reasons for prescribing drugs include infection, swelling, pain, anxiety, tooth decay, xerostomia, plaque control, inflammation, and sedation. The type, dose, duration, and instructions on how to take the drug will vary from patient to patient depending on age, weight, systemic conditions, and other considerations.

This chapter is designed to assist the dentist, dental student, and/or dental resident in the prescription of medications for the adult patient. It is not intended to be a definitive reference for the pharmacologic management of patients. This chapter does not contain indications and contraindications of medications, side effects, drug interactions, and many other important pieces of pharmacological information. Therefore, this chapter should be used in conjunction with *Pharmacology and Therapeutics for Dentistry*, an internal medicine textbook, and with consultation with the patient's physician. The focus of this chapter is to provide a rapid manner to identify potential drugs for the management of common problems experienced by dental patients.

Anxiety

It has been estimated that 14% of patients undergoing dental treatment are highly anxious about the care they will receive. Although there is a variety of nonpharmacologic anxiety management techniques, dentists can also employ pharmacologic agents to reduce dental anxiety.

Rx:	Diazepam 5 mg
Disp:	2 tablets
Sig:	Take 1 tablet in evening before going to bed and 1 tablet 1 hour before your appointment.
Proprietary:	Valium (benzodiazepine)

NOTE:	Patients should not drive themselves to or from the appointment.

Do not prescribe to pregnant women.

Rx:	Lorazepam 1 mg
Disp:	2 tablets
Sig:	Take 1 tablet in evening before going to bed and take 1 tablet 1 hour before your appointment.
Proprietary:	Ativan (benzodiazepine)
NOTE:	Patients should not drive themselves to or from appointment.

Do not prescribe to pregnant women.

Rx:	Triazolam 0.25 mg
Disp:	2 tablets
Sig:	Take 1 tablet in evening before going to bed and 1 tablet 1 hour before your appointment.
Proprietary:	Halcion (benzodiazepine)
NOTE:	Patients should not drive themselves to or from the appointment.

Do not prescribe to pregnant women.

Rx:	Oxazepam 15 mg
Disp:	2 tablets
Sig:	Take 1 tablet in evening before going to bed and take 1 tablet 1 hour before your appointment.
Proprietary:	Serax (benzodiazepine)
NOTE:	Patients should not drive themselves to or from the appointment.

Do not prescribe to pregnant women.

Rx:	Temazepam 7.5 mg

Disp:	2 tablets
Sig:	Take 1 tablet before bedtime and 1 tablet 90 minutes before dental appointment.
Proprietary:	Restoril (benzodiazepine)
NOTE:	Patients should not drive themselves to or from the appointment.

Do not prescribe to pregnant women.

General comments:	Diazepam (30 to 60) is long acting, whereas temazepam (10 to 20) lorazepam (10 to 18), oxazepam (5 to 15), and triazolam (1.5 to 5) are shorter acting.

(The numbers are the ranges of elimination $t^{1/2}$ values in hours.)

Acute Dental Pain

Acute pain evoked by disease, injury, or dental treatment often involves pain of short duration (i.e., less than 3 months). Acute pain can be attributed to pathological processes in hard tissues (e.g., dental caries) or soft tissues (e.g., lateral periodontal abscess) or dental treatment (e.g., extraction of wisdom teeth). The drugs listed below include those available over the counter (OTC) and those that need a prescription (Rx) by the dentist.

Mild Pain

OTC:	Aspirin 325 mg
Disp:	As needed to alleviate pain
Sig:	Take two tablets every 6 hours.
Ingredient:	Acetylsalicylic acid (nonsteroidal antiinflammatory drug [NSAID])
NOTE:	Do not exceed 4000 mg/day.

Do not give to children.

OTC:	Ibuprofen 200 mg
Disp:	As needed to alleviate pain
Sig:	Take one tablet every 8 hours.
Proprietary:	Motrin (NSAID)
NOTE:	Do not exceed 2400 mg/day.

Generic drugs are available OTC in 200 mg and 400 mg tablets.

OTC:	Acetaminophen 325 mg

Disp:	As needed to alleviate pain
Sig:	Two tablets every 6 hours.
Proprietary:	Tylenol (analgesic)
NOTE:	Do not exceed 4000 mg/day. In certain cases, maximum dose should not exceed 3250 mg.

For those patients for whom aspirin or other NSAIDs are contraindicated, the choice is acetaminophen.

Rx:	Lidocaine HCl 2% viscous
Disp:	100 mL or 450 mL
Sig:	Use two teaspoons to rinse around oral cavity as needed to relieve superficial pain—**expectorate rinse**. Don't use for more often than every 4 hours.
Proprietary:	Xylocaine 2% viscous (local anesthetic)
NOTE:	Viscous lidocaine (Dilocaine, Nervocaine, Xylocaine, Zilactin-L) may be prescribed to relieve pain associated with oral blisters and lesions. Use only in patients who are not at risk of swallowing the rinse.
Rx:	Diphenhydramine (12.5 mg/5 ml) syrup mixed 50/50 with bismuth subsalicylate (262 mg/15 ml). Don't use more often than every 4 hours.
Disp:	8 oz. total
Sig:	Use two teaspoons as rinse, as needed to relieve superficial pain or burning, **expectorate rinse**.
Proprietary:	Benadryl (antihistamine), mixed 50/50 with Kaopectate
Ingredients:	If Maalox is used, aluminum hydroxide, magnesium hydroxide, and simethacone are added.
NOTE:	Can be mixed with Maalox if constipation is a problem.

Moderate Pain

OTC:	Ibuprofen 400 mg
Disp:	36 tablets
Sig:	For the first 48 hours, take 1 tablet every 4 to 6 hours, then 400 mg every 4 to 6 hours as needed (prn).
Ingredient:	Ibuprofen

NOTE: Do not exceed 2400 mg ibuprofen/day.

Prescription 400 mg tablets available.

Generic ibuprofen available OTC in 200 and 400 mg tablets.

Moderate Pain and When NSAIDs Are Contraindicated

Rx: Hydrocodone/ acetaminophen (5/325)

Disp: 8 tablets

Sig: For the first 48 hours, take 1 hydrocodone/acetaminophen (5/325) tablet every 6 hours, then 650 to 1000 mg acetaminophen every 6 hours as needed (prn).

NOTE: Do not exceed maximum morphine equivalent (MME).

Severe Pain

OTC: Ibuprofen 200 mg and acetaminophen 500 mg

Disp: 36 tablets of each drug

Sig: For the first 48 hours, take 1 tablet of ibuprofen (200 mg) and 1 tablet of acetaminophen (500 mg) every 4 to 6 hours, then 1 tablet of ibuprofen (200 mg) and 1 tablet of acetaminophen (500) every 4 to 6 hours as needed (prn).

Ingredient: Ibuprofen.

NOTE: Do not exceed 2400 mg ibuprofen/day.

Do not exceed 4000 mg acetaminophen. In certain cases, maximum dose should not exceed 3250 mg.

Rx: Ibuprofen (400 mg) and hydrocodone 5 mg/acetaminophen 325 mg (5/325)

Disp: 16 ibuprofen tablets, 8 hydrocodone/ acetaminophen (5/325) tablets

Sig: For the first 48 hours, take 1 Ibuprofen (400 mg) and 1 (5 mg hydrocodone/325 mg acetaminophen) every 6 hours followed by ibuprofen (400 mg) every 4 to 6 hours as needed to alleviate pain (prn).

Proprietary: Norco 5/325 (5 mg hydrocodone/ 325 mg acetaminophen)

Ingredients: Ibuprofen (NSAID), hydrocodone (opioid), and acetaminophen (analgesic)

NOTE: Do not exceed 2400 mg ibuprofen/day.

Do not exceed MME (See above)

Rx: Oxycodone (opioid) 4.88 mg/aspirin (NSAID) 325 mg

Disp: 12 tablets

Sig: For the first 48 hours, take 1 tablet every 4-6 hours for pain, then 650 to 1000 mg acetaminophen every 6 hours as needed (prn).

Proprietary: Percodan

NOTE: Do not exceed 4000 mg acetaminophen/ day. In certain cases, maximum dose should not exceed 3250 mg.

Do not exceed MME (See above)

Severe Pain When NSAIDs Are Contraindicated

Rx: Oxycodone (5 mg)/acetaminophen (325 mg)

Disp: 12 tablets

Sig: For the first 48 hours, take 1 oxycodone/acetaminophen (5/325) tablet every 4-6 hours, then 650 to 1000 mg acetaminophen every 6 hours as needed (prn).

Proprietary: Percocet (5/325) (also Endocet [5/325], and Roxicet [5/325])

NOTE: Do not exceed 4000 mg acetaminophen/day. In certain cases, maximum dose should not exceed 3250 mg.

Do not exceed MME (See above)

Some Other Drug Combinations for Severe Pain

Rx: Hydrocodone (opioid) 5 mg/ acetaminophen (analgesic) 300 mg (5/300)

Disp: 12 tablets

Sig: For the first 48 hours, take 1 tablet every 4 to 6 hours for pain, then 650 to 1000 mg acetaminophen every 6 hours as needed (prn).

Proprietary: Vicodin

NOTE: Do not exceed 4000 mg acetaminophen/day. (See above).

Do not exceed MME (See above)

General Comments: Data have shown NSAIDs used at the correct dosage can be more effective than opioids in reducing acute pain. It is recommended that NSAIDs or acetaminophen be the first line of acute pain management.

The directions to follow by the provider to the patient (sig in prescriptions) are for patients who have received surgical or nonsurgical dental treatment. The recommendations for the patient to follow can be adjusted for other dental issues.

Opioid analgesics are narcotics that can be addictive and abused. Patients should not drive or consume alcohol or other central nervous system depressants, while using opioids.

Oxycodone is contraindicated in children and adolescents (<18 years).

Aspirin should be avoided if there is an elevated risk of bleeding. Aspirin should not be given to children or adolescents, especially with a history of chicken pox, flu, or have received a vaccine in the near past.

Opioid-naïve patients should receive the lowest opioid dose for the shortest period of time.

*Each state has a morphine milligram equivalent (MMG) that must not be exceeded for daily opioid use.

Odontogenic Infections

It has been estimated the majority of orofacial infections originate from teeth or their surrounding tissues. Odontogenic infections begin as a local infection and may spread into adjacent or distant tissues. Severe odontogenic infections are serious and can be life threatening.

Rx: Amoxicillin 500 mg

Disp: 15 tablets

Sig: 500 mg every 8 hours.

Proprietary: Amoxil (β-lactam antibiotic)

NOTE: Drug of choice for most dental infections. The drug dose can be doubled in severe infection.

Rx: Clarithromycin 500 mg

Disp: 10 tablets

Sig: 1 tablet every 12 hours.

Proprietary: Biaxin (macrolide)

Rx: Erythromycin 500 mg

Disp: 15 tablets

Sig: 1 tablet every 12 hours.

Proprietary: Ery-Tab (macrolide)

NOTE: Macrolides can be used if the patient is allergic to amoxicillin or if there is no response to amoxicillin after 48 hours.

Rx: Metronidazole 500 mg

DIsp: 10 tablets

Sig: 500 mg every 12 hours.

Proprietary: Flagyl

NOTE: May use if no response to amoxicillin after 48 hours or if allergic to amoxicillin. Metronidazole is effective against anaerobes.

Rx: Clindamycin 150 mg

Disp: 40 tablets

Sig: 1 tablet every 6 hours.

Proprietary: Cleocin (lincosamide)

NOTE: May use if no response to amoxicillin after 48 hours.

NOTE: Can be used if allergic to amoxicillin.

General Comments: Antibiotics should only be used for active infections or to prevent the spread of the infection. Dosage and duration of antibiotic will depend on location and severity of infection. Dosages and duration of treatment listed are general suggestions for a patient with cellulitis. Local intervention treatment is also important.

Oral Fungal Infections

Fungal infections in the oral cavity are superficial infections involving the mucosa. The superficial mycoses (e.g., dermatophytes, *Candida* species, etc.) are generally treated with topical drugs. *Candida albicans* is the most common fungal infection found in the oral cavity.

Rx: Nystatin (oral suspension)

Disp: 240 mL

Sig: Use 1 teaspoonful five times a day; rinse and hold in mouth as long as possible (5 minutes) before expectorating.

Proprietary: Mycostatin (antifungal polyene) 100,000 units/mL.

Vehicle contains 50% sucrose and not more than 1% alcohol.

NOTE: Has a bitter taste.

Rx: Itraconazole oral solution

Disp: Two (150 mL) bottles

Sig: Use 2 teaspoonfuls two times a day for 2 weeks; rinse and hold in mouth as long as possible (5 minutes) then expectorate.

Proprietary: Sporanx (antifungal triazole)

Rx: Clotrimazole oral troche 10 mg

Disp: 70 tablets

Sig: Dissolve one troche in mouth five times daily for 2 weeks.

Proprietary: Mycelex (antifungal imidazole)

Rx: Fluconazole tablets 100 mg

Disp: 8 tablets

Sig: Take two tablets immediately followed by one tablet per day for 6 days,

Proprietary: Diflucan (antifungal triazole)

Rx: Nystatin oral pastilles (500,000 units)

Disp: 50 tablets

Sig: Dissolve one tablet in mouth five times daily.

Proprietary: Mycostatin (antifungal polyene)

NOTE: Has bitter taste.

Rx: Iodoquinol (topical antiprotozoal, antifungal, antibacterial), hydrocortisone (steroid) cream

Disp: 1 oz. tube

Sig: Apply thin film to corners of mouth three times daily, for angular cheilitis

Proprietary: Vytone cream

Rx: Fluconazole tablets 100 mg (an alternative if the oropharyngeal fungal infection is extensive and does not respond to above treatments.)

Disp: 16 tablets

Sig: Take 2 tablets immediately, followed by 1 tablet daily for 14 days.

Proprietary: Diflucan (antifungal triazole)

General comments: Candidiasis can be treated with nystatin (Mycostatin) oral suspension, itraconazole (Sporanox) oral solution, clotrimazole (Mycelex) oral troche, Nystatin (Mycostatin) oral pastilles, or fluconazole (Diflucan) tablets. For edentulous patients prescribe Mycostatin powder (15 mg) to be sprinkled in denture. Angular chelitis can be treated with iodoquinol/hydrocortizone cream (Vytone).

Oral Viral Infections

Mild, uncomplicated oral eruptions induced by *Herpes simplex-1* or *Herpes simplex-2* can be managed with topical drug application on lips or oral cavity. Medications for oral herpes lesions will decrease the duration of the condition but is not a cure for the illness. Topical agents to anesthetize the area can relieve pain during an acute herpetic outbreak.

Herpes Simplex Virus (HSV, HHV -1 and HHV-2): Primary Infections

Rx: Valacyclovir 1000 mg/tablet

Disp: 4 tablets

Sig: Take 2 tablets followed by 2 tablets 12 hours later.

Proprietary: Valtrex (antiviral purine analog)

Rx: Acyclovir 400 mg/tablet

Disp: 15-30 tablets

Sig: Take 1 tablet three times a day for 5-10 days.

Proprietary: Zovirax (antiviral purine analog)

General comments: For medications to be effective, the signs and symptoms must be recognized within the first 3 days of onset.

Recurrent Herpes Labialis

Rx:	Acyclovir Cream 5%
Disp:	5 g tube
Sig:	Beginning with prodromal symptoms, apply thin layer to area every 4 hours for 4 days.
Proprietary:	Zovirox (antiviral purine analog)
Rx:	Penciclovir Cream 1%
Disp:	5 g tube
Sig:	Beginning with prodromal symptoms, apply thin layer to area every 2 hours, during waking hours, for 4 days.
Proprietary:	Denavir (antiviral purine analog)
Rx:	Valacyclovir 1000 mg/tablet
Disp:	4 tablets
Sig:	Take two initially followed by two 12 hours later.
Proprietary:	Valtrex (antiviral purine analog)
Rx:	Acyclovir 400 mg/tablet
Disp:	15-30 tablets
Sig:	Take 1 tablet three times per day for 5-10 days.
Proprietary:	Zovirax (antiviral purine analog)

Herpes Zoster (Shingles)

Rx:	Valacyclovir 1000 mg/tablet
Disp:	60 tablets
Sig:	Take 1 tablet three times a day for 7 days
Proprietary:	Valtrex (antiviral purine analog)

General comments: An ophthalmologic referral must be scheduled if Herpes zoster affects the tip of nose (i.e., involves nasociliary nerve and potential ocular lesions).

Ulcerative Lesions of the Oral Mucosa

These include erosive lichen planus and benign mucous membrane pemphigoid. Oral ulcerations are diverse in etiology, signs, and symptoms and as a result can be challenging to diagnose. Diagnosis of oral ulcers is dependent on history, clinical appearance, location, duration, frequency, and histopathology. A list of common drugs to treat oral ulcerations is given below.

Low Potency

Rx:	Dexamethasone elixir (0.5 mg/5 mL)
Disp:	250 mL
Sig:	Rinse with 1 teaspoon two times a day for 5 minutes and expectorate.
Proprietary:	Decadron (corticosteroid)
Dx:	Prednisolone syrup (15 mg/5 mL)
Disp:	100 mL
Sig:	Rinse with 1 teaspoon two times a day for 5 minutes and expectorate.
Proprietary:	Prelone (steroid)

Medium Potency

Rx:	Triamcinolone acetonide 0.1%
Sig:	5 g tube
Disp:	Apply to affected area four times a day.
Proprietary:	Kenalog in Orabase 0.1% (corticosteroid)

High Potency

Rx:	Fluocinonide gel 0.05%
Disp:	15 g
Sig:	Apply thin film to affected area four to six times a day.
Proprietary:	Lidex gel (corticosteroid)
General comments: Erosive lichen planus	Erosive lichen planus can be treated with fluocinonide (Lidex) gel, or other corticosteroid.

| *Aphthous Ulcers (minor or major):* | Can be treated with triamcinolone (Kenalog in Orabase), or fluocinonide (Lidex) gel. |
| *Herpetiform aphthae:* | Can be treated with dexamethsone (Decadron) elixir, or prednisolone (Prelone) syrup. |

Pain from aphthae ulcers can be managed with lidocaine 2% viscous or diphenhydramine syrup mixed with Kaopectate.

Local Anesthetics

Local anesthetics prevent acute pain by altering neural transmission. The two classes of local anesthetics are the aminoamindes and aminoesters. Local anesthetics are often combined with adrenergic agents to improve the duration of action.

Lidocaine (Xylocaine) 2% with 1:100,000 epinephrine

| Duration*: | 2.8 hours (infiltration), 3.2 hours (block) |
| Onset: | 2.5 minutes |

Mepivacaine (Iso-, Carbo- or Polocaine) 2% with 1:20,000 levonordefrin

| Duration*: | 2.5 hours (infiltration), 3.2 hours (block) |
| Onset: | 2 minutes |

Prilocaine (Citanest) 4% with 1:200,000 epinephrine

| Duration*: | 2.3 hours (infiltration), 3.4 hours (block) |
| Onset: | 3 minutes |

Articaine (Septocaine) 4% with 1:100,000 epinephrine

| Duration*: | 3.3 hours (infiltration), 3.8 hours (block) |
| Onset: | 2.5 minutes |

Bupivacaine (Marcaine) 0.5% with 1:200,000 epinephrine

| Duration*: | 5.7 hours (infiltration), 7.3 hours (block) |
| Onset: | 10 minutes |

*Duration (approximate) for soft tissue anesthesia after maxillary infiltration or inferior alveolar block.

Maximum doses per appointment for a 150 lb. person (All values are for local anesthetic without vasoconstrictor).

2% lidocaine = 3.3 mg/lb or 495 mg/150 lbs
3% mepivacaine = 2.6 mg/lb or 390 mg/150 lbs
4% prilocaine = 4.0 mg/lb or 600 mg/150 lbs
0.5% bupivacaine = 0.6 mg/lb or 90 mg/150 lbs

Calculations: For max dose of 2% Lidocaine/150 lbs
2% = 2 g/100 mL, 0.02 g/1 mL =20 mg/1 mL
20 mg/mL × 1.8 mL/cartridge = 36 mg lidocaine/cartridge
(e.g., calculation for lidocaine in a 150 lb. patient)
3.3 mg/lb (max) × 150 lb = 495 mg
495 mg max × 1 cartridge/36 mg = 13.8 cartridges
(If epinephrine is included with the lidocaine, the maximum cartridges will be less due to the maximum limit allowed for epinephrine which is 0.2mg total)

Xerostomia

Dry mouth occurs when the salivary glands do not make enough saliva to keep the mouth moist. Dry mouth can be caused by over 400 different medications, aging (often due to medications taken), radiation, or conditions that directly affect the salivary glands.

OTC:	BIOTENE ORAL BALANCE LIQUID OR SPRAY
OTC:	OASIS MOISTURIZING MOUTH SPRAY
OTC:	MEDORAL DRY MOUTH SPRAY
OTC:	ORAJEL DRY MOUTH MOISTURIZING GEL
Rx:	Pilocarpine 5 mg/tablet
Disp:	90 tablets
Sig:	Take one tablet three times a day.
Proprietary:	Salagen (antimuscarinic)
NOTE:	May be increased to 2 tablets three times a day.
Rx:	Cevimeline 30 mg
Disp:	90 capsules
Sig:	Take 1 tablet three times a day.
Proprietary:	Evoxac (antimuscarinic)
General Comments:	You may need to avoid eating or drinking for a time after using pilocarpine or cevimeline. *OTC*, over the counter

Oral Hemorrhage

There is a need for therapeutic agents that can accelerate blood coagulation following surgical procedures in the oral cavity. Since bleeding from an oral surgical site may not be easily controlled with pressure, pharmacologic agents may be considered.

Tranexamic Acid

Applied topically to areas where bleeding is not easily controlled. The medication has a short duration of action and pressure must be applied to the area in question.

Proprietary: Cyklokapron (antifibrinolytic agent)

Periodontal Regeneration

Periodontal regeneration restores the alveolar bone, periodontal ligament, and cementum. There have been only a few biologic agents approved for regeneration of the periodontium.

Amelogenin

Amelogenin is an enamel matrix derivative extracted from porcine fetal tooth material to stimulate growth of soft and hard tissues. The average amount of regeneration is 1.33 mm.

Proprietary:Emdogain

GEM 21 S (Human Platelet-Derived Growth Factor-BB and β-Tricalcium Phosphate)

GEM 21 S uses human recombinant platelet-derived growth factor- BB (rhPDGF) combined with a carrier β-tricalcium phosphate (β-TCP). rhPDGF is a glycoprotein that regulates cell growth and division while β-TCP is a calcium salt of phosphoric acid. The average amount of periodontal regeneration is limited.

Ingredient: human recombinant platelet-derived growth factor-BB

Platelet-Rich Plasma

Platelet-rich plasma is blood plasma with an enriched amount of platelets. The platelets from blood can be selectively collected in a pellet after centrifugation and then applied to the site. Average gain in attachment levels is 1.22 mm.

Ingredients: It has been reported that there are more than 30 growth factors associated with platelets (e.g., platelet derived growth factor, fibroblast growth factor, epidermal growth factor, etc.).

Guided Bone Regeneration

Guided bone regeneration (GBR) directs the production of new alveolar bone to specific sites using a variety of materials (e.g., barrier membrane, freeze dried bone, recombinant human bone morphogenic protein-2, etc.).

Infuse Bone Graft

Bone morphogenic proteins are a family of growth factors that have the ability to induce the growth of bone and cartilage. Recombinant human bone morphogenic protein-2 (rhBMP-2) has been used off-label to regenerate bone in the maxilla or mandible. Infuse bone graft consists of two components: rhBMP-2 that is placed on an absorbable collagen sponge when implanted. rhBMP-2 does not produce a gain in attachment of the gingiva and may cause ankyloses of the tooth to bone.

Ingredient: recombinant human bone morphogenic protein-2.

Dental Caries

Fluorides

Dentinbloc dentin desensitizer
GEL-KAM FLUOROCARE DUAL RINSE KIT
Colgate Gel-Kam Gel
PREVIDENT PLUS TOPICAL GEL
'THIXO-FLUR TOPICAL GEL

Silver Diamine Fluoride

A liquid applied topically to treat dental caries. Once brushed onto an active caries lesion, it has been shown to stop cavity development. It will cause black staining around areas to which it is applied.

Plaque Control

Chlorhexidine
Proprietary: Periogard

Sedation

Moderate sedation (conscious sedation) is a minimally depressed level of consciousness produced by a variety of pharmacologic agents. Although cognitive function and coordination is modestly impaired, there is a regular breathing pattern and response to physical stimuli (e.g., spoken to or touched). The drugs should render a level of consciousness to carry a wide margin of safety and must never induce a completely unconscious state. States require additional education prior to the administration of agents that induce moderate sedation in the dental office. The tables below outline characteristics of some drugs used in moderate sedation, and also an antagonist for benzodiazepines and an antagonist for opioids.

Drug	Class	Onset	Peak Effect	$T_{1/2}$ (hr)
Midazolam	benzodiazepine	1 min	3–5 min	2.5
Diazepam	benzodiazepine	1–5 min	3–5 min	30–60
Fentanyl	opioid	<1 min	5–15 min	3–4
Dexmedetomidine	alpha-2 adrenergic receptor agonist	<5 min	15–20 min	2–3

Drug	Class	Peak Effect
Flumazenil	benzodiazepine antagonist	6–10 min
Naloxone	opioid antagonist	5–15 min

Appendix A

Drugs Used to Treat Parkinson Disease

The treatment of Parkinson disease targets the underlying pathogenesis of the disease. Parkinsonism is a progressive neurodegenerative disease with significant motor impairment. Therapy for the disease is based on correcting the effects of dopamine deficiency in the basal ganglia of the brain. Dopaminergic agonists are used to make up for the loss of dopaminergic neurons.

This figure is useful in visualizing the opposing effects of dopaminergic neurons and cholinergic neurons on a motor pathway in the basal ganglia. Figure A shows the desired balance between the two pathways, with dopamine controlling motor output. Figure B shows the degeneration of the dopaminergic pathway, where the effect on the motor pathway is overstimulated by the cholinergic pathway.

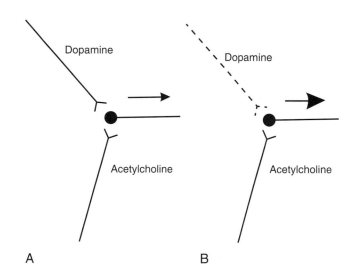

A Summary of Major Drugs Used to Treat Parkinsonism

Drug	Mechanism of Action	Comments
Levodopa (L-dopa)	Converted to dopamine in the brain	L-dopa is able to pass the blood-brain barrier
Carbidopa	Protects L-dopa from metabolism outside the brain	Increases the net L-dopa entering the brain
Tolcapone, entacapone	Inhibit COMT	Inhibit peripheral metabolism of L-dopa
Selegiline	Blocks MOA-B	Increases dopamine at presynaptic sites
Pramipexole, ropinirole, rotigotine	Dopamine receptor agonists	Stimulate dopamine receptors directly
Trihexyphenidyl, benztropine	Inhibit muscarinic receptors in the brain	See figure for effect on motor output.
Amantadine	Increases release of dopamine	Has anticholinergic action and blocks NMDA glutamate receptors

COMT, Catechol-O-methyl transferase; *MOA-B*, monoamine oxidase type B; *NMDA*, n-methyl D-aspartate.

Appendix B

Antiseizure Medications

Seizure disorders can be classified as follows:
- Generalized onset
  - Tonic-clonic
  - Absence
  - Others
- Focal onset (three types), also known as partial onset

Antiseizure medications act by a variety of mechanisms, including action on ion channels, gamma aminobutyric acid–related mechanisms, and inhibiting synaptic release proteins.

Summary of Some Antiseizure Medications

Drug	Mechanism of Action	Seizure Indications	Comments
Carbamazepine	Na^+ channel blocker	Tonic-clonic, focal	Also used for neuropathic pain, induces liver enzymes
Oxcarbazepine	Na^+ channel blocker	Focal	Also used for neuropathic pain
Phenytoin	Na^+ channel blocker	Tonic-clonic, focal	Gingival hyperplasia and hirsutism are typical
Phenobarbital	Activates Cl^- channels	Tonic-clonic, focal	Sedation is common, induces liver enzymes
Gabapentin	Inhibits action of $\alpha2\delta$ protein	Focal	Also used for neuropathic pain
Pregabalin	Inhibits action of $\alpha2\delta$ protein	Focal	Also used for neuropathic pain
Lamotrigine	Na^+ channel blocker	Tonic-clonic, absence	Also useful in bipolar disorder
Lacosamide	Na^+ channel blocker	Focal	Dizziness and nausea my occur
Levetiracetam	Inhibits the action of SV2A protein	Focal, tonic-clonic	Broad indications, diplopia and ataxia may occur
Clonazepam	Enhances the effect of $GABA_A$ on its receptor	Absence, others	Sedation is likely
Ethosuximide	Blocks T-type Ca^{++} channels	Absence	Often the first drug used for absence seizures
Valproic acid	May block T-type Ca^{++} channels and Na^+ channels	Tonic-clonic, absence	Broad indications, can cause neuro-tube defects in first trimester of pregnancy

$\alpha2\delta$, Cell surface protein involved in secretion at the cell membrane; *SV2A protein*, intracellular protein involved in secretion; *GABA*, gamma aminobutyric acid.

Appendix C

Autacoids

Autacoids are chemicals released by cells throughout the body. The effects of those chemicals are typically located close to the cells that release the substance. Autacoids are sometimes referred to as "local hormones," but this term does not universally apply to all autacoids.

Table C.1 shows a classification of autacoids. Within most classes, receptors have been identified for which agonists and antagonists have been produced. An example of a drug that acts at each autacoid receptor site is given in Table C.1.

Histamine is one of the oldest known autacoids and histamine receptor antagonists are commonly used.

Table C.2 lists representative histamine receptor blockers. The two most studied histamine receptors are histamine$_1$ (H$_1$) and histamine$_2$ (H$_2$). Stimulation of H$_1$ receptors mediates bronchoconstriction, smooth muscle contraction, allergic rhinitis, hives, pain, vasodilation, and neuronal effects, and a "triple response." Effects in the central nervous system include satiety, motion sickness, regulation of sleep-wake cycles, memory, and others. Stimulation of H$_2$ receptors leads to gastric acid secretion and vasodilation.

TABLE C.1 **Autacoids and Examples of Receptor Ligands[a]**

Autacoid	Agonist	Antagonist
Histamine	Histamine	Diphenhydramine
Serotonin (5-HT)	Sumatriptan	Ketanserin
Angiotensin II	Angiotensin II	Losartan
Prostaglandins	Misoprostol	
Kinins	Bradykinin	Icatibant
Leukotrienes	Leukotrienes	Montelukast
Nitric oxide[a]	Nitroglycerin[b,c]	

[a]Nitric oxide activates guanylyl cyclase in the cytoplasm leading to an increase in cyclic guanosine monophosphate (GMP).
[b]Most autacoids act at several types of receptor subclasses. This table gives only an example within each autacoid class.
[c]Nitroglycerin generates nitric oxide.

TABLE C.2 **Histamine Receptors and Blockers**

Receptor Blocker	Examples	Indications	Adverse Effects
H$_1$ (traditional antihistamines)	Diphenhydramine, chlorpheniramine, hydroxyzine	Nasal allergies, common cold, sedation, allergic dermatitis	Sedation, tremors, nervousness, dry mouth
H$_1$ (non-sedating)	Loratadine, cetirizine, fexofenadine	Allergic reactions, urticaria	Dry mouth, dizziness
H$_2$	Cimetidine,[a] famotidine, nizatidine, ranitidine,	Duodenal and gastric ulcers, gastroesophageal reflux disease	Dizziness, fatigue, mental confusion

[a]Cimetidine, by inhibiting several cytochrome p450 enzymes, can interact with several drugs.

Appendix D

Gastrointestinal Drugs

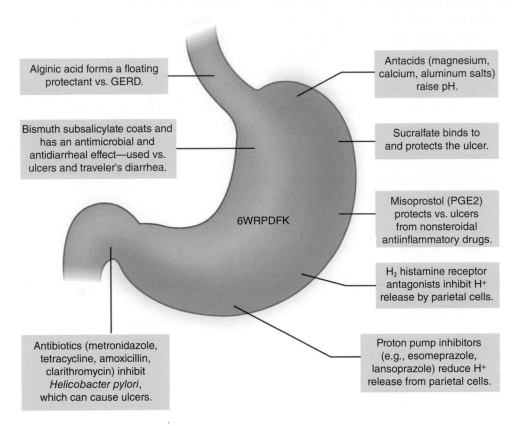

Alginic acid forms a floating protectant vs. GERD.

Antacids (magnesium, calcium, aluminum salts) raise pH.

Bismuth subsalicylate coats and has an antimicrobial and antidiarrheal effect—used vs. ulcers and traveler's diarrhea.

Sucralfate binds to and protects the ulcer.

Misoprostol (PGE2) protects vs. ulcers from nonsteroidal antiinflammatory drugs.

H_2 histamine receptor antagonists inhibit H^+ release by parietal cells.

Antibiotics (metronidazole, tetracycline, amoxicillin, clarithromycin) inhibit *Helicobacter pylori*, which can cause ulcers.

Proton pump inhibitors (e.g., esomeprazole, lansoprazole) reduce H^+ release from parietal cells.

The above figure shows the actions of several classes of drugs used to protect the stomach from various disorders. The H_2 histamine antagonists are cimetidine, famotidine, nizatidine, and ranitidine. *GERD*, Gastroesophageal reflux disease.

In the lower gastrointestinal (GI) tract, a common disorder is constipation. The figure below shows the action of four classes of drugs to treat constipation.

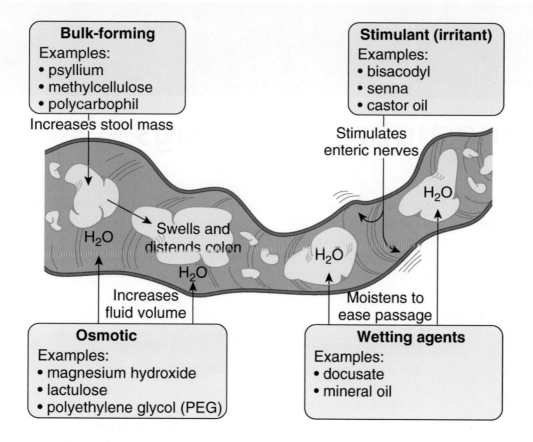

Methylnaltrexone and alvimopan, by blocking opioid receptors in the GI tract, are used to treat constipation caused by opioids. Methylnaltrexone and alvimopan do not cross the blood-brain barrier at therapeutic doses.

Diarrhea can be treated with several choices of drugs. The table below gives a summary.

Drug	Mechanism	Comments
Bismuth subsalicylate	Inhibits prostaglandin and Cl⁻ secretion	Commonly used, may blacken the stool.
Diphenoxylate, loperamide	Stimulate opioid receptors in lower GI tract	Loperamide does not enter the brain. Atropine is added to diphenoxylate.
Antibiotics (fluoroquinolones, azithromycin)	Antibacterial effect in lower GI tract	Use if other drugs are not effective.

Appendix **E**

Immunosuppressant Drugs

This appendix lists agents that are used to suppress the immune system. Immunopharmacology is a broad subject that includes drugs to treat immunodeficiencies and drugs used to suppress the immune system. This table is limited to some drugs that are used to reduce the immune response in autoimmune diseases, to prevent rejection in transplant patients, and three other disorders. Refer to the eighth edition of *Pharmacology and Therapeutics for Dentistry* for a discussion of these and other drugs used in immunotherapy.

Immunosuppressant Drugs

Drug Class	Mechanism of Action	Examples
Corticosteroids	Alter gene expression, reduce cell-mediated and humoral immunity	Prednisone
Cytotoxic drugs	Purine antagonists, block cell proliferation	Azathioprine, mycophenolate mofetil
	Alkylating agents	Cyclophosphamide
	Inhibit pyrimidine synthesis	Leflunomide, teriflunomide
	Increase pH of endosomes and lysosomes, decreasing T-cell function	Hydroxychloroquine
Immunophilin ligands	Bind to cyclophilin and block effect of calcineurin	Cyclosporine[a]
	Bind to tacrolimus-binding protein and inhibit calcineurin	Tacrolimus, sirolimus
Miscellaneous	Inhibit TNF-α production, modulate ubiquitin ligase	Thalidomide, lenalidomide
Monoclonal antibodies (mAb)	Inhibit cytokines such as tumor necrosis factor and various interleukins	Adalimumab, infliximab, canakinumab, siltixamab, Guselkumab
Other cytokine inhibitors	Interleukin-1 receptor antagonists	Anakinra, rilonacept
Anti-IgE mAb	Binds IgE and prevents symptoms of allergies due to IgE	Omalizumab
Anti-RANK ligand mAb	Inhibits maturation of osteoclasts	Denosumab
Antiplatelet (anti-clotting) mAb	Prevents platelets from binding to factors important in blood clotting	Abciximab
Anti-cholesterol mAb	Prevents cell uptake and breakdown of LDL receptor	Alirocumab, evolocumab

[a]Associated with gingival hyperplasia.
IgE, Immunoglobulin E; *LDL*, low-density lipoprotein; *RANK*, receptor activator of nuclear factor *kappa* B; *TNF*, tumor necrosis factor.

Anticancer Drugs

Numerous classes of drugs and individual drugs within each class are used to treat cancer. Different cancers require different drugs based on the presence of specific drug targets in each cancer. Moreover, combinations of drugs, which act by different mechanisms and act at different phases of the cell cycle, are often used to attack the cancer at different targets to increase the effectiveness of the chemotherapy. Newer and more specific targeting of specific cancer cells is a more recent addition to the strategy for treating cancer. Anticancer drugs, being toxic to noncancer cells, cause significant toxicities in most cases. Refer to the eighth edition of *Pharmacology and Therapeutics for Dentistry* for a much more extensive coverage of these drugs.

Representative Anticancer Drugs

Class	Mechanism	Examples
Alkylating agents	Alkylate DNA, RNA, or proteins essential to the cell	Cyclophosphamide, chlorambucil, busulfan, thiotepa, dacarbazine, carmustine
Antimetabolites (resemble folic acid or a purine or pyrimidine base)	Provide a "fraudulent" substrate for reactions important for cell division.	Methotrexate, mercaptopurine, 5-fluorouracil
Antibiotics	Bind to DNA and block production of nucleotides, or cause DNA strand breaks	Doxorubicin, daunorubicin, idarubicin, mitomycin, bleomycin
Vinca alkaloids	Bind to microtubules and cause arrest of cell division	Vinblastine, vincristine, vinorelbine
Platinum compounds	Cross-link DNA	Cisplatin, carboplatin
Taxanes	Block microtubule function	Paclitaxel, docetaxel
Topoisomerase inhibitors	Induce DNA strand breaks	Etoposide, teniposide
Enzyme	Inhibits protein synthesis	Asparaginase
Inhibitor of key enzyme in DNA synthesis	Inhibits ribonucleoside diphosphate reductase	Hydroxyurea
Hormone agonist	Useful in certain cancers and supportive care	Prednisone, dexamethasone
Sex hormone antagonists	Prevent production or effect of sex hormones	Anastrozole, tamoxifen, flutamide, bicalutamide
Tyrosine kinase inhibitors	Inhibit cell division	Imatinib, sunitinib, ceritinib
Growth factor inhibitors (monoclonal antibodies)	Bind to growth factors or growth factor receptors, preventing downstream signaling	Panitumumab, trastuzumab, bevacizumab, ramucirumab
Proteosome inhibitors	Prevent recycling of amino acids for protein synthesis	Bortezomib, carfilzomib
Check point inhibitors (monoclonal antibodies)	Allow T cells to attack cancer cells	Ipilimumab, nivolumab

Appendix G

Emergency Drugs

Medical emergencies occurring in a dental office require diagnosis and treatment. Most emergencies will present as loss of consciousness, respiratory distress, or altered patient status (e.g., nausea, anxiety, pain, rash, etc.). The general treatment protocol for a medical emergency is to maintain the airway, terminate the procedure, reposition the patient, take vital signs and administer oxygen, provide proper emergency drugs, and, when appropriate, activate the emergency medical system. The therapeutic choices for management of office emergencies are constantly increasing, and each office should have appropriate medical supplies to deal with common medical emergencies. Listed below are a minimum number of drugs that can be used for an office emergency kit. What drugs you choose and which route of administration you use for your emergency kit will depend on what you do in the office and how well educated you are in the management of medical emergencies. Detailed information regarding drugs for medical emergencies can be found in Chapter 41 of the eighth edition of *Pharmacology and Therapeutics for Dentistry*.

Indication	Drug	Name	How Supplied	Dose/Route
Allergy	Sympathomimetic amine	Epinephrine	1:1000 ampule	0.1–0.3 cc subQ injection, may repeat in 15 min
	β_2 agonist	Albuterol	Inhaler	Metered puffs from albuterol inhaler
	Antihistamine	Diphenhydramine	Elixir (oral) or 50 mg/mL, IM	25–50 mg orally, IM
	Glucocorticoid	Hydrocortisone	Liquid	100 mg IV
Chest pain	Vasodilator	Nitroglycerin	Tablet/Sublingual spray	0.4 mg sublingual
	NSAID	Aspirin	325 mg tablet	Chewable in mouth
Hypoglycemia	Glucose	Orange juice	Bottle	Oral
		Dextrose 5% in water	50 mL IV bag	IV
All	Oxygen	Oxygen	Tank	Delivery mask

IM, Intramuscular; *IV*, intravenous; *NSAID*, nonsteroidal antiinflammatory drugs; *SubQ*, subcutaneous.

Appendix H

Prescription Writing

A complete, ideal prescription is comprised of several parts, each of which provides specific information about the prescriber, the patient, and the drug. The patient's full name, age, and address are required on prescriptions for Drug Enforcement Administration (DEA)-controlled substances.

The symbol Rx, known as the *superscription*, is generally understood to be an abbreviation of the Latin *recipe*, meaning "take thou."

The *inscription* provides specific information about the drug preparation: (1) the name of the drug, which can be either the nonproprietary or the proprietary name; and (2) the unit dosage or amount of the drug in milligrams or other appropriate units of measure and the dosage form.

The next part of the prescription is the *subscription*. The subscription is the prescriber's directions to the pharmacist regarding fulfilling the inscription. The subscription is usually brief and includes the following:

1. The quantity (and dosage form) of the drug to be dispensed (i.e., the number of tablets or capsules or the volume of a liquid preparation needed for a course of therapy).
2. Instruction to the pharmacist if the prescription can be refilled without the prescriber writing a new prescription.
3. Dispensing characteristics of the drug.

The transcription, or signature—from the Latin signa, meaning "label" or "let it be labeled" and indicated on the prescription by "Label: or Sig:"—is the prescriber's directions to the patient that appear on the medicine container. At one time, such directions were uniformly written in Latin, but modern practice is to use English. Latin abbreviations are still used by many clinicians in prescriptions and progress notes to save time.

The handwritten signature and professional degree of the prescriber convey the authority of the prescriber to order the medication and of the pharmacist to fill the prescription. Finally, the prescriber's DEA registration number must appear on any prescription for a controlled or scheduled drug in compliance with the Controlled Substances Act of 1970.

Prescription pads should also be kept secured in a locked drawer or under a similar cover when not in use to avoid loss or theft. Inventories of prescription pads and drug stocks should be performed regularly to detect theft and diversion of prescription forms and drugs. Sequentially numbered prescription blanks make detection of diversion easier.

John R. Brown, D.M.D
123 Main st.
Metropolis, N.J.
Phone: 625-7846

For _____ Age _____
_____ Date _____

R

Substitution
☐ permitted
☐ not permitted
Refill 0 1 2 3

Signature _____
DEA # _____

INDEX

Page numbers followed by "*f*" indicate figures, "*t*" indicate tables, and "*b*" indicate boxes.